DISSECTIONS

DISSECTOR FOR

Netter's ATLAS OF HUMAN ANATOMY

DISSECTIONS   Volume I

SHARON OBERG, Ph.D.

CIBA-GEIGY CORPORATION · SUMMIT, NEW JERSEY

To my wingman and consort

ISBN 0-914168-20-7
Library of Congress Catalog No: 94-070108

First Printing
Printed in U.S.A.

Offset printing by The Case-Hoyt Corporation
Binding by The Riverside Group
Laser-scanned separations by Page Imaging, Inc.
Design by Philip Grushkin

FOREWORD

It is fitting that Sharon Oberg should write a dissection guide to accompany Netter's ATLAS OF HUMAN ANATOMY because she worked closely with Dr. Netter on a day-by-day basis to complete the ATLAS. At that time, she was known as Dr. Sharon Colacino. The joint effort resulted in the most complete collection of Frank Netter's renowned medical-anatomical illustrations under one cover. DISSECTIONS, Volume I of the DISSECTOR, is comprehensive and well illustrated. DISCUSSIONS, Volume II, conceptualizes the observations of each dissection and is designed as preparatory reading for each dissection.

One of the major strengths in the organization of these two volumes is that each dissection stands on its own merits. Any gross anatomy course, even one that is not sequenced the same way, can be suitably accommodated to this two-volume set. However, the sequence in the DISSECTOR is as logical as any I have seen in a human anatomical dissection guide. The two volumes plus Netter's ATLAS OF HUMAN ANATOMY could form the basis for an entire gross anatomy experience.

Our course in human anatomy at the University of Wisconsin adopted Netter's ATLAS OF HUMAN ANATOMY several years ago, and both the staff and students are delighted with it. The DISSECTOR will enhance the use of this monumental piece of work and, together with the ATLAS, will provide the basis for a well-organized, exciting experience in the anatomy laboratory.

JAMES C. PETTERSEN, Ph.D.
Alumni Professor of Anatomy
University of Wisconsin Medical School

ACKNOWLEDGMENTS

These volumes were not conceived or assembled alone. My sincere gratitude is extended to all of the following:

To Frank Netter, who overflowed with knowledge, talent, and love of the human body, for teaching me that the Great Wall of China was built one brick at a time, and to Phil Flagler, for giving me the green light to try my own voice and design these volumes the way I chose.

To all the people who so humbly donated their bodies to be studied as cadavers, for helping us learn the wonders of God's work; to all students of anatomy, for telling me what they wanted to have in a dissector; and to my own honored teachers, for helping me learn not to match the body to the book. Special thanks go to Lewis Dickinson, for performing each dissection in order to verify the sequence of the steps; to Paul Hayes, for tackling the "dissection" of my original draft; and to my colleagues, for supporting my efforts to collect these words. Thanks also go to the Medical University of South Carolina and to the University of Saskatchewan, Canada.

To Ciba-Geigy Corporation, for sponsoring the publication of this DISSECTOR; to Phil Grushkin, a dear friend and valued team player, for bringing his calm, careful attention to detail and beauty to these pages; to Karen Phillips, for patiently correcting my noun and verb tenses and helping me condense my original text; to Nicole Friedman, for researching Dr. Frank Netter's original art to locate illustrations; to Ed Jones, for carefully transforming and adapting original Netter art into computer illustrations; to Jeffie Lemons, for typing much of the original discussions manuscript; to Kristine Jordan Bean and unsung proofreaders, for adding their editorial efforts to this enormous undertaking; and to Maria Erdélyi-Brown, who brought the strength of her intelligence and wit to this project, for being a charming slave driver and making these two volumes work for the students.

To my two sons, Anthony and Nicholas, who scrambled to live their own lives, for drawing me into writing in order to fill the absence of their laughter, and to my husband, Bob, for the gift of his music and for his sense of humor throughout the publication process.

I thank you all for your support and enthusiasm.

SHARON OBERG, Ph.D.
Associate Professor
Department of Cell Biology and Anatomy
Medical University of South Carolina

INTRODUCTION

The DISSECTOR FOR NETTER'S ATLAS OF HUMAN ANATOMY comprises two volumes: DISSECTIONS, Volume I, and DISCUSSIONS, Volume II. DISSECTIONS is organized by regions and is designed to accompany Netter's ATLAS OF HUMAN ANATOMY. The relevant sections of DISCUSSIONS, which are organized by systems, should be read before each dissection.

Directives

Each dissection begins with a reminder to *Complete* the previous dissections and to *Read* the appropriate discussion before proceeding. (The discussion on Bones should be read before the first dissection in each section.) This preparation is essential.

The directives for each dissection are given in step-by-step commands, expressed in boldface capital letters (e.g., **REMOVE, CUT, REFLECT**). Like the items in a pilot's checklist, these instructions must be followed in the sequence indicated. While most of the directives used in DISSECTIONS are self-explanatory, some require particular attention:

CLEAN Although the student is not specifically directed to clean every structure, all body parts are better visualized when fascia and fat have been carefully removed. This meticulous preparation may seem tedious, but it will greatly enhance the student's observations.

CAUTION These statements are intended to alert the student to a structure that may be damaged by the dissection procedures that follow.

LOCATE and **LOOK** These directives suggest that the structures indicated may not be easily identified. The student should probably not spend too much time trying to visualize these structures unless specifically directed by the laboratory instructor.

Terms

Important terms are printed in **boldface** at their first important mention. (Osteologic terms, however, are not in boldface in DISSECTIONS.) Boldface terms in the text appear as **red** labels on the accompanying plates.

Structures that are discussed in the text of DISSECTIONS but are not illustrated on an accompanying plate are followed by the qualifier (*not shown*). Structures illustrated on a plate but not labeled are designated (*not labeled*) in the text.

<u>Underlined</u> terms are used throughout the text for emphasis (e.g., "During these steps, do <u>not</u> cut serratus posterior superior and rhomboideus muscles.") and clarity (e.g., "**CUT** through <u>right</u> lamina..."). Cranial nerves are designated by roman numerals, and some eponyms are used.

Plates and Figures

The DISSECTOR is designed to be used in conjunction with Netter's ATLAS OF HUMAN ANATOMY, and nearly all the plates reproduced in black and white in DISSECTIONS correspond to full-color plates in the ATLAS. DISSECTIONS is not a miniature ATLAS in black and white; some of the plates in DISSECTIONS represent only a detail of the original plate in the ATLAS.

During dissection, the student should consult the ATLAS OF HUMAN ANATOMY frequently. To facilitate cross-referencing, the plate numbers appearing in DISSECTIONS correspond to the original plate numbers in the ATLAS. Plate numbers appearing in parentheses in the text refer to ATLAS plates that have not been reproduced in DISSECTIONS.

Illustrations in DISSECTIONS that do not appear in the ATLAS are labeled **Figures**. These figures are simplified versions of existing or adapted Netter plates used here for a specific purpose (e.g., to show incision lines).

The labels on the plates in DISSECTIONS are not always identical to the corresponding labels in the ATLAS. In the DISSECTIONS plates, only the structures referred to in text are labeled, and some structures not specifically identified in the ATLAS plate have been labeled in DISSECTIONS. Labels that have been added are printed in **black**.

During the preparation of the DISSECTOR, the author and editors discovered inadvertent mistakes in some labels in the ATLAS OF HUMAN ANATOMY. They would appreciate any errors being brought to their attention.

The index for ATLAS OF HUMAN ANATOMY should be used to locate other plates in the ATLAS that depict structures identified on the DISSECTIONS plates as well as structures designated as (*not shown*) or (*not labeled*) in the text.

Although the ATLAS should be consulted to help locate and identify structures, the student should not try to reproduce the appearance of the plates during the dissection but rather should follow the text of DISSECTIONS as a guide through the dissection process.

DISSECTION TECHNIQUES

Dissection is the careful and thoughtful separation of body parts. Examination of the structure of the body in the laboratory gives the student an opportunity to learn by direct observation. The anatomical details observed during dissection establish the foundation on which to build an understanding of the general organizational concepts of the human body.

The cadaver is the student's most valued teacher. The student must remember that the cadaver is the remains of a human being and must be treated with respect at all times. The cadaver is also the medical student's first patient and deserves proper care. Only the part of the body being dissected should be undraped. The cadaver must be kept moist with preservation fluid and covered when the dissection session is over. The parts of the body most likely to dry out (hands, feet, head, and genitalia) should be inspected periodically.

At the end of each dissection session, the student should remove all scraps of tissue from the table or tank and dispose of these parts in the containers provided. The laboratory must be kept as clean as an operating room.

The medical curriculum of the 1990s limits the time available for preparation and dissection. To make economical use of time, the student should prepare for each dissection by reading the relevant discussions, reviewing the previous laboratory session and dissections, and previewing the upcoming dissection before entering the laboratory. DISSECTIONS and the ATLAS OF HUMAN ANATOMY must be brought to each dissection session in the laboratory. The student should also refer to skeletal material often during the dissection period.

Since the sequence of dissections differs from school to school, DISSECTIONS provides space (when possible) at the end of each section for directions and notes, specifically changes in dissection procedures. DISSECTIONS makes no attempt to direct the student to preserve structures for practical examinations. The author does, however, indicate the tool that should be used for cutting; e.g., the Stryker saw is a rotating saw used to remove orthopedic casts.

Each student must bring 1 blunt-nosed pair of thumb forceps, 1 scalpel handle with an adequate supply of blades, and 1 pair of sharp-pointed scissors for dissection. The three figures on the following page show how to hold these instruments.

The student should properly clean all instruments after each laboratory session and dispose of scalpel blades in the appropriate containers.

During separation of tissue planes or removal of skin, traction should be applied to keep the field exposed. Forceps or fingers may be used for pulling tissues aside. Use of hemostats is optional.

In most regions of the body, body parts are separated by blunt dissection. In this technique, the closed points of scissors are pushed into the tissue. As the scissor blades are opened, the outer dull edges of the blades gently separate the tissues. Fingers can also be used for blunt dissection.

In dissection, the scalpel is used primarily for removing skin. The scalpel incisions may extend beyond the internal layer of skin through subcutaneous tissue to the outer layer of deep fascia encasing the muscles. To help protect the inner tissue, the student should direct the scalpel blade toward the inner surface of the skin, not toward the structures of the deeper body wall.

Careful dissection takes time. Since each dissection takes about 2 hours, the student should conduct the dissection in the most comfortable position, using the best possible lighting. Dissection technique improves with time and effort. Patience, practice, and pride will be rewarded with good results.

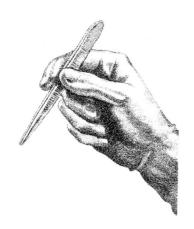

The forceps is held between the index finger and the thumb.

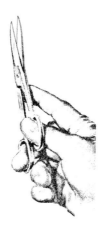

The thumb and middle finger are inserted into the handles, while the scissor blades are supported and directed by the index finger.

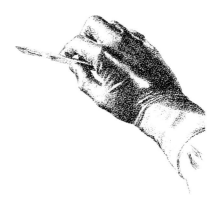

The scalpel handle may be held as a kitchen knife or as a pencil.

CONTENTS

Section 1

BACK

DISSECTIONS

DISSECTION 1.1
SUPERFICIAL BACK

Read DISCUSSIONS **1.1** Surface Anatomy, **1.2** Bones, and **1.4** Superficial Muscles.

PLACE cadaver in prone position with chest on wooden block so that head is <u>not</u> touching table.

MARK location of **dorsal cutaneous nerves** on skin with felt-tip marker.

INCISE skin of back (**Figure 1**). Begin by creating flap over T8–L2, and work both ways.

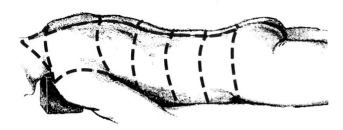

Figure 1

REFLECT skin flaps laterally, removing subcutaneous tissue with skin.

DISCARD skin flaps and subcutaneous tissue.

LOCATE several dorsal cutaneous nerves and their accompanying arteries and veins. Note that they are in segmental series, piercing superficial muscles of back near midline in cervical and upper thoracic regions. In lower thoracic and lumbar regions, dorsal cutaneous nerves are found 3 finger-widths from midline.

CAUTION Preserve greater occipital nerve (dorsal ramus of C2) and occipital artery as they pierce trapezius muscle inferior lateral to external occipital protuberance.

CLEAN trapezius muscle, moving blade in direction of muscle fibers. Do <u>not</u> dissect anterior to lateral border of upper part of trapezius muscle now. Clavicular attachment of trapezius muscle will be examined in DISSECTION **8.1**.

CLEAN latissimus dorsi muscle, leaving **thoracolumbar fascia** intact. Humeral insertion of latissimus dorsi muscle will be studied in DISSECTION **5.2**.

PLATE 163

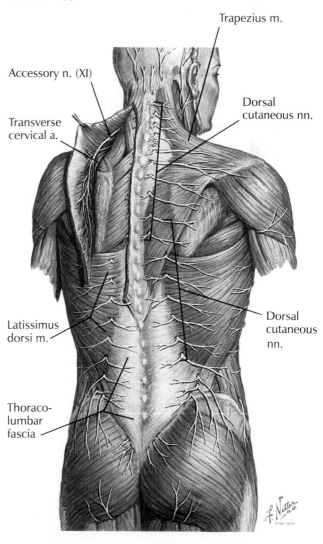

DEFINE boundaries of **triangle** of **auscultation** as superior border of latissimus dorsi muscle, lateral border of trapezius muscle, and medial border of scapula.

DEFINE boundaries of **lumbar triangle** as lateral border of latissimus dorsi muscle, posterior border of external abdominal oblique muscle, and iliac crest.

DEFINE lateral margin of lower part of trapezius muscle.

CAUTION During next steps, do <u>not</u> cut serratus posterior superior and rhomboideus muscles.

BLUNT DISSECT deep to trapezius muscle, separating it from underlying tissue.

INSERT fingers or closed scissors deep to vertebral origin of trapezius muscle, beginning at its most inferior attachment.

Figure 2

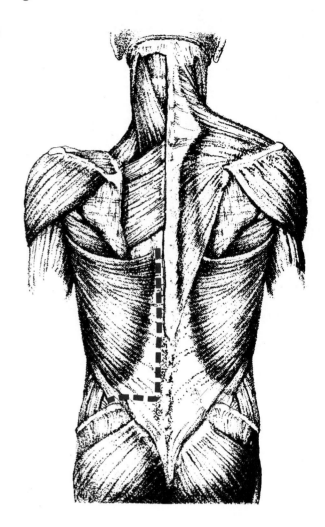

Triangle of auscultation

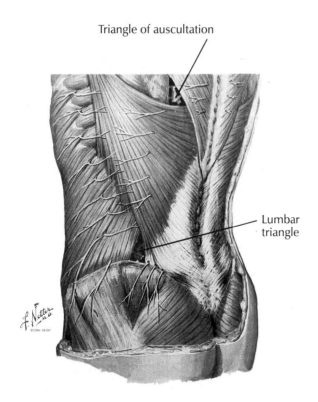

Lumbar triangle

PLATE 237

CUT trapezius muscle progressively along each side of vertebral column. Cut trapezius muscle from spine of scapula, continuing incision along vertebral column. Continue vertical incision to greater occipital protuberance.

INSERT closed scissors deep to occipital attachment of trapezius muscle. Retraction of shoulder or extension of head may facilitate this step.

CUT upper fibers of trapezius muscle from its occipital attachment.

REFLECT trapezius muscle laterally. Note that nerves and blood vessels entering deep surface of trapezius muscle are to be cut.

LOCATE accessory nerve (XI) and descending branch of **transverse cervical artery** along vertebral border on deep surface of trapezius muscle.

LOOK for branches from spinal nerves C3, 4 to trapezius muscle.

INSERT closed scissors deep to posterior layer of thoracolumbar fascia to establish safe plane for cutting (**Figure 2**).

INCISE vertically through posterior layer of thoracolumbar fascia medial to origin of muscle fibers of latissimus dorsi muscle.

PLATE 160

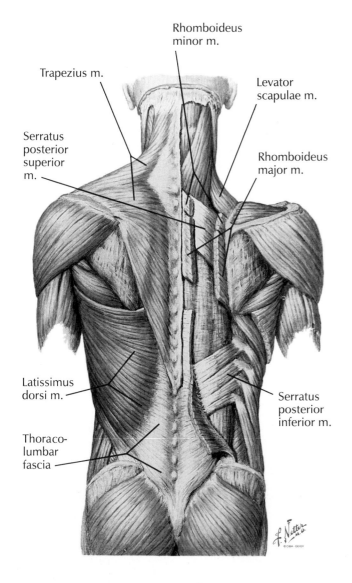

Trapezius m.

Rhomboideus minor m.

Levator scapulae m.

Serratus posterior superior m.

Rhomboideus major m.

Latissimus dorsi m.

Serratus posterior inferior m.

Thoraco-lumbar fascia

INCISE horizontally through thoracolumbar fascia from lower border of preceding vertical incision to lateral border of latissimus dorsi muscle.

REFLECT latissimus dorsi muscle laterally, blunt dissecting deep to muscle as reflection progresses.

IDENTIFY serratus posterior inferior muscle, which may easily be reflected with latissimus dorsi muscle.

CLEAN levator scapulae and **rhomboideus major** and **minor muscles**.

INSERT fingers or closed scissors deep to superior vertebral attachment of rhomboideus muscles to establish plane between rhomboideus muscles and underlying **serratus posterior superior muscle**.

CAUTION Preserve dorsal scapular nerve and dorsal scapular artery (*not shown*) along vertebral border on deep surface of rhomboideus muscles.

CUT rhomboideus muscles as close to spinous processes as possible.

REFLECT both rhomboideus major and minor muscles laterally.

CUT levator scapulae muscle from its scapular insertion.

CAUTION During next 3 steps, do <u>not</u> cut serratus posterior inferior muscle.

REFLECT levator scapulae muscle superiorly.

PRESERVE branches of **dorsal scapular nerve** (*not shown*) to levator scapulae muscle.

CLEAN serratus posterior superior and posterior inferior muscles.

CUT both serratus posterior muscles from their vertebral attachments, and reflect them laterally.

LOOK for branches of intercostal nerves innervating serratus posterior muscles.

5

DISSECTION 1.2
DEEP BACK

Complete DISSECTION **1.1** Superficial Back.

Read DISCUSSION **1.5** Deep Muscles.

PLACE cadaver in prone position.

CLEAN splenius capitis muscle to define medial and lateral borders. Note that additional skin may need to be reflected, but do <u>not</u> discard, because replacement of skin will help preserve structures of neck for later DISSECTION **8.1**.

PLATE 399 detail

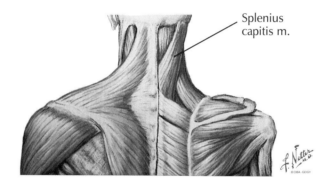

Splenius capitis m.

BLUNT DISSECT deep to vertebral origin of splenius capitis muscle.

CUT splenius capitis muscle from its vertebral attachment.

REFLECT splenius capitis muscle superiorly toward mastoid process and transverse processes of cervical vertebrae.

TRACE occipital artery medially to space between splenius capitis and semispinalis capitis muscles. Note that occipital artery is accompanied by **greater occipital nerve**.

CLEAN semispinalis capitis muscle.

LOCATE occipital artery passing deep to mastoid insertion of longissimus capitis muscle.

BLUNT DISSECT deep to mastoid attachment of **longissimus capitis muscle** to determine muscle thickness for cutting plane.

CUT longissimus capitis muscle as close to its mastoid insertion as possible.

REFLECT longissimus capitis muscle inferiorly.

COMPLETE vertical cut inferiorly through posterior layer of **thoracolumbar fascia** lateral to spinous processes of vertebrae.

CLEAN erector spinae muscle. Note that additional skin may need to be reflected inferiorly to inspect inferior attachments of erector spinae muscle.

PLATE 164

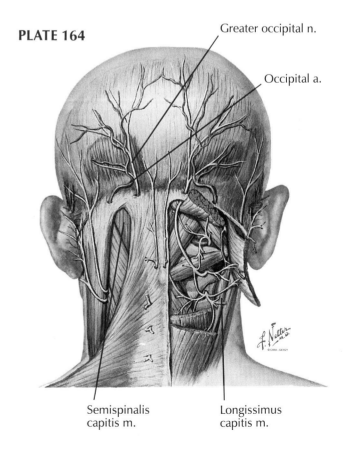

Greater occipital n.

Occipital a.

Semispinalis capitis m.

Longissimus capitis m.

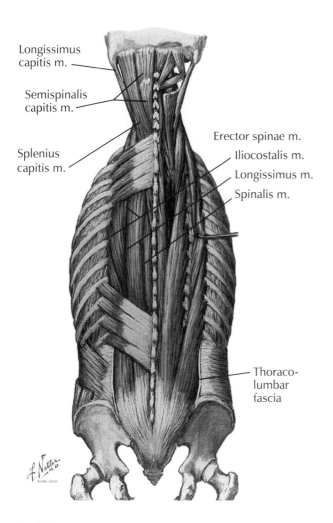

Longissimus capitis m.

Semispinalis capitis m.

Splenius capitis m.

Erector spinae m.

Iliocostalis m.

Longissimus m.

Spinalis m.

Thoraco-lumbar fascia

PLATE 161

NOTE that detailed dissections of each individual muscle slip are <u>not</u> encouraged for following steps.

SEPARATE erector spinae muscle into 3 parallel longitudinal columns, beginning from dorsal sacrum and medial edge of posterior part of iliac crest.

IDENTIFY parts of **erector spinae muscle**: **iliocostalis** laterally, **spinalis** medially, and **longissimus** between these 2 columns of muscle.

LOCATE dorsal cutaneous nerves (*not shown*) piercing between iliocostalis and longissimus muscles.

OBSERVE that each column may be named regionally.

BLUNT DISSECT erector spinae muscle from vertebral and costal attachments.

TRANSECT bulk of erector spinae muscle midway in small of back.

CUT individual muscle slips from their attachments to vertebrae and ribs, as erector spinae muscle is reflected superiorly.

REMOVE erector spinae muscle progressively to expose **transversospinalis muscles** (*labeled by individual names*).

IDENTIFY representative muscle slips for remaining **transversospinalis muscles** (**multifidus, semispinalis,** and **rotatores**) and **levatores costarum, interspinalis,** and **intertransverse muscles**.

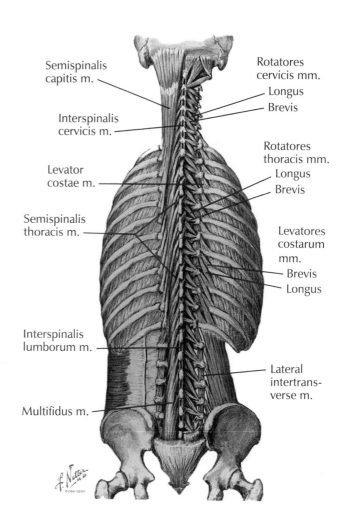

Semispinalis capitis m.

Interspinalis cervicis m.

Levator costae m.

Semispinalis thoracis m.

Interspinalis lumborum m.

Multifidus m.

Rotatores cervicis mm.

Longus

Brevis

Rotatores thoracis mm.

Longus

Brevis

Levatores costarum mm.

Brevis

Longus

Lateral intertransverse m.

PLATE 162

7

DISSECTION 1.3
SUBOCCIPITAL REGION

Complete DISSECTION **1.2** Deep Back.

Read DISCUSSION **1.6** Suboccipital Region.

PLACE cadaver in prone position.

CAUTION During next step, preserve greater occipital nerve.

BLUNT DISSECT deep to occipital insertion of **semispinalis capitis muscle** at medial border of muscle.

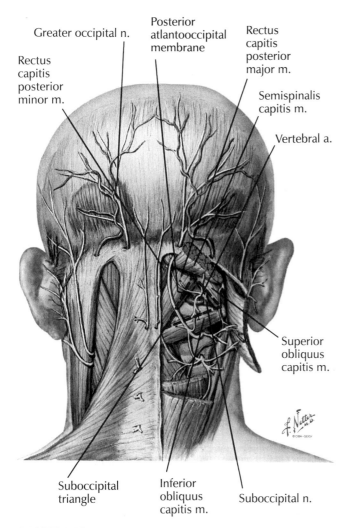

Greater occipital n.

Posterior atlantooccipital membrane

Rectus capitis posterior major m.

Rectus capitis posterior minor m.

Semispinalis capitis m.

Vertebral a.

Superior obliquus capitis m.

Suboccipital triangle

Inferior obliquus capitis m.

Suboccipital n.

PLATE 164

CUT semispinalis capitis muscle from its occipital attachment inferior to greater occipital nerve.

REFLECT semispinalis capitis muscle inferiorly.

LOOK for branches of dorsal primary rami (C1–3), which supply semispinalis capitis muscle on its deep surface.

IDENTIFY superior and **inferior obliquus capitis muscles** and **rectus capitis posterior major** and **minor muscles**.

TRACE greater occipital nerve around inferior border of inferior obliquus capitis muscle.

CAUTION During next step, preserve suboccipital nerve.

REMOVE fat and venous plexus from suboccipital triangle.

DEFINE borders of **suboccipital triangle** as rectus capitis posterior major and superior and inferior obliquus capitis muscles.

IDENTIFY suboccipital nerve (dorsal ramus of C1) within suboccipital triangle.

LOCATE branches of suboccipital nerve to rectus capitis posterior major and minor and superior and inferior obliquus capitis muscles.

LOCATE vertebral artery passing over posterior arch of atlas and through **posterior atlanto-occipital membrane**. Note that inferior obliquus capitis muscle may be reflected to expose vertebral artery.

REMOVE remaining deep muscles of back from spinous processes and laminae from entire length of vertebral column between C1–L5 with scalpel or chisel, as completely as possible. This procedure will prepare vertebral column for DISSECTION **1.4**.

DISSECTION 1.4

SPINAL CORD

Complete DISSECTIONS **1.2** Deep Back and
1.3 Suboccipital Region.

Read DISCUSSIONS **1.2** Bones, **1.3** Joints and
Ligaments, and **1.7** Spinal Cord and Meninges.

PLACE cadaver in prone position.

EXAMINE width of **lamina** of vertebrae from
different regions of vertebral column on skeleton.

CUT through right and left laminae of every
vertebra C2–L5, as far laterally on each lamina as
possible. Cut is to be approximately 1/2 inch
lateral to spinous process. Use either Stryker
saw or chisel and mallet.

REMOVE laminae with attached spinous
processes from entire length of vertebral column
below C1. Note that cutting vertebral column into
segments of 5 or 6 vertebrae may facilitate this
procedure.

IDENTIFY ligamentum flavum on deep surface of
removed vertebrae between adjacent laminae.
Note that some fat may need to be removed to
expose ligament.

CAUTION During next step, preserve gluteal
muscles.

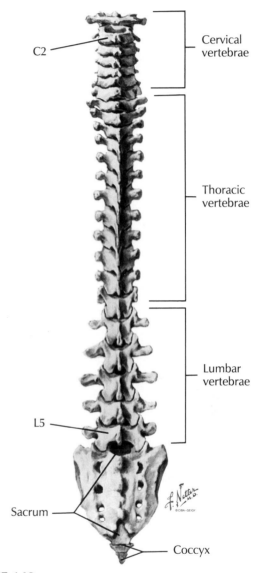

C2

Cervical
vertebrae

Thoracic
vertebrae

Lumbar
vertebrae

L5

Sacrum

Coccyx

PLATE 142

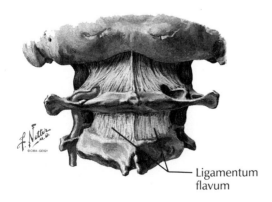

Ligamentum
flavum

PLATE 14

CUT through length of right and left sides of thin
dorsal surface of **sacrum** vertically between
posterior sacral foramina and median sacral crest
with Stryker saw or chisel and mallet.

REMOVE posterior wall of sacrum.

CLEAN exposed **epidural space** of fat and **internal
vertebral venous plexus** to expose **dura mater**.

IDENTIFY external filum terminale of dura mater extending from S2 to internal end of coccyx.

OBSERVE dura mater enclosing roots of spinal nerves.

CAUTION During next step, preserve arachnoid layer of meninges.

CUT dura mater vertically in its posterior midline for its entire length.

RETRACT dura mater with dissection pins to expose spinal cord and other meninges.

IDENTIFY arachnoid collapsed on spinal cord.

PLATE 148

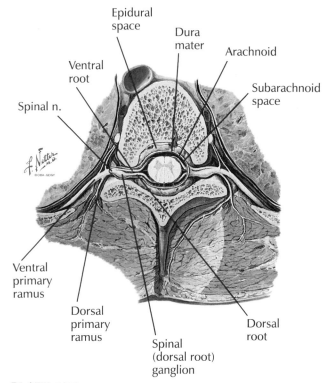

PLATE 156

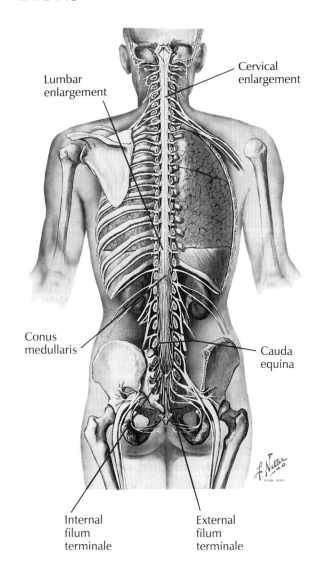

INJECT subarachnoid space with water from 50-mL syringe by carefully slipping 3-inch, 16-gauge needle through arachnoid.

IDENTIFY paired **posterior spinal arteries** deep to arachnoid.

TRACE 1 posterior spinal artery laterally to its origin from **posterior radicular artery**.

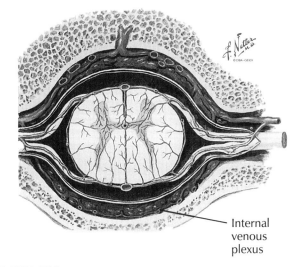

PLATE 159

CAUTION During next step, preserve pia mater and spinal cord.

CUT arachnoid vertically its entire length.

OBSERVE pia mater and its more than 20 serial serrations extending between dorsal and ventral rootlets of each spinal nerve to impale dura mater. Note that these **denticulate ligaments** end at **conus medullaris**, which is spinal cord level S5, located at vertebral level L1.

IDENTIFY conus medullaris, **internal filum terminale** of pia mater, **cauda equina**, and **cervical** and **lumbar enlargements**.

LOCATE spinal rootlets of **accessory nerve (XI)** (*not shown*), between dorsal and ventral rootlets of C1–6, passing posterior to denticulate ligaments, and follow this nerve superiorly to foramen magnum.

REMOVE adjacent inferior and superior articular processes with rongeur forceps from 1 intervertebral articulation to expose **spinal (dorsal root) ganglion** lying in intervertebral foramen. Note that previous laminectomy may have destroyed all articular processes.

PLATE 155

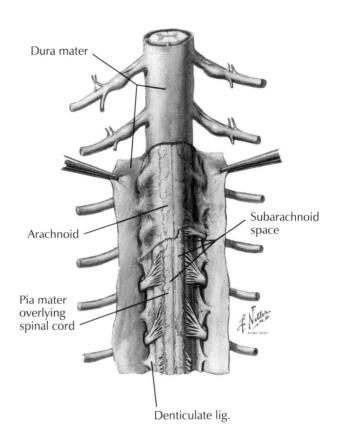

Dura mater

Arachnoid

Subarachnoid space

Pia mater overlying spinal cord

Denticulate lig.

PLATE 158

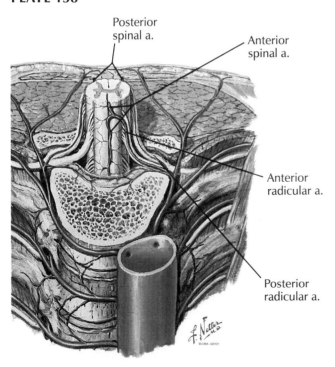

Posterior spinal a.

Anterior spinal a.

Anterior radicular a.

Posterior radicular a.

IDENTIFY 1 **spinal nerve, ventral root, dorsal root, dorsal primary ramus**, and origin of **ventral primary ramus**.

CAUTION During next step, preserve anterior dura mater.

TRANSECT spinal cord at midthoracic level.

REFLECT both cut ends about 3 inches to expose anterior surface of spinal cord.

IDENTIFY single **anterior spinal artery**.

LOCATE origin of ventral rootlets of 1 spinal nerve, and trace it to its passage through dural sheath. Note that dorsal and ventral roots have separate dural sheaths.

TRACE 1 anterior spinal artery laterally as it passes with ventral root of spinal cord to its origin from **anterior radicular artery**.

Section 2

ANTERIOR BODY WALL

DISSECTIONS

DISSECTION 2.1

PECTORAL REGION

Read DISCUSSIONS **2.1** Surface Anatomy,
2.2 Mammary Gland (Female), **2.3** Bones of
Thoracic Wall, **2.6** Pectoral Region, **5.2** Bones
(Shoulder Girdle and Arm), **5.5** Axilla, **5.6** Brachial
Plexus, and **6.2** Bones (Pelvic Girdle).

PLACE cadaver in supine position.

ABDUCT arms until resistance is felt. Arms may
be secured in abducted position with ropes or by
continuous retraction by lab partner.

MARK location of anterior cutaneous branches of
intercostal nerves.

CAUTION   During next step, preserve origin of
superficial muscle fibers of platysma muscle over
clavicle, cephalic vein in area of anterior shoulder
and axillary fold, and intercostobrachial nerve in
axilla.

INCISE skin and subcutaneous tissue of pectoral
and axillary regions (**Figure 3**). Note that
mammary tissue is to be removed with
subcutaneous tissue in female.

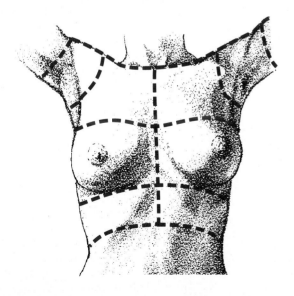

Figure 3

REFLECT skin flaps laterally. Fascial strands
attached to axillary skin may make this task
difficult. Note that although skin of axilla is being
reflected now, cleaning will be completed during
DISSECTION **5.1**.

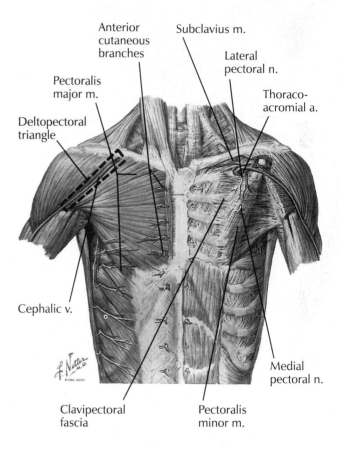

PLATE 174

DISCARD skin and subcutaneous tissue.

LOCATE anterior cutaneous branches of at least
2 intercostal nerves and their accompanying
arteries and veins. These small branches pierce
pectoralis major muscle in series of 1 per rib, and
are found 1 finger-width lateral to sternum.

LOCATE termination of **cephalic vein** in groove
(**deltopectoral triangle**) between pectoralis major
muscle and deltoid muscle.

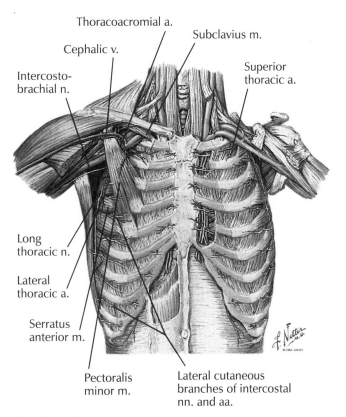

Thoracoacromial a.

Cephalic v.

Subclavius m.

Intercosto-
brachial n.

Superior
thoracic a.

Long
thoracic n.

Lateral
thoracic a.

Serratus
anterior m.

Pectoralis
minor m.

Lateral cutaneous
branches of intercostal
nn. and aa.

PLATE 175

LOOK for **deltopectoral lymph nodes** (*not shown*) and **deltoid branch** of **thoracoacromial artery** accompanying cephalic vein.

IDENTIFY pectoralis major muscle, moving scalpel blade parallel to direction of fibers.

BLUNT DISSECT deep to clavicular attachment of pectoralis major muscle. Begin where cephalic vein passes anterior axillary fold.

CUT attachment of pectoralis major muscle to clavicle with scissors along inferior border of bone.

BLUNT DISSECT deep to sternal attachment of pectoralis major muscle. Arm may be adducted to facilitate this step.

CUT sternocostal head of pectoralis major muscle with scissors 2 finger-widths parallel to lateral edge of sternum.

REFLECT pectoralis major muscle laterally, locating branches of **medial** and **lateral pectoral nerves** as they enter muscle on its deep surface.

CLEAN undersurface of pectoralis major muscle to identify medial pectoral nerve, which either pierces pectoralis minor muscle or passes lateral to it, and to identify lateral pectoral nerve, which passes medial border of **pectoralis minor muscle.**

IDENTIFY pectoral branches of **thoracoacromial artery** and **vein**, which accompany lateral pectoral nerve.

OBSERVE clavipectoral fascia and its component parts. Note that this fascia will be removed as dissection progresses.

CLEAN subclavius muscle of fat deposits.

LOCATE superior thoracic artery as it passes medial border of pectoralis minor muscle.

CLEAN pectoralis minor muscle.

DETACH pectoralis minor muscle from ribs 2–5.

REFLECT pectoralis minor muscle superiorly.

IDENTIFY acromial and **clavicular branches** of **thoracoacromial artery**.

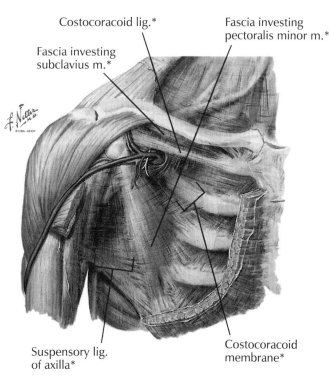

Costocoracoid lig.*

Fascia investing
pectoralis minor m.*

Fascia investing
subclavius m.*

Suspensory lig.
of axilla*

Costocoracoid
membrane*

*Clavipectoral fascia

PLATE 403

16

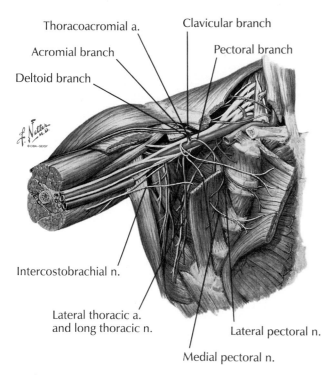

Thoracoacromial a.

Clavicular branch

Acromial branch

Pectoral branch

Deltoid branch

Intercostobrachial n.

Lateral thoracic a. and long thoracic n.

Lateral pectoral n.

Medial pectoral n.

PLATE 404

TRACE branches of thoracoacromial trunk retrograde to their common source from axillary artery.

LOCATE origin of **lateral thoracic artery** deep to pectoralis minor muscle.

REMOVE fat and fascia in axilla with forceps, fingers, and blunt-scissor dissection, taking care not to injure structures embedded in fat.

LOCATE axillary lymph nodes, but do not preserve them.

IDENTIFY lateral cutaneous branches of **intercostal nerve** and **artery** between serrations of serratus anterior muscle.

IDENTIFY intercostobrachial nerve as it crosses axilla from lateral cutaneous branch of 2nd intercostal nerve.

IDENTIFY long thoracic nerve as it accompanies lateral thoracic artery to pass external to **serratus anterior muscle**.

CLEAN serratus anterior muscle.

DIRECT attention to breast embedded in discarded skin of female (**Figure 4**).

SECTION removed breast sagittally through subcutaneous tissue and nipple.

REMOVE fat from breast around 1 **gland lobule**.

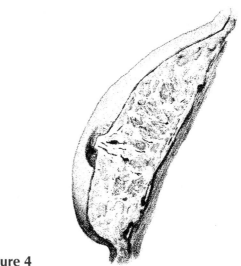

Figure 4

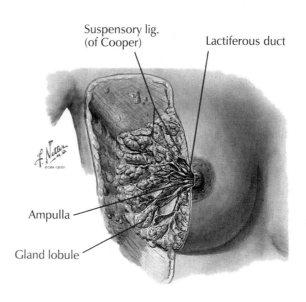

Suspensory lig. (of Cooper)

Lactiferous duct

Ampulla

Gland lobule

PLATE 167

IDENTIFY ampulla and **lactiferous duct**, which extend from isolated gland lobule to nipple.

LOCATE several dense, fibrous suspensory ligaments.

DISSECTION 2.2
ANTERIOR THORACIC WALL

Complete DISSECTION 2.1 Pectoral Region.

Read DISCUSSIONS 2.4 Joints of Thoracic Wall, 2.7 Muscles of Thoracic Wall, 2.8 Muscles of Anterior Abdominal Wall, 2.9 Nerves, and 2.10 Arteries and Veins.

PLACE cadaver in supine position.

IDENTIFY perforating branches of internal thoracic artery and anterior cutaneous branches of intercostal nerves as they pierce intercostal spaces 1 finger-width from both sides of sternum.

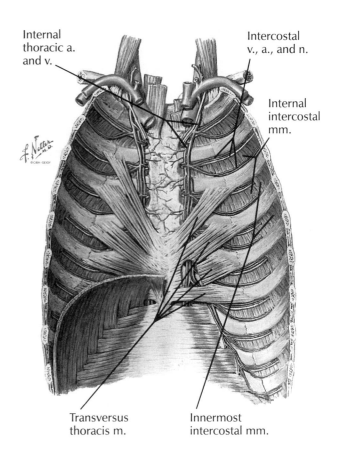

Internal thoracic a. and v.

Intercostal v., a., and n.

Internal intercostal mm.

Transversus thoracis m.

Innermost intercostal mm.

PLATE 176

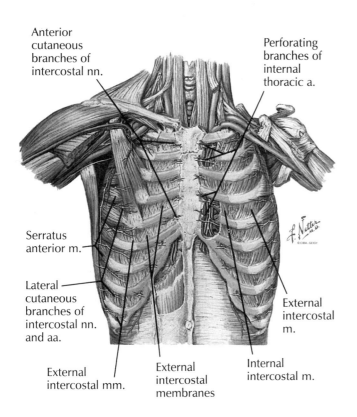

Anterior cutaneous branches of intercostal nn.

Perforating branches of internal thoracic a.

Serratus anterior m.

Lateral cutaneous branches of intercostal nn. and aa.

External intercostal mm.

External intercostal membranes

Internal intercostal m.

External intercostal m.

PLATE 175

REMOVE remaining sternocostal attachments of pectoralis major muscle with scalpel in preparation for inspection of intercostal muscles.

IDENTIFY lateral cutaneous branches of intercostal nerve and artery piercing intercostal spaces anterior to digitations of serratus anterior muscle.

IDENTIFY external intercostal muscles and external intercostal membranes of intercostal spaces 2–5.

BLUNT DISSECT deep to external intercostal membrane, using underlying fiber direction of internal intercostal muscles as guide.

CONTINUE blunt dissection deep to muscle fibers of external intercostal muscles.

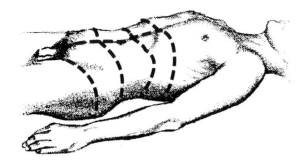

Figure 5

CUT inferior attachment of external intercostal muscle from superior border of ribs 3–6.

REFLECT external intercostal muscles superiorly to expose **internal intercostal muscles**.

BLUNT DISSECT deep to anterior fibers of **serratus anterior muscle**.

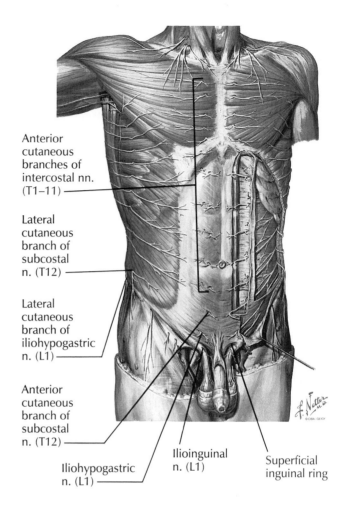

Anterior cutaneous branches of intercostal nn. (T1–11)

Lateral cutaneous branch of subcostal n. (T12)

Lateral cutaneous branch of iliohypogastric n. (L1)

Anterior cutaneous branch of subcostal n. (T12)

Iliohypogastric n. (L1)

Ilioinguinal n. (L1)

Superficial inguinal ring

PLATE 240

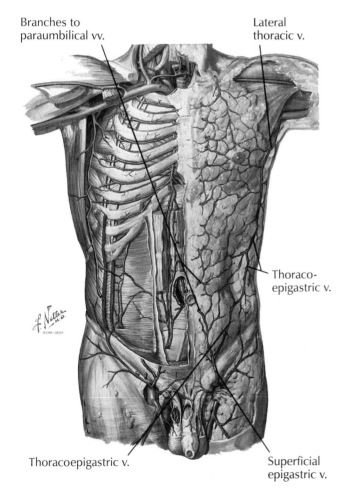

Branches to paraumbilical vv.

Lateral thoracic v.

Thoraco-epigastric v.

Thoracoepigastric v.

Superficial epigastric v.

PLATE 239

REFLECT serratus anterior muscle toward its scapular origin by freeing its attachments to ribs with scalpel. Continue reflection to expose ribs and intercostal spaces as far lateral as midaxillary line.

CAUTION During next step, preserve internal thoracic artery and vein and intercostal veins, arteries, and nerves.

CUT internal intercostal muscle from its attachments to both inferior and superior margins of cartilaginous part of ribs 1–6 as far lateral as costochondral junction on both sides.

CAUTION Preserve internal thoracic artery and vein by using fingers to free internal thoracic artery and vein from deep surface of muscle as incised part of internal intercostal muscle is removed lateral to sternum.

BLUNT DISSECT transversus thoracis muscle free from its attachment to ribs deep to **internal thoracic artery** and **vein**. Use fingers and closed scissors.

LOCATE intercostal vein, artery, and **nerve** in inferior groove of 1 rib. Forceps may be used to reach these structures.

DIRECT attention to anterior abdominal wall.

INCISE skin of anterior abdominal wall (**Figure 5**).

CAUTION   During next steps, preserve superficial inguinal ring.

REFLECT skin flaps laterally, removing subcutaneous fat with skin.

DISCARD skin flaps and subcutaneous tissue.

LOOK for superficial veins, but do not preserve them.

LOCATE some **anterior** and **lateral cutaneous branches** of **thoracoabdominal nerves** (T7–11) and subcostal nerve (T12).

IDENTIFY anterior cutaneous branch of iliohypogastric nerve (L1), which pierces aponeurosis of external abdominal oblique muscle above inguinal ligament.

IDENTIFY superficial inguinal ring. External spermatic fascia will be studied in DISSECTION **2.4**. Do not dissect inguinal region now.

IDENTIFY anterior cutaneous branch of ilio-inguinal nerve (L1), which exits from superficial inguinal ring.

DISSECTION 2.3
ANTERIOR ABDOMINAL WALL

Complete DISSECTION **2.2** Anterior Thoracic Wall.

Read DISCUSSIONS **2.5** Fasciae, **2.7** Muscles of Thoracic Wall, **2.8** Muscles of Anterior Abdominal Wall, **2.9** Nerves, and **2.10** Arteries and Veins.

PLACE cadaver in supine position.

CLEAN superior attachments of **anterior layer** of **rectus sheath**.

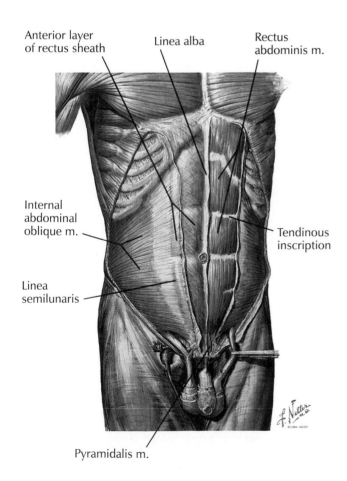

Anterior layer of rectus sheath

Linea alba

Rectus abdominis m.

Internal abdominal oblique m.

Tendinous inscription

Linea semilunaris

Pyramidalis m.

PLATE 233

BLUNT DISSECT deep to superior fibers of both **rectus abdominis muscles** and anterior layer of rectus sheath.

CAUTION   During next step, preserve medial fibers of external abdominal oblique muscle.

REFLECT superior part of <u>both</u> rectus abdominis muscles inferiorly by freeing their attachments to ribs with scalpel. Continue reflection to expose ribs.

IDENTIFY linea alba as vertical line where anterior and posterior layers of rectus sheath fuse in midline.

IDENTIFY linea semilunaris demarcated by lateral border of rectus abdominis muscle.

CUT vertical incision in anterior layer of rectus sheath 1 finger-width lateral to linea alba its entire length on <u>both</u> sides.

CAUTION   During next step, preserve inguinal region.

MAKE 2 horizontal incisions in anterior layer of rectus sheath on <u>both</u> sides, 1 at xiphoid end and 1 at pubic end, each from vertical incision to linea semilunaris. Inspection of rectus sheath is to be completed later in this dissection.

CUT ribs 2–7 in midaxillary line, using Stryker saw, rongeur forceps, or chisel and mallet (**Figure 6**).

CAUTION   During next step, do not damage lungs by inserting scissors too deeply.

CUT muscles in intercostal spaces along same midaxillary line, using scissors.

TRANSECT cartilaginous part of ribs 6, 7. Additional muscle fibers of external abdominal oblique and rectus abdominis muscles may be freed from ribs with scalpel to locate costochondral junctions.

TRANSECT body of sternum above xiphoid process with Stryker saw or chisel and mallet.

TRANSECT manubrium below costosternal joint of rib 1 with Stryker saw or chisel and mallet.

CUT muscles in intercostal space 7 along inferior border of rib 7.

CUT muscles in intercostal space 1 along inferior border of rib 1.

BLUNT DISSECT deep to ribs, using fingers to free parietal pleura from breastplate.

REMOVE anterior breastplate.

DIRECT attention to internal surface of breastplate.

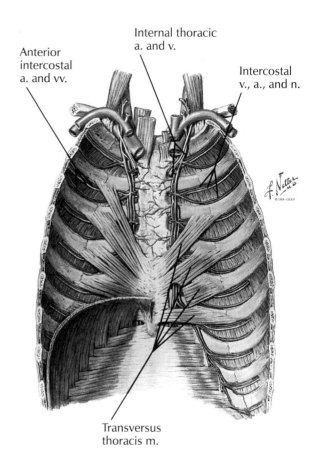

Anterior intercostal a. and vv.

Internal thoracic a. and v.

Intercostal v., a., and n.

Transversus thoracis m.

PLATE 176

Figure 6

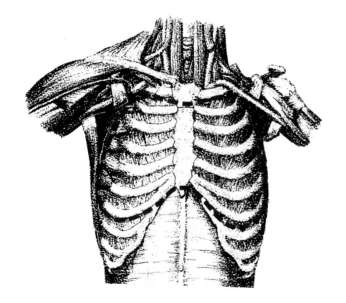

EXAMINE intercostal vein, artery, and **nerve** in costal grooves of ribs of anterior breastplate.

EXAMINE internal thoracic artery and **vein** as they pass 1 finger-width on either side of sternum. Note how these vessels supply **anterior intercostal arteries** and **veins.**

IDENTIFY remaining attachments of **transversus thoracis muscle** on deep surface of breastplate.

REDIRECT attention to anterior abdominal wall.

LOCATE anterior branches of **thoracoabdominal nerves** and **branches** of **superior** and **inferior epigastric arteries** and **veins** as they pierce anterior layer of rectus sheath.

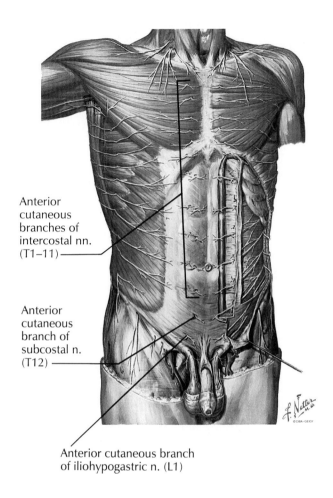

Anterior
cutaneous
branches of
intercostal nn.
(T1–11)

Anterior
cutaneous
branch of
subcostal n.
(T12)

Anterior cutaneous branch
of iliohypogastric n. (L1)

PLATE 240

REFLECT anterior layer of rectus sheath laterally on <u>both</u> sides. Note that **tendinous inscriptions** may need to be severed to free anterior layer.

IDENTIFY inconstant **pyramidalis muscle.**

BLUNT DISSECT rectus abdominis muscle from linea alba and linea semilunaris.

NOTE that remaining dissection should be restricted to just 1 side of cadaver to preserve inguinal region for examination in DISSECTION **2.4.**

TRANSECT <u>right</u> rectus abdominis muscle 2 finger-widths above umbilicus.

REFLECT inferior cut end of <u>right</u> rectus abdominis muscle inferiorly. Reflect superior cut end of <u>right</u> rectus abdominis muscle to remove it. Note that branches of nerves and arteries serving rectus abdominis muscle will be cut to do so.

EXAMINE posterior layer of **rectus sheath.**

LOOK for **arcuate line.**

CLEAN right **external abdominal oblique muscle.**

BLUNT DISSECT small area between <u>right</u> external abdominal oblique and **internal abdominal oblique muscles** to establish plane between muscles. Begin near linea semilunaris intersection with costal margin.

CUT <u>right</u> external abdominal oblique muscle along midaxillary line from costal margin to anterior superior iliac spine (**Figure 7**).

Figure 7

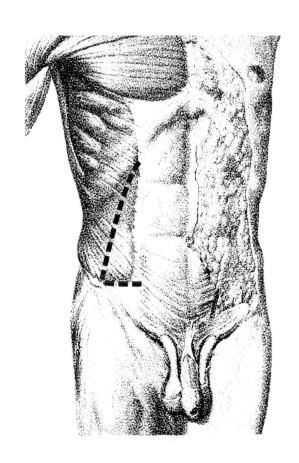

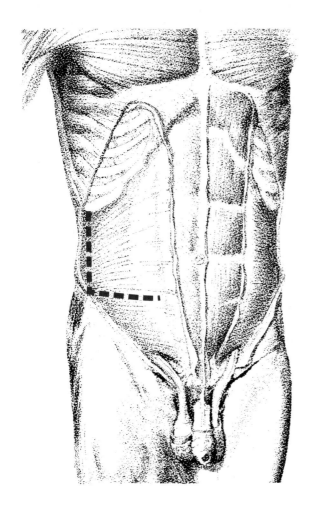

Figure 8

CAUTION During next step, preserve iliohypogastric nerve by not cutting too far inferior.

MAKE horizontal incision in aponeurosis of <u>right</u> external abdominal oblique muscle from anterior superior iliac spine to linea semilunaris.

BLUNT DISSECT deep to <u>right</u> external abdominal oblique muscle between vertical incision and linea semilunaris.

REFLECT medial flap of <u>right</u> external abdominal oblique muscle toward rectus abdominis muscle.

BLUNT DISSECT deep to remaining lateral part of <u>right</u> external abdominal oblique muscle, freeing attachment to ribs.

LOCATE cutaneous branch of **iliohypogastric nerve**, freeing it from external abdominal oblique muscle so it may be traced later.

CAUTION During next step, do not tear muscle layers.

REFLECT lateral part of <u>right</u> external abdominal oblique muscle to expose internal abdominal oblique muscle.

TRACE iliohypogastric nerve to establish its passage between internal abdominal oblique and transversus abdominis muscles.

PLATE 238

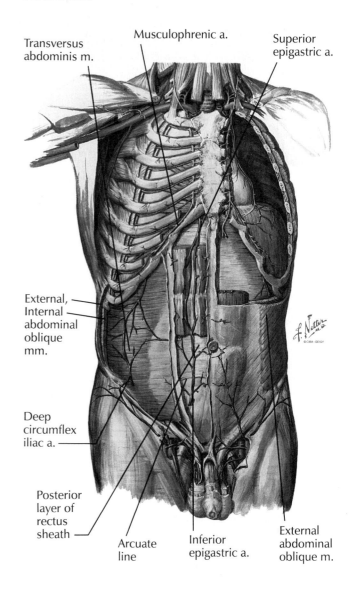

Transversus abdominis m.

Musculophrenic a.

Superior epigastric a.

External, Internal abdominal oblique mm.

Deep circumflex iliac a.

Posterior layer of rectus sheath

Arcuate line

Inferior epigastric a.

External abdominal oblique m.

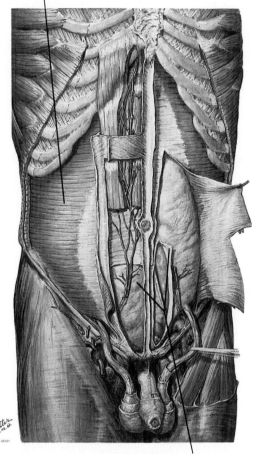

Transverse
abdominis m.

Transversalis
fascia

PLATE 234

CUT <u>right</u> internal abdominal oblique aponeurosis close to anterior superior iliac spine, carrying incision through muscle toward costochondral junction of rib 10 (**Figure 8**).

BLUNT DISSECT deep to <u>right</u> internal abdominal oblique muscle to establish plane for next cut.

MAKE horizontal incision in <u>right</u> internal abdominal oblique muscle from anterior superior iliac spine to linea semilunaris.

BLUNT DISSECT deep to <u>right</u> internal abdominal oblique muscle between vertical incision and linea semilunaris.

REFLECT medial flap of <u>right</u> internal abdominal oblique muscle toward rectus abdominis muscle.

LOCATE deep circumflex iliac artery medial to anterior superior iliac spine between internal abdominal oblique muscle and **transversus abdominis muscle**.

LOCATE passage of thoracoabdominal nerves between internal abdominal oblique and transversus abdominis muscles.

INSPECT transversus abdominis muscle on <u>right</u> side.

DISSECTION 2.4
INGUINAL REGION

Complete DISSECTION **2.3** Anterior Abdominal Wall.

Read DISCUSSION **2.11** Inguinal Region.

PLACE cadaver in supine position.

BLUNT DISSECT deep to transversalis fascia by cutting small opening in posterior layer of rectus sheath immediately inferior to umbilicus and continue to free between parietal peritoneum and transversalis fascia.

MAKE transverse incision from initial opening inferior to umbilicus to anterior superior iliac spine on <u>both</u> sides (**Figure 9**). Extend incision through <u>right</u> side of abdominal wall, which was previously dissected, and then through <u>left</u> (undisturbed) side. Note that rectus abdominis muscle is to be cut on <u>left</u> (undisturbed) side and transversus abdominis muscle on <u>both</u> sides.

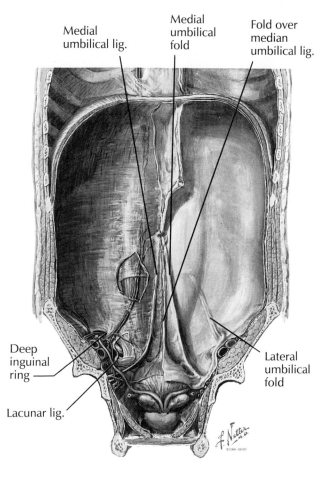

Medial umbilical lig.
Medial umbilical fold
Fold over median umbilical lig.
Deep inguinal ring
Lateral umbilical fold
Lacunar lig.

PLATE 236

ELEVATE lower part of anterior abdominal wall by running hand between **parietal peritoneum** and transversalis fascia.

CAUTION During next steps, preserve fundiform ligament (in male), and do not damage lateral aspects of abdominal wall.

CUT vertical incision from umbilicus to pubic bone. Make incision just to <u>left</u> of linea alba on <u>left</u> side.

REFLECT both triangular flaps of lower abdominal wall as far laterally as possible so internal surface may be examined.

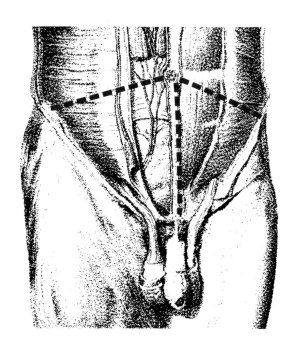

Figure 9

IDENTIFY median, **medial**, and **lateral umbilical folds**.

REFLECT superior portion of abdominal wall to examine convergence of umbilical folds toward umbilicus.

NOTE that next steps are to be carried out unilaterally on <u>right</u> side.

DIRECT attention to internal surface of inguinal region of anterior abdominal wall.

IDENTIFY inguinal ligament as it extends from anterior superior iliac spine to pubic tubercle, and **lacunar ligament** as it extends posteriorly to pectineal line on superior ramus of pubic bone.

IDENTIFY deep inguinal ring. Note that there is usually dimple in parietal peritoneum indicating its location just lateral to lateral umbilical fold.

NOTE that next 3 inspections will be repeated in DISSECTION **4.3**. Do not clean structures now.

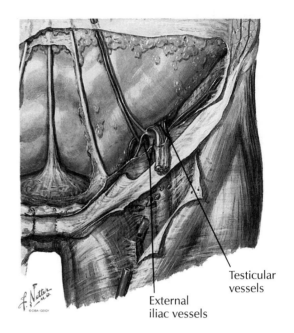

PLATE 244

IDENTIFY external iliac vessels as they pass deep to inguinal ligament.

IDENTIFY ductus (vas) deferens and **testicular vessels** passing over external iliac vessels toward deep inguinal ring (in male).

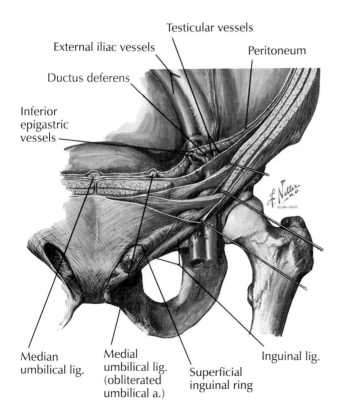

PLATE 245

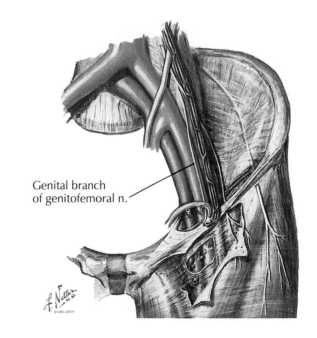

PLATE 244

IDENTIFY (in female) **round ligament** of **uterus** (*not shown*) passing over external iliac vessels toward deep inguinal ring (**Plate 343**).

CAUTION   During next step, do not damage structures just identified.

REMOVE parietal peritoneum from reflected flap on <u>right</u> side to expose **obliterated urachus**, **obliterated umbilical artery**, and **inferior epigastric vessels**, which form median, medial, and lateral umbilical folds, respectively.

FOLLOW either ductus deferens and testicular vessels (in male) or round ligament of uterus (in female) to deep inguinal ring.

LOOK for **genital branch** of **genitofemoral nerve** as it enters deep inguinal ring (in male).

INSERT finger through **inguinal canal** from deep inguinal ring to **superficial inguinal ring**. Note that walls of inguinal canal will stretch because finger is larger than diameter of canal. In females, note that round ligament of uterus fans out as it exits superficial inguinal ring.

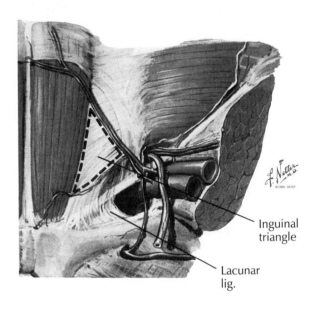

Inguinal triangle

Lacunar lig.

PLATE 243

BLUNT DISSECT between **transversalis fascia** and **transversus abdominis muscle**.

IDENTIFY falx inguinalis as it forms superior and inferior walls of inguinal canal.

DIRECT attention to external surface of inguinal region.

REVIEW boundaries of inguinal canal. Canal is formed by aponeurosis of external abdominal oblique muscle anteriorly and by transversus abdominis muscle and falx inguinalis posteriorly. Note that falx inguinalis also contributes to roof of inguinal canal and lacunar ligament contributes to its floor.

DEFINE boundaries of **inguinal triangle** as inguinal ligament inferiorly, lateral edge of rectus abdominis muscle medially, and inferior epigastric artery laterally. Note that superficial inguinal ring is located within inguinal triangle.

Female

Labia majora will be inspected in DISSECTION **7.1**. Therefore, join dissection group to study scrotum in male.

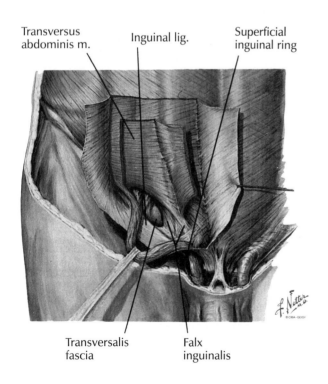

Transversus abdominis m.   Inguinal lig.   Superficial inguinal ring

Transversalis fascia   Falx inguinalis

PLATE 243

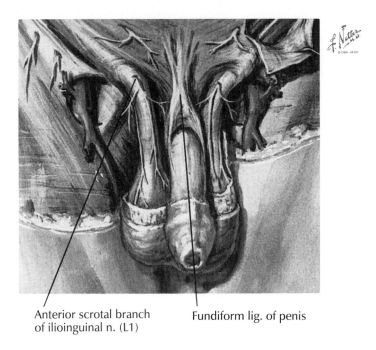

Anterior scrotal branch
of ilioinguinal n. (L1)

Fundiform lig. of penis

PLATE 240 detail

Male

CAUTION During next steps, preserve fundiform ligament of penis.

FOLLOW anterior scrotal branch of **ilioinguinal nerve** from superficial inguinal ring to anterior skin of scrotum.

INCISE skin of scrotum, from superficial inguinal ring vertically to inferior limit of scrotum, and skin around root of penis (**Figure 10**).

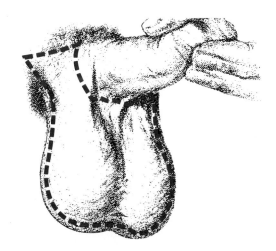

Figure 10

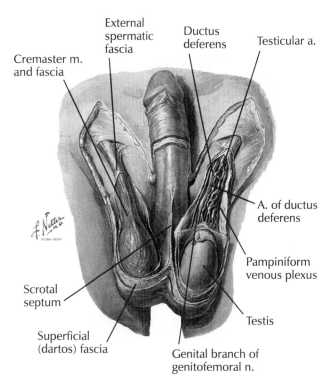

Cremaster m.
and fascia

External
spermatic
fascia

Ductus
deferens

Testicular a.

A. of ductus
deferens

Pampiniform
venous plexus

Testis

Scrotal
septum

Superficial
(dartos) fascia

Genital branch of
genitofemoral n.

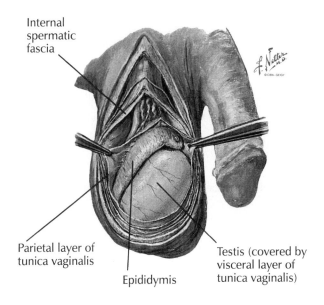

Internal
spermatic
fascia

Parietal layer of
tunica vaginalis

Epididymis

Testis (covered by
visceral layer of
tunica vaginalis)

PLATE 365

IDENTIFY fundiform ligament of **penis**, which extends from linea alba encircling root of penis to attach to median scrotal septum.

REFLECT skin and **superficial (dartos) fascia** of anterior scrotum laterally and inferiorly to expose fascial coverings of spermatic cord and testis. Note that scrotal skin is thin and dartos tunic is firmly attached to it.

29

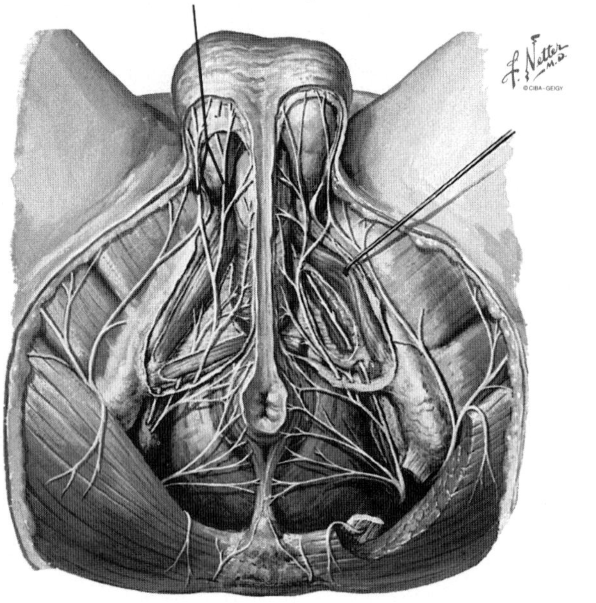

Posterior scrotal
branches of perineal n.

PLATE 386

LOCATE median scrotal septum as it divides scrotum into halves.

LOCATE scrotal ligament (*not shown*), which is derived from gubernaculum.

LOCATE posterior scrotal branches of **perineal nerve** in fascia of posterior scrotum.

CUT scrotal ligament and posterior scrotal skin as close to root of penis as possible.

DISCARD anterior scrotal skin with dartos tunic and scrotal septum.

NOTE that separation of fascial layers of spermatic cord and testis is difficult to achieve. Attempt to dissect them to help understand derivation of those layers. Use scissors and forceps to tease structures apart.

BLUNT DISSECT between **external spermatic fascia** (derived from external abdominal oblique muscle layer) and **cremaster muscle** and **fascia** (derived from internal abdominal oblique muscle layer). Continue to open between these layers around testis.

BLUNT DISSECT between cremaster muscle and **internal spermatic fascia** (derived from transversalis fascia layer). Continue to open between these layers around testis.

IDENTIFY ductus deferens and its **artery** on its surface.

IDENTIFY testicular artery and **pampiniform plexus** of **veins**.

IDENTIFY genital branch of **genitofemoral nerve**, which serves cremaster muscle.

OPEN parietal layer of **tunica vaginalis** to expose testis and epididymis. Use scissors to make initial incision; continue this incision by pulling parts away from each other. Note that coverings cannot be reflected completely. Cut away reflected part of tunica vaginalis, and discard.

IDENTIFY testis and **epididymis**, **sinus** of **epididymis** (*not shown*), and **mediastinum** of **testis** (*not shown*).

Section 3

THORAX

DISSECTIONS

DISSECTION 3.1
PLEURA AND LUNGS

Complete DISSECTIONS **2.2** Anterior Thoracic Wall and **2.3** Anterior Abdominal Wall.

Read DISCUSSION **3.1** Lungs.

PLACE cadaver in supine position.

OPEN exposed **parietal pleura** on both sides with vertical incision along costochondral line between ribs 1–7. Note that removal of breastplate may have already torn parietal pleura.

EXPLORE pleural cavity by placing hands between parietal and **visceral pleura**. Take care not to cut hands on ragged ends of ribs. There may be adhesions between parietal and visceral pleura. Separate adhesions as necessary to proceed.

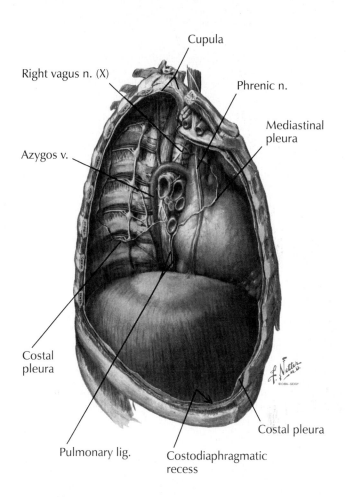

Cupula

Right vagus n. (X)

Phrenic n.

Mediastinal pleura

Azygos v.

Costal pleura

Costal pleura

Pulmonary lig.

Costodiaphragmatic recess

PLATE 218

NOTE that right and left pleural cavities are not in communication with each other.

RELATE regional naming of parietal pleura during exploration to become comfortable with distinctions of **mediastinal**, **apical** (**cupula**), **costal**, and **diaphragmatic pleura**.

EXPLORE reflections of pleura, which are clefts formed between 2 layers of parietal pleura. Run fingers between costal and mediastinal pleura to establish extent of **costomediastinal recess** (*not shown*). Run fingers between costal and diaphragmatic pleura to establish extent of **costodiaphragmatic recess**.

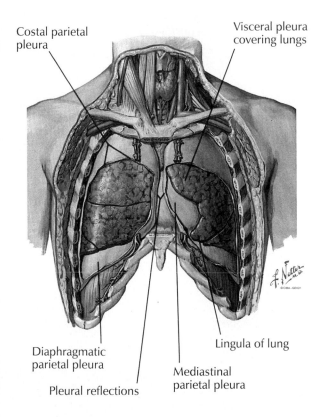

Costal parietal pleura

Visceral pleura covering lungs

Diaphragmatic parietal pleura

Pleural reflections

Mediastinal parietal pleura

Lingula of lung

PLATE 186

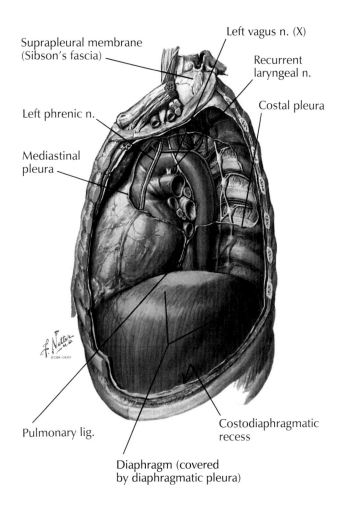

Suprapleural membrane (Sibson's fascia)

Left vagus n. (X)

Recurrent laryngeal n.

Left phrenic n.

Costal pleura

Mediastinal pleura

Pulmonary lig.

Costodiaphragmatic recess

Diaphragm (covered by diaphragmatic pleura)

PLATE 219

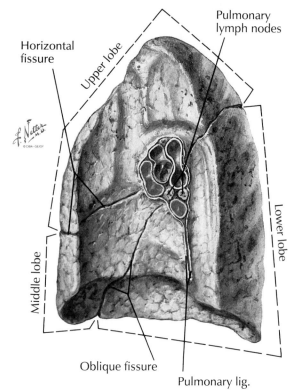

Horizontal fissure

Pulmonary lymph nodes

Upper lobe

Middle lobe

Lower lobe

Oblique fissure

Pulmonary lig.

PLATE 187

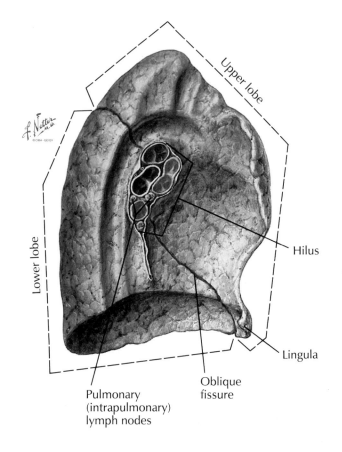

Upper lobe

Lower lobe

Hilus

Lingula

Pulmonary (intrapulmonary) lymph nodes

Oblique fissure

PLATE 187

NOTE inferior pleural margin extends from rib 8 at costochondral line to rib 10 in midaxillary line and rib 12 in scapular line.

EXPLORE root of **lung** (*not labeled*) where visceral pleura from surface of lung becomes continuous with mediastinal pleura. Double fold of pleura inferior to root of lung is called **pulmonary ligament**. It may be seen more easily later, after lungs have been removed.

RETRACT right lung at its root, as far laterally as possible, by having 1 student pull on lung from around **hilus**.

CAUTION During following transection, preserve vagus nerve (*not shown*) and azygos vein, which pass posterior to root of lung, and phrenic nerve, which passes anterior to root of lung.

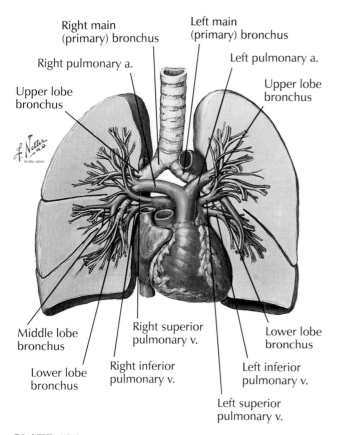

Right main (primary) bronchus
Left main (primary) bronchus
Right pulmonary a.
Left pulmonary a.
Upper lobe bronchus
Upper lobe bronchus
Middle lobe bronchus
Right superior pulmonary v.
Lower lobe bronchus
Lower lobe bronchus
Right inferior pulmonary v.
Left inferior pulmonary v.
Left superior pulmonary v.

PLATE 194

TRANSECT root of <u>right</u> lung at hilus close to where pulmonary vessels exit from pericardium. Attempt to cut proximal to division of **right main (primary) bronchus** into **lobar (secondary) bronchi.**

REPEAT retraction and transection on <u>left</u> lung, again taking care to preserve **vagus** and **phrenic nerves**.

REMOVE both lungs from thorax, freeing any remaining adhesions as necessary.

IDENTIFY pulmonary ligament at inferior pole of hilus of lung.

EXAMINE internal surface of thorax.

CAUTION During next step, preserve sympathetic trunk along inner surface of heads of ribs and sides of vertebral bodies.

STRIP entire extent of costal pleura from interior of right and left sides of rib cage.

CAUTION During next step, preserve phrenic nerve and pericardiacophrenic artery and vein. They will be examined further in DISSECTION **3.2**.

BLUNT DISSECT diaphragmatic and mediastinal pleura free from diaphragm and pericardium.

DIRECT attention to examination of lungs.

IDENTIFY bronchopulmonary lymph nodes at hilus of lung and **tracheobronchial lymph nodes** around root of lung. Do not preserve them.

EXPLORE oblique and **horizontal fissures** of **right lung** and **oblique fissure** of **left lung**, separating adhesions as necessary.

IDENTIFY upper, middle, and **lower lobes** of **right lung**.

IDENTIFY upper and **lower lobes** and **lingula** of **left lung**.

IDENTIFY bronchi by presence of cartilaginous rings. Note that bronchi are posterior to pulmonary vessels at hilus of lung.

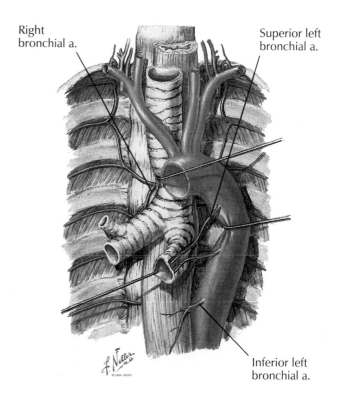

Right bronchial a.
Superior left bronchial a.
Inferior left bronchial a.

PLATE 196

35

IDENTIFY pulmonary veins by thin wall and anterior position at hilus of lung and **pulmonary artery** by its more substantial wall.

EXAMINE veins, artery, and bronchi on lung and on cut root of lung in thorax.

CAUTION During next step, preserve branches of pulmonary artery and vein.

TRACE main (primary) bronchus of each lung to its division into **lobar (secondary) bronchi**, and then trace 1 lobar bronchus into its division into **segmental (tertiary) bronchi**. Perform this dissection by picking away substance of lung with forceps in each hand. Use one forceps to protect structure being traced, and other forceps to remove lung tissue.

OBSERVE that branches of pulmonary artery accompany intrasegmental bronchi and that branches of pulmonary vein travel intersegmentally between bronchopulmonary segments.

IDENTIFY bronchopulmonary segments on surface of lung or model of lung (see DISCUSSION **3.1**).

LOOK for branches of **bronchial arteries** on posterior surfaces of primary bronchi. Note that there are usually 2 bronchial arteries to left primary bronchus and 1 bronchial artery to right primary bronchus. Their origins will be examined in DISSECTION **3.4**.

NOTE that lungs may be stored in separate container for later review.

DISSECTION 3.2
SUPERIOR MEDIASTINUM

Complete DISSECTION **3.1** Pleura and Lungs.

Read DISCUSSION **3.3** Anterior and Superior Mediastinum.

PLACE cadaver in supine position.

LOCATE pericardiacophrenic artery, which branches from **internal thoracic artery** to accompany phrenic nerves to diaphragm.

CAUTION   During following steps, do not damage structures entering axilla. These steps will permit retraction of manubrium and medial parts of clavicle and rib 1.

RETRACT mediastinal pleura as far posteriorly as possible.

CUT costochondral junction of rib 1 on <u>both</u> sides with bone cutters (**Figure 11**).

CUT soft tissue around chondral part of rib 1 with scissors to free rib and allow for retraction.

BLUNT DISSECT deep to clavicle to remove any soft tissue from inferior surface of clavicle.

CUT middle 1/3 of clavicle just lateral to clavicular attachment of sternocleidomastoid muscles. Use rongeur forceps or Stryker saw, and stop cutting immediately after clavicle is severed. Note that some skin may need to be reflected to expose superior edge of clavicle.

ELEVATE manubrium of sternum with medial ends of clavicle and chondral part of rib 1 attached, and retract them as far superiorly as possible. Take care not to cut hands on ragged ends of bones. With scissors, free any underlying fascia attached to bones.

IDENTIFY and **REMOVE thymus gland** or its adipose tissue replacement.

CLEAN great vessels as dissection progresses. To prevent damage, use 2 pairs of forceps or blunt scissors to tease fascia away from vessels.

IDENTIFY right brachiocephalic vein formed by **right internal jugular** and **right subclavian veins** deep to <u>right</u> sternoclavicular joint. This union is very high in superior mediastinum.

IDENTIFY left brachiocephalic vein formed by **left internal jugular** and **left subclavian veins** deep to <u>left</u> sternoclavicular joint.

Figure 11

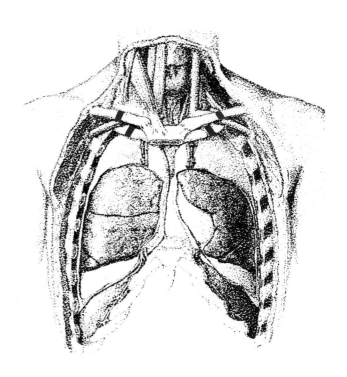

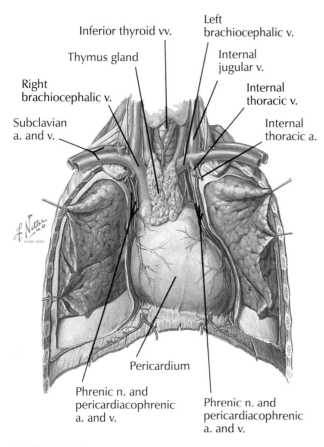

Inferior thyroid vv.

Thymus gland

Right brachiocephalic v.

Subclavian a. and v.

Left brachiocephalic v.

Internal jugular v.

Internal thoracic v.

Internal thoracic a.

Pericardium

Phrenic n. and pericardiacophrenic a. and v.

Phrenic n. and pericardiacophrenic a. and v.

PLATE 200

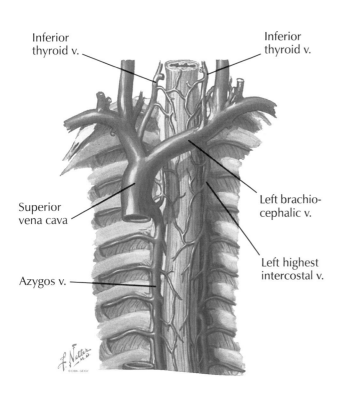

Inferior thyroid v.

Inferior thyroid v.

Superior vena cava

Azygos v.

Left brachio-cephalic v.

Left highest intercostal v.

PLATE 226 detail

IDENTIFY right phrenic nerve as it passes anterior to right subclavian artery and lateral to right brachiocephalic vein and superior vena cava. It passes anterior to root of lung and lateral to right pericardium.

IDENTIFY left phrenic nerve as it passes left of left brachiocephalic vein and arch of aorta, anterior to root of left lung, and then lies on left anterior surface of pericardium.

LOCATE site where **right** and **left internal thoracic veins** drain into respective right and left brachiocephalic veins.

LOCATE site where **inferior thyroid veins** (separately or by common trunk) drain into <u>left</u> brachiocephalic vein.

PLATE 220 detail

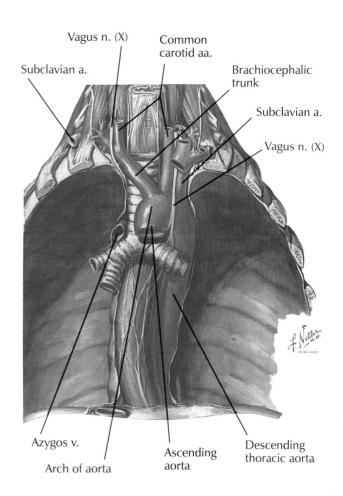

Vagus n. (X)

Subclavian a.

Common carotid aa.

Brachiocephalic trunk

Subclavian a.

Vagus n. (X)

Azygos v.

Arch of aorta

Ascending aorta

Descending thoracic aorta

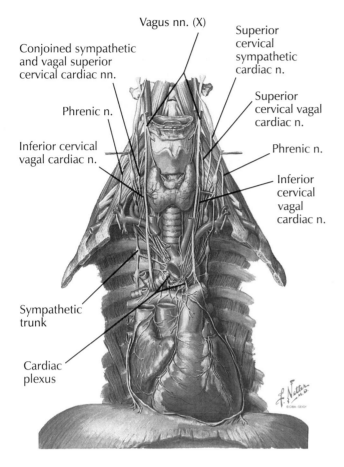

Vagus nn. (X)

Conjoined sympathetic and vagal superior cervical cardiac nn.

Superior cervical sympathetic cardiac n.

Phrenic n.

Superior cervical vagal cardiac n.

Inferior cervical vagal cardiac n.

Phrenic n.

Inferior cervical vagal cardiac n.

Sympathetic trunk

Cardiac plexus

PLATE 214

LOCATE site where **left highest intercostal vein** drains into left brachiocephalic vein. Note that highest intercostal vein may have been damaged during removal of rib cage or cutting of rib 1. Drainage of highest intercostal vein should still be found on posterior surface of brachiocephalic vein.

IDENTIFY superior vena cava formed by right and left brachiocephalic veins deep to <u>right</u> costal cartilage 1.

LOCATE drainage of **azygos vein** into superior vena cava after it loops over superior pole of root of right lung.

CUT entrance of <u>left</u> highest intercostal vein into <u>left</u> brachiocephalic vein.

CAUTION   During next step, preserve right vagus nerve (**X**) in its position medial to azygos vein and lateral to trachea.

CUT entrance of azygos vein into superior vena cava.

CUT right and left brachiocephalic veins medial to entrance of inferior thyroid veins.

REFLECT superior vena cava and both brachiocephalic veins inferiorly to expose **ascending aorta** and **arch** of **aorta**.

CAUTION   During next step, preserve <u>right</u> vagus nerve.

CLEAN origins of branches of arch of aorta.

IDENTIFY brachiocephalic trunk and its division into **right subclavian** and **right common carotid arteries** deep to <u>right</u> sternoclavicular joint.

LOCATE right vagus nerve (**X**) as it passes between right brachiocephalic artery and vein.

IDENTIFY left common carotid artery and **left subclavian artery**. Note that both arteries pass deep to <u>left</u> sternoclavicular joint. Left subclavian artery then crosses anterior to cupula of left pleura.

PLATE 201

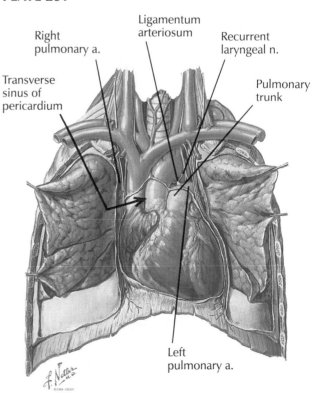

Right pulmonary a.

Ligamentum arteriosum

Recurrent laryngeal n.

Transverse sinus of pericardium

Pulmonary trunk

Left pulmonary a.

LOCATE left vagus nerve (X) as it passes between left subclavian and common carotid arteries and left brachiocephalic vein to lie on anterior surface of arch of aorta where arch becomes **descending aorta.**

LOOK for **superior cervical cardiac branch** of **right** and **left sympathetic trunks** and **inferior cervical cardiac branch** of **right** and **left vagus nerves (X)**, both of which pass anterior to arch of aorta between location of phrenic and vagus nerves. Note that both these cardiac branches join **cardiac (superficial) plexus**, which is located beneath arch of aorta.

LOOK for inconstant **lowest thyroid artery** (*not shown*) as small branch of arch of aorta between brachiocephalic and left common carotid arteries. Note that when present (10%), lowest thyroid artery ascends anterior to trachea.

IDENTIFY pulmonary trunk and its right and left branches, which lie inferior and deep to arch of aorta. Note that **right pulmonary artery** (*not shown*) passes toward right lung under arch of aorta and posterior to superior vena cava. It continues inferior to azygos vein.

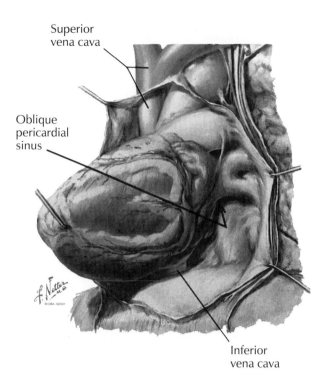

Superior
vena cava

Oblique
pericardial
sinus

Inferior
vena cava

PLATE 203

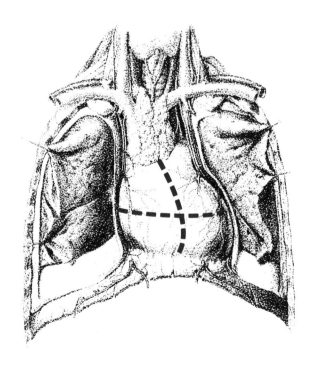

Figure 12

CAUTION   During next step, preserve <u>left</u> recurrent laryngeal nerve.

LOCATE ligamentum arteriosum, which connects beginning of **left pulmonary artery** to arch of aorta. Blunt dissection is required to clean and expose ligamentum arteriosum.

LOCATE left recurrent laryngeal nerve as it passes beneath arch of aorta, held in place by ligamentum arteriosum. Free fascia from recurrent laryngeal nerve by protecting it with one forceps and removing fascia with other forceps.

EXAMINE pericardium in situ.

INCISE anterior pericardium with vertical cut and transverse cut with blunt scissors (**Figure 12**).

REFLECT 4 triangular flaps of pericardium laterally to expose anterior surface of heart.

NOTE pericardial reflections onto both aorta and pulmonary trunk.

CLEAN pericardial cavity with damp towel or gauze if necessary. Do not clean surface of heart now.

REIDENTIFY pulmonary trunk and **ascending aorta**.

REIDENTIFY superior vena cava.

RETRACT apex of heart.

IDENTIFY inferior vena cava.

LOCATE pulmonary veins by examining **oblique pericardial sinus**. Move hand posterior to surface of heart, pushing fingers as far superiorly as possible. Reflection of pericardium that obstructs course of fingers is called oblique sinus.

LOCATE transverse pericardial sinus by placing finger between pulmonary artery and ascending aorta.

NOTE that examination of heart and its vessels will continue in DISSECTION **3.3**.

DISSECTION 3.3
HEART

Complete DISSECTIONS **3.1** Pleura and Lungs and **3.2** Superior Mediastinum.

Read DISCUSSION **3.2** Heart.

PLACE cadaver in supine position.

NOTE that, periodically, directions will suggest returning heart to its in situ orientation.

IDENTIFY anterior coronary sulcus and **anterior interventricular sulcus**. Note that sulci are usually filled with fat and can be identified by presence of coronary vessels traveling in them.

IDENTIFY surface of **right atrium** and its **auricle**.

IDENTIFY left auricle. Note that surface of left atrium will be examined after heart is removed.

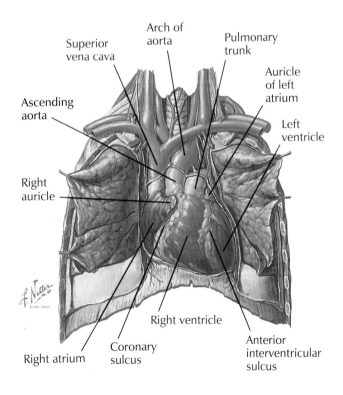

PLATE 201

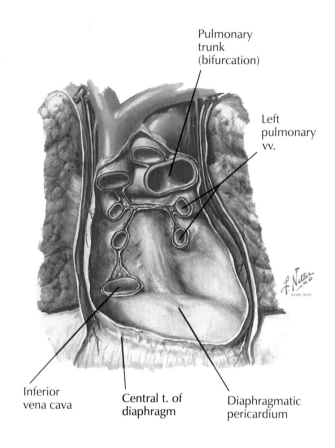

PLATE 203

IDENTIFY surfaces of **right** and **left ventricles**.

CUT ascending aorta just inferior to its pericardial reflection with scissors.

CUT pulmonary trunk just inferior to its pericardial reflection with scissors.

BLUNT DISSECT superior vena cava free from its pericardial reflection with fingers.

CUT inferior vena cava superior to its passage through diaphragm.

BLUNT DISSECT pulmonary arteries and **veins** free from their pericardial reflections.

42

REMOVE heart from pericardial cavity. Note that pulmonary veins must be freed from their pericardial attachments as heart is pulled out.

EXAMINE interior of posterior pericardium and attachment of pericardium to **central tendon** of **diaphragm**.

DIRECT attention to posterior surface of heart.

IDENTIFY surface of **left atrium** and **left ventricle**.

IDENTIFY posterior coronary sulcus and **posterior interventricular sulcus**.

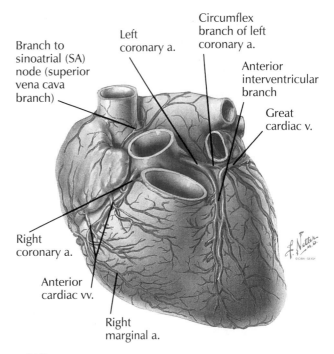

Branch to sinoatrial (SA) node (superior vena cava branch)

Left coronary a.

Circumflex branch of left coronary a.

Anterior interventricular branch

Great cardiac v.

Right coronary a.

Anterior cardiac vv.

Right marginal a.

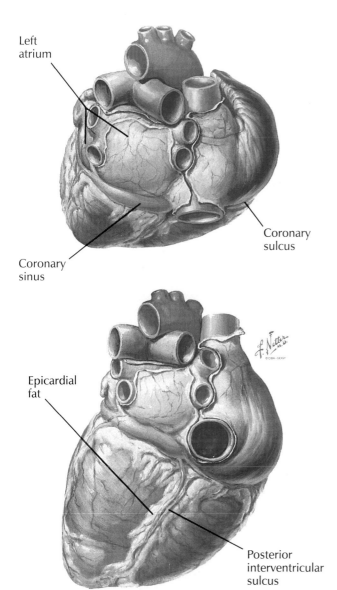

Left atrium

Coronary sinus

Coronary sulcus

Epicardial fat

Posterior interventricular sulcus

PLATE 202

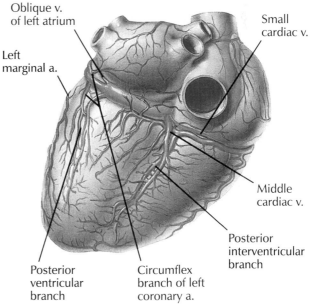

Oblique v. of left atrium

Small cardiac v.

Left marginal a.

Posterior ventricular branch

Circumflex branch of left coronary a.

Middle cardiac v.

Posterior interventricular branch

PLATE 204

REMOVE **epicardial fat** to expose coronary arteries and cardiac veins.

DIRECT attention to anterior surface of heart.

IDENTIFY **right coronary artery, right marginal artery**, and **posterior interventricular artery**.

IDENTIFY **left coronary artery, anterior interventricular artery, left marginal artery**, and **circumflex artery**.

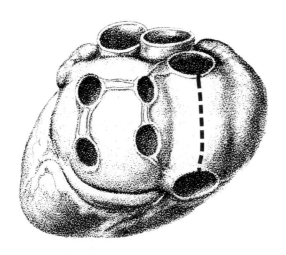

Figure 13

LOOK for **artery** to **sinoatrial (SA) node** as it branches from right coronary artery very close to origin of right coronary artery from ascending aorta.

NOTE that origins of right and left coronary arteries will be examined later in this dissection.

IDENTIFY great, **middle**, and **small cardiac veins** and **coronary sinus**.

LOOK for **anterior cardiac veins** and **oblique vein**.

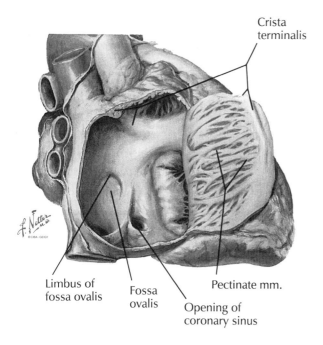

Crista
terminalis

Limbus of
fossa ovalis

Fossa
ovalis

Pectinate mm.

Opening of
coronary sinus

PLATE 208

NOTE that cleaning coronary vessels will remove **cardiac plexus** (*not shown*) that serves them.

INCISE posterior surface of **right atrium** vertically from superior vena cava to inferior vena cava with scissors (**Figure 13**).

CLEAN interior of right atrium by removing any clotted blood or fixative with running water.

IDENTIFY crista terminalis and **pectinate muscles**.

LOCATE site of **sinoatrial node** by finding area where crista terminalis meets superior vena cava. Confirm its location on external surface of heart by locating artery of sinoatrial node.

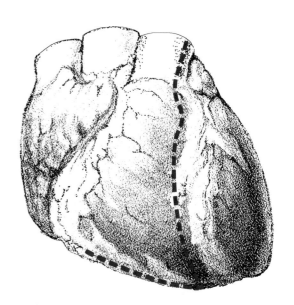

Figure 14

IDENTIFY fossa ovalis and **limbus** of **fossa ovalis**.

LOCATE valve of **inferior vena cava** below fossa ovalis. Note that limbus is continuous with valve of inferior vena cava.

LOCATE opening of **coronary sinus** and its valve. Insert probe into opening and confirm that it enters coronary sinus on posterior surface of heart.

IDENTIFY cusps of **tricuspid valve**.

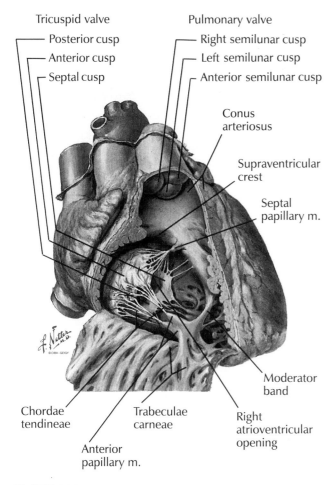

Tricuspid valve
— Posterior cusp
— Anterior cusp
— Septal cusp

Pulmonary valve
— Right semilunar cusp
— Left semilunar cusp
— Anterior semilunar cusp

Conus arteriosus

Supraventricular crest

Septal papillary m.

Moderator band

Chordae tendineae

Trabeculae carneae

Right atrioventricular opening

Anterior papillary m.

PLATE 208

INSERT probe through **right atrioventricular opening** for orientation of next cut.

INCISE anterior surface of heart to <u>right</u> of anterior interventricular sulcus from pulmonary trunk to inferior margin of heart with scissors (**Figure 14**). Continue this incision laterally along <u>right</u> acute margin of heart to gain access to interior of right ventricular chamber.

NOTE that **annulus fibrosus** (*not shown*) may be identified as tough structure sensed during previous cut.

CLEAN interior of right ventricle by removing any clotted blood or fixative with running water.

IDENTIFY trabeculae carneae, conus arteriosus (infundibulum), and **supraventricular crest**.

EXAMINE 3 cusps of tricuspid valve from ventricular view.

RETURN heart to its *in situ* position to understand that **septal cusp** relates to interventricular septum medially, **posterior cusp** relates to diaphragmatic wall inferiorly, and **anterior cusp** relates to anterior wall of heart.

REMOVE heart from thorax for continued inspection.

IDENTIFY chordae tendineae and **papillary muscles** as they anchor all 3 cusps to walls of heart.

LOCATE anterior papillary and **septal papillary muscles**. Note that **posterior papillary muscle** may be too deep to identify.

IDENTIFY moderator band as trabeculum extending from interventricular septum to anterior papillary muscle. Note that moderator band may have been cut during opening of right ventricle.

EXAMINE valve of **pulmonary trunk**.

IDENTIFY anterior, **right**, and **left semilunar cusps** of **valve** of **pulmonary trunk**. Note that anterior cusp may have been cut during opening of right ventricle.

LOCATE nodule in free edge of each semilunar cusp.

RETURN heart to its *in situ* position to understand that anterior cusp lies anterior left, right cusp lies anterior right, and left cusp lies posterior.

REMOVE heart from thorax for continued inspection.

INCISE posterior surface of **left atrium** from 1 <u>right</u> pulmonary vein to 1 <u>left</u> pulmonary vein with scissors (**Figure 15**). Make 2nd incision vertically from midpoint of 1st incision to superior edge of coronary sinus.

CLEAN interior of left atrium by removing any clotted blood or fixative with running water.

EXAMINE smooth interior of left atrium.

LOCATE pectinate muscle in left auricle. Note that these muscles may be difficult to see without cutting auricle open.

PALPATE atrial septum by placing finger of <u>right</u> hand against it from right atrium and finger of <u>left</u> hand against it from left atrium.

INVESTIGATE patency of foramen ovale.

IDENTIFY cusps of **mitral valve.**

INSERT probe through **left atrioventricular opening** for orientation of next cut.

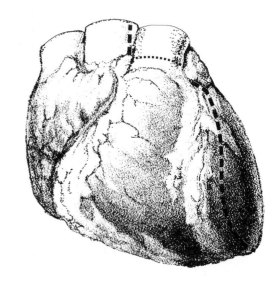

Figure 16

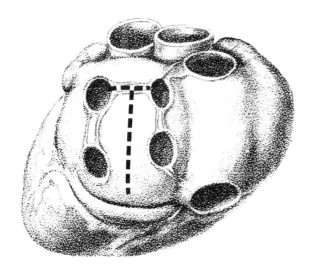

Figure 15

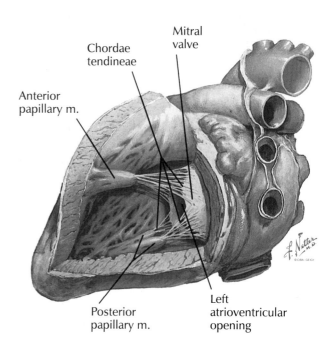

Chordae tendineae — Mitral valve

Anterior papillary m.

Posterior papillary m. — Left atrioventricular opening

PLATE 209

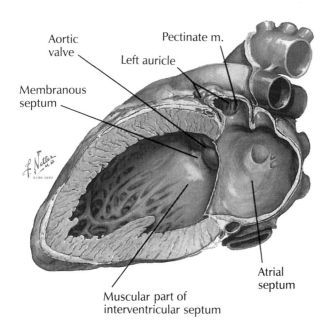

Aortic valve — Pectinate m.

Left auricle

Membranous septum

Muscular part of interventricular septum

Atrial septum

PLATE 209

INCISE anterior surface of left ventricle to <u>left</u> of anterior interventricular sulcus from aorta to apex of heart (**Figure 16**). Note that circumflex branch of left coronary artery will be cut by this incision. Control scissors so that orientation of incision can be altered during cut.

CLEAN interior of left ventricle by removing any clotted blood or fixative with running water.

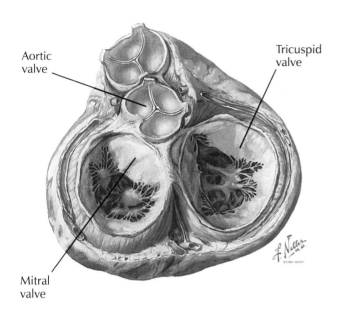

Aortic valve

Tricuspid valve

Mitral valve

PLATE 210

NOTE that wall of left ventricle is approximately 3 times as thick as wall of right ventricle.

EXAMINE 2 cusps of mitral valve from ventricular view. Note that anterior cusp separates left atrioventricular opening from opening of aorta.

IDENTIFY chordae tendineae and papillary muscles.

LOCATE anterior papillary muscle attached to interventricular septum and **posterior papillary muscle** attached to diaphragmatic wall.

PALPATE muscular part of **interventricular septum** and **membranous part** of **interventricular septum**. Place finger of <u>right</u> hand against atrial septum from right atrium and finger of <u>left</u> hand against membranous part of interventricular septum from left ventricle. Note that fingers touch right and left sides of same structure; i.e., membranous interventricular septum is really atrioventricular.

EXAMINE valve of **aorta.**

IDENTIFY right, left, and **posterior semilunar cusps** of **valve** of **aorta.** Note that anterior cusp may have been cut during opening of left ventricle.

LOCATE opening of **right coronary artery** just distal to right aortic semilunar cusp and **opening** for **left coronary artery** just distal to left aortic semilunar cusp.

LOCATE nodule in free edge of each semilunar cusp.

RETURN heart to its *in situ* position to understand that left cusp lies anterior left, right cusp lies anterior right, and posterior cusp lies posterior.

NOTE that heart may be stored in separate container for later review.

PLATE 211

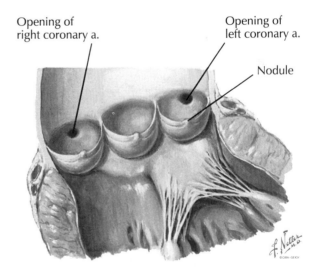

Opening of right coronary a.

Opening of left coronary a.

Nodule

DISSECTION 3.4
POSTERIOR MEDIASTINUM

Complete DISSECTIONS **3.2** Superior Mediastinum and **3.3** Heart.

Read DISCUSSION **3.4** Posterior Mediastinum.

PLACE cadaver in supine position.

CAUTION   During next step, preserve vagus nerves (X) and esophageal plexus.

REMOVE posterior pericardium carefully, blunt dissecting it free from cut ends of aorta and pulmonary trunk. Note that margin of pericardium is to be cut around central tendon of diaphragm.

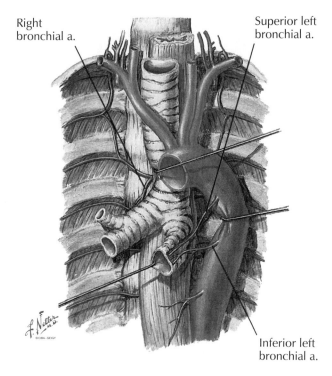

Right bronchial a.

Superior left bronchial a.

Inferior left bronchial a.

PLATE 196

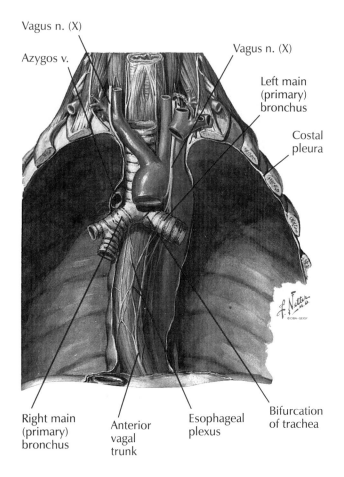

Vagus n. (X)

Azygos v.

Vagus n. (X)

Left main (primary) bronchus

Costal pleura

Right main (primary) bronchus

Anterior vagal trunk

Esophageal plexus

Bifurcation of trachea

PLATE 220 detail

CUT brachiocephalic trunk at its origin from arch of aorta.

RETRACT aorta and pulmonary trunk to <u>left</u>. Note that these vessels are to be cleaned to facilitate reflection.

LOOK for **cardiac (deep) plexus**, which lies posterior to right pulmonary artery in bifurcation of trachea.

IDENTIFY tracheal and **bronchial lymph nodes** but do not save them.

CLEAN bifurcation of **trachea** and note that bifurcation occurs deep to sternal angle at level of vertebra T5.

IDENTIFY carina (*not shown*) at bifurcation of trachea by palpation.

NOTE that **right main bronchus** is in more direct vertical line with trachea than **left main bronchus**.

ELEVATE main bronchi to expose origin of **right bronchial artery** from either proximal descending aorta or upper intercostal arteries, and **2 left bronchial arteries** from proximal descending aorta.

CAUTION During next step, preserve left recurrent laryngeal nerve.

RETRACT main bronchi and bifurcation of trachea as far superiorly as possible. Note that bronchial arteries need to be cut to do so.

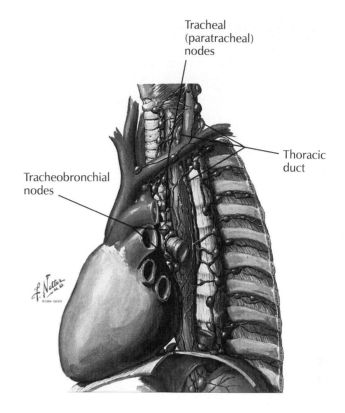

PLATE 227 detail

PLATE 225

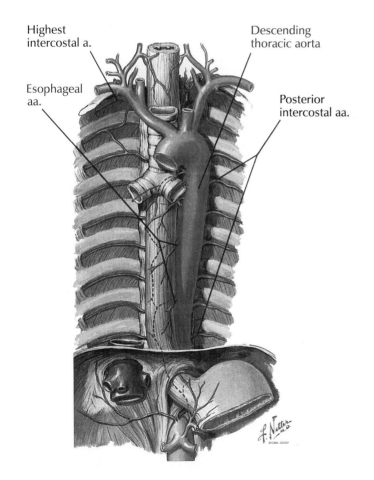

Highest intercostal a.

Descending thoracic aorta

Esophageal aa.

Posterior intercostal aa.

LOOK for **esophageal plexus** on surface of esophagus.

RETRACT esophagus to right and clean it.

LOCATE left vagus nerve (**X**) as it passes anterior to arch of aorta to contribute to esophageal plexus on anterior surface of esophagus.

TRACE anterior esophageal plexus to formation of **anterior trunk** of **vagus nerve**, which lies on anterior left surface of distal esophagus.

RETRACT esophagus to left.

LOCATE right vagus nerve (**X**) as it passes anterior to arch of azygos vein to contribute to esophageal plexus on posterior surface of esophagus.

TRACE posterior esophageal plexus to formation of **posterior trunk** of **vagus nerve** (**X**), which lies on posterior right surface of distal esophagus.

LOOK for **esophageal branches** of descending aorta.

CLEAN descending aorta in posterior mediastinum.

ELEVATE descending aorta to expose origins of paired **posterior intercostal arteries**.

LOCATE thoracic duct by reflecting descending aorta to left as far as possible. Note that this vessel's walls are very thin. Attempt to preserve it as dissection proceeds.

BLUNT DISSECT both vagal trunks on surface of esophagus to preserve them during following steps.

TRANSECT esophagus in thorax as closely as possible to its exit through **esophageal hiatus** of **diaphragm** (*not labeled*).

TRANSECT esophagus second time at level of bifurcation of trachea.

REMOVE esophagus and incise its anterior wall vertically to examine its lumen. Note that esophageal arteries must be cut to remove esophagus.

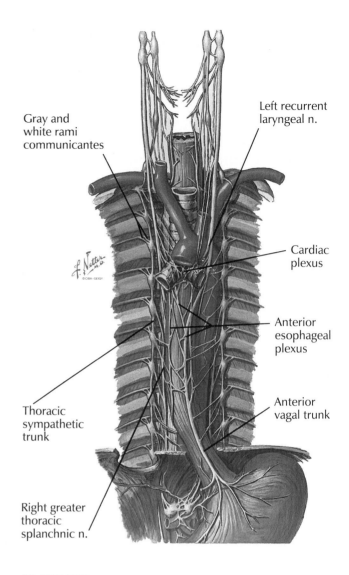

Gray and white rami communicantes

Left recurrent laryngeal n.

Cardiac plexus

Anterior esophageal plexus

Thoracic sympathetic trunk

Anterior vagal trunk

Right greater thoracic splanchnic n.

PLATE 228

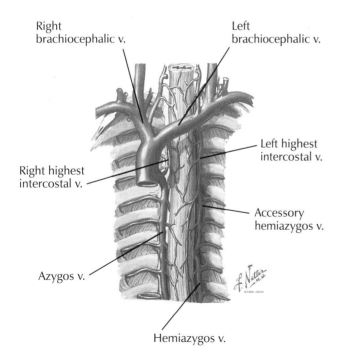

Right brachiocephalic v.

Left brachiocephalic v.

Right highest intercostal v.

Left highest intercostal v.

Accessory hemiazygos v.

Azygos v.

Hemiazygos v.

PLATE 226 detail

BLUNT DISSECT around circumference of descending aorta where it exits from thorax through **aortic hiatus** of **diaphragm** (*not shown*). Use finger to free aorta from all surrounding tissue.

TRANSECT descending aorta at aortic hiatus with scissors.

CUT origins of paired posterior intercostal arteries as cut end of descending aorta is progressively reflected superiorly.

RETRACT descending aorta to expose **azygos, hemiazygos**, and **accessory hemiazygos veins**, and their **tributaries**.

TRACE thoracic sympathetic trunks along necks of ribs in upper thorax to sides of vertebral bodies in lower thorax.

CLEAN thoracic sympathetic trunks, taking care to preserve rami communicantes between intercostal nerves and sympathetic trunks. Note that ganglia of sympathetic trunks are located superiorly on heads of ribs.

IDENTIFY gray rami communicantes, which lie lateral to sympathetic trunk and proximal to white rami communicantes.

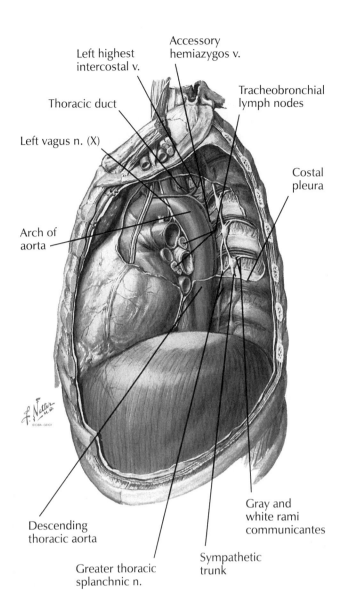

Left highest intercostal v.
Accessory hemiazygos v.
Thoracic duct
Tracheobronchial lymph nodes
Left vagus n. (X)
Costal pleura
Arch of aorta
Descending thoracic aorta
Greater thoracic splanchnic n.
Gray and white rami communicantes
Sympathetic trunk

PLATE 219

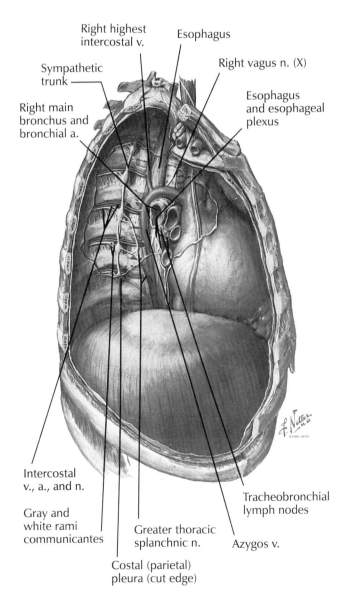

Right highest intercostal v.
Esophagus
Sympathetic trunk
Right vagus n. (X)
Right main bronchus and bronchial a.
Esophagus and esophageal plexus
Intercostal v., a., and n.
Gray and white rami communicantes
Greater thoracic splanchnic n.
Costal (parietal) pleura (cut edge)
Tracheobronchial lymph nodes
Azygos v.

PLATE 218

IDENTIFY white rami communicantes, which lie lateral to sympathetic trunk and distal to gray rami communicantes.

NOTE that color of both rami communicantes will not be evident in dissection.

IDENTIFY greater thoracic splanchnic nerve, which lies medial to thoracic sympathetic trunk and has contributions from T5–9. Note that lesser (T10, 11) and least (T12) thoracic splanchnic nerves will be traced in DISSECTION **4.6** after liver has been removed. Likewise, exit of splanchnic nerves and sympathetic trunk from thorax will be established then.

REMOVE any remnants of costal pleura to expose passage of intercostal vessels and nerves, first on internal surfaces of external intercostal muscles and then between innermost and internal intercostal muscles. Note that within costal grooves, **posterior intercostal veins** are located superior to **posterior intercostal arteries**, which are located superior to **intercostal nerves**.

TRACE posterior intercostal arteries of intercostal spaces 1–2 to their origin from **highest intercostal artery**. Note that highest intercostal artery is branch of costocervical trunk, which is branch of subclavian artery.

TRACE remaining posterior intercostal arteries to cut ends of origin from descending aorta. Note that posterior intercostal arteries usually pass posterior to structures in posterior mediastinum.

TRACE posterior intercostal veins to site of drainage into azygos system of veins. Note that hemiazygos vein usually crosses vertebral body T8 to drain into azygos vein, and accessory hemi-azygos vein usually crosses vertebral body T6 to drain into azygos vein.

NOTE that vein from right intercostal space 1 drains into **right brachiocephalic vein** and veins from right intercostal spaces 2–4 form **right highest intercostal vein**, which drains into azygos vein.

NOTE that vein from left intercostal space 1 drains into **left brachiocephalic vein** as **left highest intercostal vein**, which itself usually receives drainage from veins from left intercostal spaces 2–4. Left intercostal veins not drained by highest intercostal and hemiazygos veins drain into accessory hemiazygos vein.

Section 4

ABDOMEN

DISSECTIONS

DISSECTION 4.1

PERITONEUM

Complete DISSECTIONS **2.2** Anterior Thoracic Wall, **2.3** Anterior Abdominal Wall, and **2.4** Inguinal Region.

Read DISCUSSIONS **4.1** Peritoneum, **4.2** Topographic Regions, **4.3** Stomach, **4.9** Liver, and **4.11** Spleen.

PLACE cadaver in supine position.

CUT vertical incision from just <u>left</u> of umbilicus to xiphoid process of sternum.

EXTEND incision through cartilage of <u>left</u> costal margin from xiphoid process to margin of removed breastplate (**Figure 17**).

CAUTION   During following step, preserve falciform ligament with superior right flap.

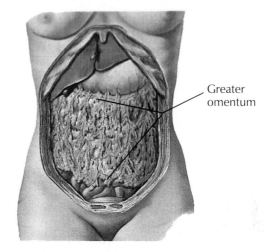

Greater omentum

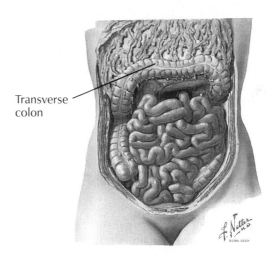

Transverse colon

PLATE 252

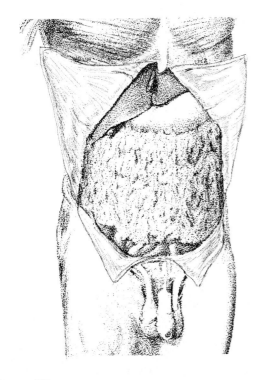

Figure 17

REFLECT 4 triangular flaps of abdominal wall to expose abdominal cavity, using fingers to free any adhesions between abdominal wall and viscera.

CUT through anterior part of diaphragm from xiphoid process, extending 1 hand-width into muscle fibers of diaphragm if more space is needed to examine abdominal cavity.

RETRACT left costal margin to left for following inspection.

EXPLORE peritoneal cavity by following limits of **parietal peritoneum** (*not labeled*) lining abdominal cavity and by placing hands between parietal peritoneum and **visceral peritoneum** (*not labeled*) reflecting onto organs. Hands will be in **greater peritoneal sac** (*not labeled*).

NOTE that there may be adhesions between different regions of peritoneum. Separate adhesions as dissection proceeds.

OBSERVE greater omentum overlapping small intestine. Note that greater omentum is attached to greater curvature of stomach.

REFLECT greater omentum superiorly, and observe that its posterior attachment is to **transverse colon**.

IDENTIFY regions of greater omentum that relate to stomach by flipping omentum back and forth as needed. **Gastrocolic ligament** (*not labeled*) is broad connection between greater curvature of stomach and transverse colon. **Gastrophrenic ligament** is short fold of peritoneum extending from superior end of greater curvature of stomach to diaphragm.

IDENTIFY duodenojejunal flexure as it appears at top left side of diagonal line where mesentery begins. Duodenum to be studied in DISSECTION **4.4**.

INSPECT mesentery by pulling up on small intestine to expose expansion of mesentery. Note that double layer of peritoneum suspends jejunoileal part of small intestine from posterior wall of abdomen along diagonal line.

EXAMINE arcades (loops of arteries) found within mesentery if fat deposited between layers of peritoneum allows inspection. Note that number of arcades increases distally from proximal end of jejunum (1 or 2 tiers) to distal end of ileum (4–6 tiers).

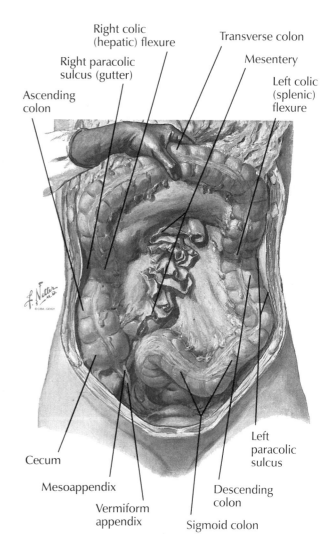

Right colic (hepatic) flexure

Transverse colon

Right paracolic sulcus (gutter)

Mesentery

Ascending colon

Left colic (splenic) flexure

Cecum

Mesoappendix

Vermiform appendix

Left paracolic sulcus

Descending colon

Sigmoid colon

PLATE 254

IDENTIFY cecum of large intestine and **vermiform appendix**.

NOTE that cecum usually has short mesentery and that there is **mesoappendix**.

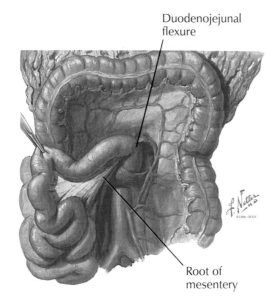

Duodenojejunal flexure

Root of mesentery

PLATE 253

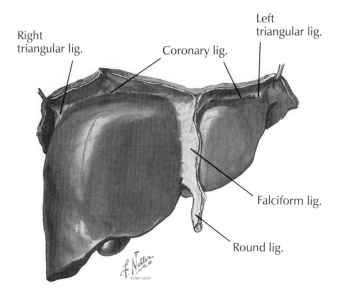

Right triangular lig.

Coronary lig.

Left triangular lig.

Falciform lig.

Round lig.

PLATE 270

FOLLOW ascending colon superiorly to **right colic (hepatic) flexure**, noting attachment of ascending colon to posterior abdominal wall.

INSPECT transverse colon, and follow it to **left colic (splenic) flexure**, continuing to **descending colon**. Transverse mesocolon will be inspected later in this dissection. Note that descending colon is attached to posterior abdominal wall.

RETRACT small intestine to right and superiorly.

FOLLOW sigmoid colon to its entry to pelvis. Note that **sigmoid mesocolon** is double layer of peritoneum suspending sigmoid colon from posterior wall of pelvis along diagonal line between distal descending colon and proximal rectum.

IDENTIFY right and **left paracolic sulci** (**gutters**). Note that space between root of mesentery and descending colon is continuous with pelvic cavity.

NOTE that parietal peritoneum follows structures into pelvis, draping over contents of pelvis.

RETRACT small intestine to left and inferiorly.

DIRECT attention to peritoneum associated with liver and stomach.

IDENTIFY falciform ligament of **liver** between liver and umbilicus in anterior abdominal wall.

PALPATE round ligament of **liver** (obliterated umbilical vein) within free margin of falciform ligament.

EXPLORE coronary ligament of **liver** by placing hands between diaphragm and liver on either side of falciform ligament. Follow contour of liver upward and backward until peritoneal reflections inhibit inspection.

IDENTIFY right and **left triangular ligaments** as double-layered reflections of peritoneum on lateral edges of coronary ligament.

ELEVATE inferior margin of liver superiorly.

IDENTIFY right, **left**, and **quadrate lobes** of **liver**, and locate **gallbladder**. Note that **caudate lobe** will be inspected in DISSECTION **4.4**.

RETRACT left lobe of liver superiorly, and stomach inferiorly and to <u>left</u>, to observe **lesser curvature** of **stomach** and **1st part** of **duodenum**.

IDENTIFY fundus and **body** as well as **cardiac** and **pyloric parts** of **stomach**.

IDENTIFY lesser omentum. Note region of lesser omentum designated as **hepatoduodenal ligament**, which extends from liver to duodenum, and region designated as **hepatogastric ligament**, which extends from liver to stomach.

PLATE 271

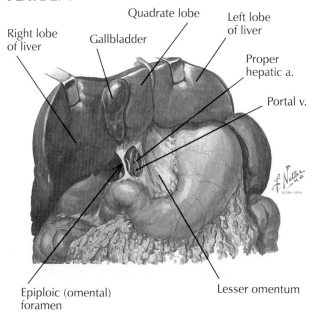

Right lobe of liver

Gallbladder

Quadrate lobe

Left lobe of liver

Proper hepatic a.

Portal v.

Epiploic (omental) foramen

Lesser omentum

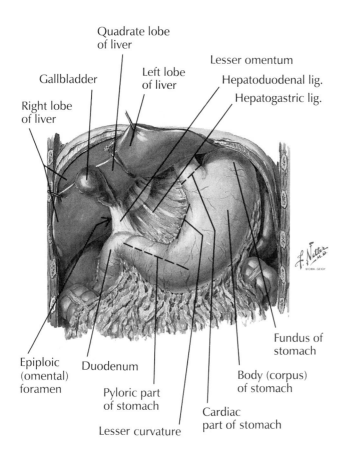

Quadrate lobe of liver

Gallblader

Left lobe of liver

Lesser omentum

Hepatoduodenal lig.

Hepatogastric lig.

Right lobe of liver

Epiploic (omental) foramen

Duodenum

Pyloric part of stomach

Lesser curvature

Cardiac part of stomach

Body (corpus) of stomach

Fundus of stomach

PLATE 258

PALPATE vessels within free edge of lesser omentum (hepatoduodenal ligament).

PLACE finger in **epiploic (omental) foramen** deep to free margin of lesser omentum.

CAUTION During following steps, preserve portal vein, hepatic artery, and common bile duct contained within hepatoduodenal ligament.

BLUNT DISSECT deep to lesser omentum by inserting closed scissors through epiploic foramen.

PLACE rolled paper towel through epiploic foramen into **omental bursa (lesser peritoneal sac,** *not labeled)* for reference during dissection.

CAUTION During next step, preserve left and right gastric arteries along lesser curvature of stomach, and avoid cutting into structures in posterior wall of omental bursa.

INCISE hepatogastric ligament of lesser omentum along and superior to lesser curvature of stomach.

RETRACT stomach inferiorly to expose posterior wall of omental bursa.

PALPATE extent of omental bursa with fingers.

LOCATE superior recess of **omental bursa** posterior to stomach.

LOOK for patency between anterior (double peritoneal) layer and posterior (double peritoneal) layer of greater omentum, or for their fusion.

IDENTIFY transverse mesocolon, which suspends entire length of transverse colon to posterior wall of parietal peritoneum just below pancreas.

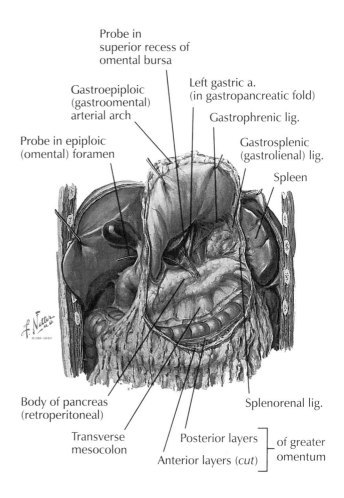

Probe in superior recess of omental bursa

Gastroepiploic (gastroomental) arterial arch

Left gastric a. (in gastropancreatic fold)

Gastrophrenic lig.

Probe in epiploic (omental) foramen

Gastrosplenic (gastrolienal) lig.

Spleen

Body of pancreas (retroperitoneal)

Transverse mesocolon

Splenorenal lig.

Posterior layers

Anterior layers (*cut*)

of greater omentum

PLATE 255

IDENTIFY left gastropancreatic fold covering left gastric artery. Note that this fold may be difficult to see if stomach is insufficiently mobile.

PALPATE pancreas as it lies deep to stomach. Note that only **body** of pancreas is visible now.

IDENTIFY regions of greater omentum that relate to spleen by placing <u>left</u> hand in omental bursa and <u>right</u> hand around hilus of spleen. **Gastrosplenic (gastrolienal) ligament** is short fold of peritoneum extending from left end of greater curvature of stomach to hilus of spleen. Reach deeper with hands to palpate anterior surface of left kidney. **Splenorenal (lienorenal) ligament** is short fold of peritoneum extending from hilus of spleen posteriorly to left kidney.

PALPATE spleen under <u>left</u> rib cage, examining its surfaces and margins with hands.

ELEVATE spleen to <u>left</u>.

LOCATE hilus of spleen by palpating splenic vessels within splenorenal ligament.

CAUTION   During next step, preserve gastroepiploic (gastroomental) arteries and veins.

INCISE both anterior and posterior layers of greater omentum along and inferior to greater curvature of stomach. Note that part of greater omentum attached to transverse colon is to be incised.

DISCARD excised part of greater omentum.

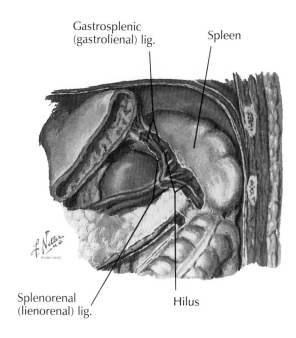

Gastrosplenic (gastrolienal) lig.

Spleen

Splenorenal (lienorenal) lig.

Hilus

PLATE 281

DISSECTION 4.2
ABDOMINAL VISCERA 1

Complete DISSECTION **4.1** Peritoneum.

Read DISCUSSIONS **4.4** Small Intestine, **4.6** Arteries and Veins of GI Tract, **4.10** Gallbladder and Biliary Ducts, and **4.13** Nerves of GI Tract and Accessory Organs.

PLACE cadaver in supine position.

NOTE that structures are usually inspected before studying neurovascular supply; in the abdomen, however, arteries, veins, and nerves are to be studied before opening viscera. Exposure of arteries and veins will be completed in DISSECTIONS **4.3** and **4.4** after GI tract has been removed. To appreciate relationships, clean vessels as much as possible *in situ*.

CLEAN arteries and veins that pass along lesser and greater curvatures of stomach, as far as hepatoduodenal ligament. Use one forceps to protect vessels and other forceps to remove peritoneum, fat, and fascia. Examine origins of vessels as dissection proceeds.

PLATE 255

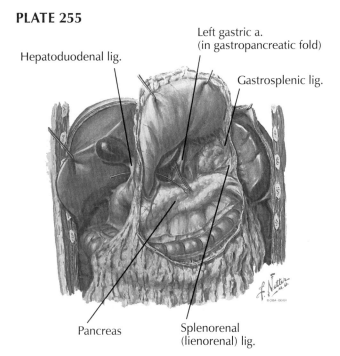

Hepatoduodenal lig.

Left gastric a. (in gastropancreatic fold)

Gastrosplenic lig.

Pancreas

Splenorenal (lienorenal) lig.

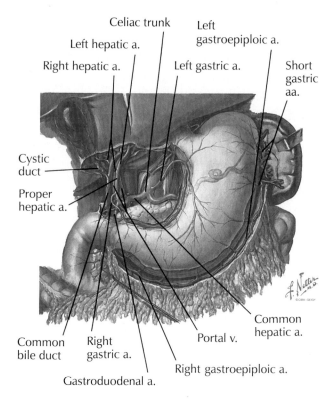

Celiac trunk

Left hepatic a.

Right hepatic a.

Left gastroepiploic a.

Left gastric a.

Short gastric aa.

Cystic duct

Proper hepatic a.

Common bile duct

Right gastric a.

Gastroduodenal a.

Portal v.

Right gastroepiploic a.

Common hepatic a.

PLATE 282

RETRACT stomach inferiorly and to left to expose **left gastropancreatic fold**, which contains left gastric vessels, and **gastrosplenic (gastrolienal) ligament**, which contains short gastric vessels.

REMOVE peritoneum of left gastropancreatic fold from **left gastric artery**, and follow this artery from **celiac trunk** to lesser curvature of stomach.

CAUTION   During next step, preserve left gastroepiploic, pancreatic, and short gastric veins for inspection in DISSECTION **4.3**.

REMOVE peritoneum of gastrosplenic ligament from **left gastroepiploic artery** and **short gastric arteries**, and follow these arteries to left side of greater curvature of stomach.

RETRACT stomach inferiorly and to right to expose **right gastropancreatic fold** (*not shown*) covering right gastric artery.

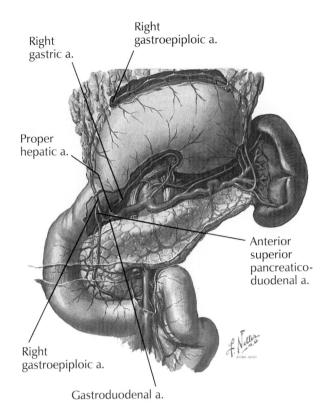

Right gastric a.

Right gastroepiploic a.

Proper hepatic a.

Right gastroepiploic a.

Anterior superior pancreatico- duodenal a.

Gastroduodenal a.

PLATE 283

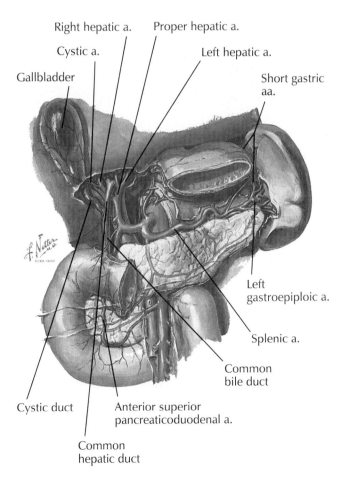

Right hepatic a.   Proper hepatic a.

Cystic a.   Left hepatic a.

Gallblader

Short gastric aa.

Left gastroepiploic a.

Splenic a.

Common bile duct

Cystic duct

Anterior superior pancreaticoduodenal a.

Common hepatic duct

PLATE 284

CAUTION During removal of peritoneum and fascia, preserve all vessels. Cleaning is essential for learning abdominal arteries, but it takes patience and time.

REMOVE peritoneum of right gastropancreatic fold from **right gastric artery**, and follow this artery from **proper hepatic artery** to lesser curvature of stomach.

REMOVE peritoneum of **hepatoduodenal ligament** (free margin of lesser omentum) from proper hepatic artery.

TRACE common hepatic artery retrograde to its origin from celiac trunk.

FOLLOW branching of common hepatic artery into proper hepatic artery and **gastroduodenal artery**. Note that branching is proximal to origin of right gastroepiploic artery.

FOLLOW branching of proper hepatic artery first into right gastric artery and then into **right** and **left hepatic arteries**, which enter right and left lobes of liver.

REVIEW branching pattern of celiac trunk.

IDENTIFY common bile duct, which lies in hepatoduodenal ligament (free margin of lesser omentum) to right of common hepatic artery, and **portal vein**, which also lies in hepatoduodenal ligament, posterior to common hepatic artery and common bile duct.

FOLLOW common bile duct retrograde to its formation by **common hepatic duct** and **cystic duct**. Note that cystic duct empties **gallbladder** and is supplied by **cystic artery**. These structures will be examined further in DISSECTION **4.4**.

FOLLOW division of portal vein into **right** and **left lobar branches**, which enter liver. Note that **left gastric vein** drains into portal vein before lobar branches are formed.

RETRACT stomach superiorly.

BLUNT DISSECT deep to **1st part** of **duodenum** with fingers.

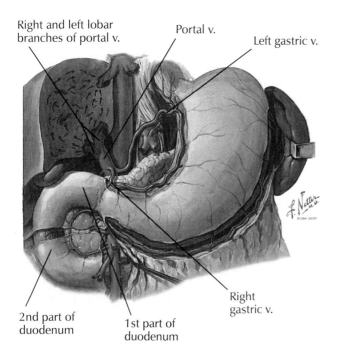

Right and left lobar branches of portal v.

Portal v.

Left gastric v.

Right gastric v.

2nd part of duodenum

1st part of duodenum

PLATE 294

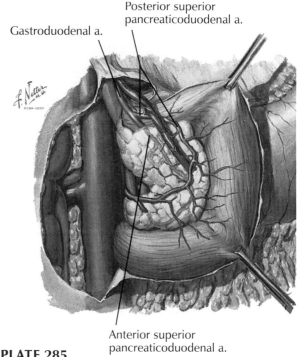

Gastroduodenal a.

Posterior superior pancreaticoduodenal a.

Anterior superior pancreaticoduodenal a.

PLATE 285

RETRACT 1st part of duodenum inferiorly by blunt dissection deep to **2nd part** of **duodenum**.

LOCATE gastroduodenal artery deep to 1st part of duodenum, and trace it retrograde to its origin from common hepatic artery.

TRACE branching of gastroduodenal artery into **right gastroepiploic artery** and **superior pancreaticoduodenal artery**. Note that superior pancreaticoduodenal artery will be examined in DISSECTION **4.3**.

FOLLOW right gastroepiploic artery to right side of greater curvature of stomach. Note that it anastomoses with left gastroepiploic artery.

RETRACT stomach either superiorly or inferiorly to expose **pancreas** and **splenorenal (lienorenal) ligament**.

CAUTION During next step, preserve vessels at hilus of spleen.

REMOVE peritoneum of splenorenal ligament from **splenic artery** at hilus of spleen.

FOLLOW left gastroepiploic artery and **short gastric arteries** back to their origins from splenic artery.

CAUTION During next step, preserve pancreatic branches of splenic artery.

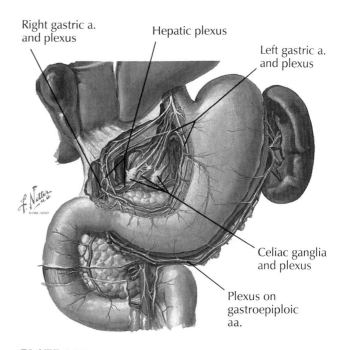

Right gastric a. and plexus

Hepatic plexus

Left gastric a. and plexus

Celiac ganglia and plexus

Plexus on gastroepiploic aa.

PLATE 305

FOLLOW and clean course of splenic artery along and superior to tail of pancreas. Confirm its origin from celiac trunk.

NOTE that **autonomic nerve plexuses** follow all branches of celiac trunk.

IDENTIFY celiac ganglia surrounding celiac trunk.

DISSECTION 4.3

ABDOMINAL VISCERA 2

Complete DISSECTION **4.2** Abdominal Viscera 1.

Read DISCUSSIONS **4.5** Large Intestine, **4.6** Arteries and Veins of GI Tract, **4.8** Pancreas, and **4.13** Nerves of GI Tract and Accessory Organs.

CONTINUE inspection of neurovascular supply to abdominal viscera.

REFLECT transverse colon and mesocolon either superiorly or inferiorly to expose **pancreas**.

REFLECT jejunoileum inferiorly and to left.

REMOVE exposed layer of mesentery and contiguous **transverse mesocolon** and parietal peritoneum from right side of posterior abdominal wall.

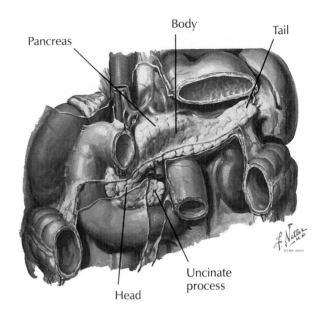

PLATE 279

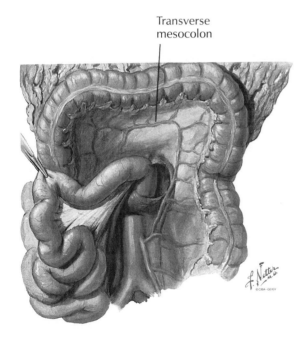

Transverse mesocolon

PLATE 253

CAUTION During following steps, preserve pancreatic tissue. Experience helps student distinguish between pancreatic and adipose tissue.

REMOVE fat from around pancreas.

IDENTIFY head, neck and **uncinate process** of **pancreas**.

CAUTION During next step, preserve connection of pancreatic ducts with 2nd part of duodenum.

BLUNT DISSECT and RETRACT pancreas superiorly with fingers to perform following steps.

CLEAN origin of **superior mesenteric artery** as it appears inferior to neck of pancreas. Note that superior mesenteric artery passes anterior to 4th part of duodenum. This space is sufficiently confined that fingers may be required as guide.

NOTE autonomic nerve plexus that follows branches of superior mesenteric artery as dissection proceeds.

LOCATE superior mesenteric ganglia around superior mesenteric artery.

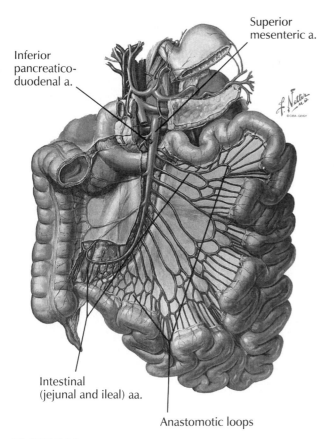

Inferior
pancreatico-
duodenal a.

Superior
mesenteric a.

Intestinal
(jejunal and ileal) aa.

Anastomotic loops

PLATE 286

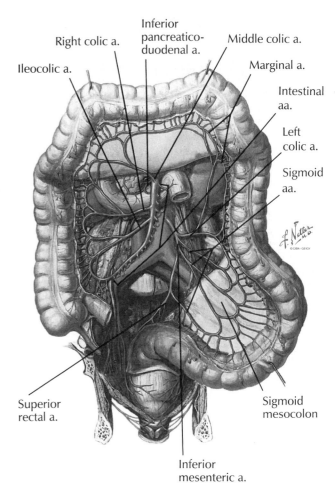

Right colic a.

Ileocolic a.

Inferior
pancreatico-
duodenal a.

Middle colic a.

Marginal a.

Intestinal
aa.

Left
colic a.

Sigmoid
aa.

Superior
rectal a.

Sigmoid
mesocolon

Inferior
mesenteric a.

PLATE 287

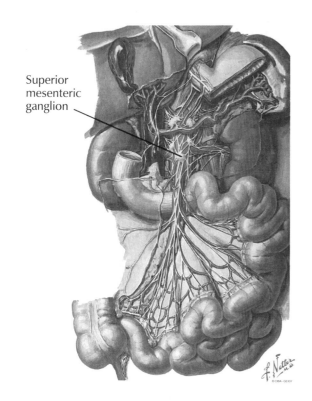

Superior
mesenteric
ganglion

PLATE 308

ORIENT branches of superior mesenteric artery to its termination near distal end of ileum by fanning out mesentery.

NOTE that tributaries of superior mesenteric vein may be removed as dissection proceeds, but identifiable superior mesenteric venous trunk should be tagged and preserved to study when portal vein is examined later. Tributaries of superior mesenteric vein lie anterior to and right of branches of superior mesenteric artery.

NOTE that inferior pancreaticoduodenal artery (1st branch of superior mesenteric artery) will be examined later in this dissection when it is exposed.

CLEAN middle colic artery from its origin inferior to pancreas into its right and left branches as they supply transverse colon.

CLEAN right colic artery from its origin distal to origin of middle colic artery to its ascending and descending branches as they supply ascending colon.

CLEAN ileocolic artery from its origin distal to origin of right colic artery to its ileal, cecal, and appendicular branches as they supply those structures.

CLEAN series of **intestinal branches** of superior mesenteric artery as they supply jejunum and ileum. This procedure may take substantial time. Note that each intestinal branch divides into 2 arteries that anastomose with adjacent arteries to form arcades (loops).

OBSERVE that number of arcades increases distally in small intestine. There may be 4–6 tiers of arcades in distal ileum and 1 or 2 tiers in proximal jejunum.

Posterior superior
pancreaticoduodenal a.

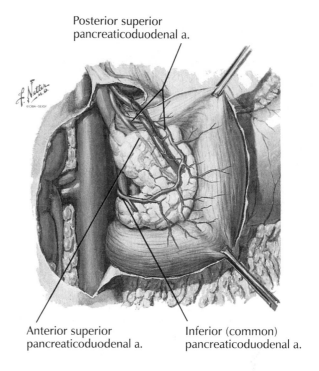

Anterior superior
pancreaticoduodenal a.

Inferior (common)
pancreaticoduodenal a.

PLATE 285

PLATE 309

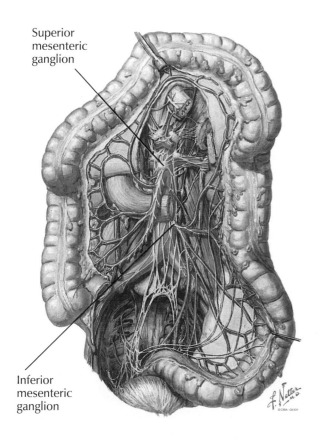

Superior
mesenteric
ganglion

Inferior
mesenteric
ganglion

RETRACT jejunum and ileum to right.

CLEAN exposed layer of mesentery, **sigmoid mesocolon**, and contiguous parietal peritoneum from side of posterior abdominal wall.

CLEAN inferior mesenteric artery from its origin superior to bifurcation of aorta.

NOTE autonomic nerve plexus that follows branches of inferior mesenteric artery.

LOCATE inferior mesenteric ganglia around inferior mesenteric artery.

CLEAN left colic artery and its ascending and descending branches to descending colon.

IDENTIFY marginal artery as it forms anastomotic connection around mesenteric border of large intestine from ileum to sigmoid colon.

CLEAN sigmoid branches of inferior mesenteric artery to sigmoid colon.

CLEAN superior rectal artery (distal end of inferior mesenteric artery), and trace it for short distance into pelvis.

DIRECT attention to pancreas.

BLUNT DISSECT deep to pancreas to expose following anastomoses.

LOCATE inferior pancreaticoduodenal artery between head of pancreas and 3rd part of duodenum.

TRACE inferior pancreaticoduodenal artery from its origin from superior mesenteric artery to its anastomosis with **superior pancreaticoduodenal artery**. Note that origin of superior pancreatico-duodenal artery from gastroduodenal artery was examined in DISSECTION **4.2.**

LOOK for anterior and posterior branches of both superior and inferior pancreaticoduodenal arteries.

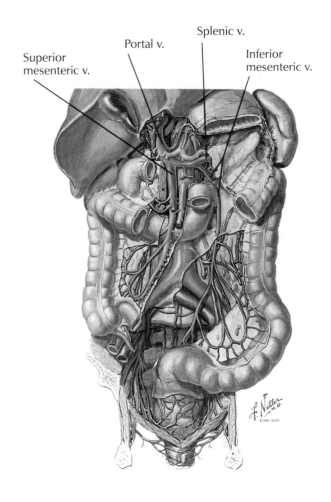

PLATE 296

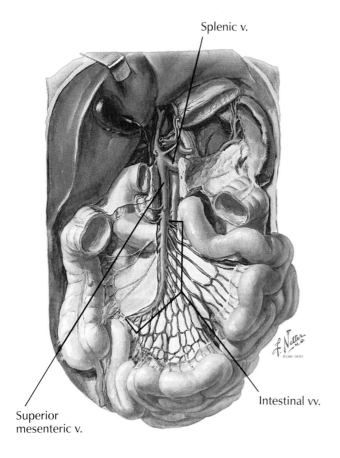

PLATE 295

DIRECT attention to formation of **portal vein**.

RETRACT pancreas from posterior abdominal wall to expose **splenic vein** and its formation by left gastroepiploic vein, short gastric veins, and pancreatic veins.

LOCATE union of **superior mesenteric vein** with splenic vein, which occurs posterior to neck of pancreas.

LOCATE union of **inferior mesenteric vein** with splenic vein, superior mesenteric vein, or both, which forms portal vein.

DISSECTION 4.4
REMOVAL OF ABDOMINAL VISCERA

Complete DISSECTIONS **4.2** and **4.3** Abdominal Viscera 1 and 2.

Read DISCUSSIONS **4.1** Peritoneum, **4.4** Small Intestine, **4.5** Large Intestine, **4.6** Arteries and Veins of GI Tract, **4.7** Lymph Drainage of GI Tract, **4.8** Pancreas, **4.9** Liver, **4.10** Gallbladder and Biliary Ducts, and **4.12** Lymph Drainage of Accessory Organs.

PLACE cadaver in supine position.

CUT left triangular ligament of **liver** and anterior layer of coronary ligament through to **right triangular ligament**.

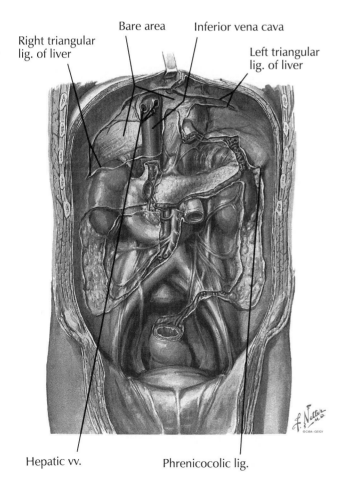

Right triangular lig. of liver

Bare area

Inferior vena cava

Left triangular lig. of liver

Hepatic vv.

Phrenicocolic lig.

PLATE 257

Duodenum

Superior (1st) part

Descending (2nd) part

Horizontal (3rd) part

Ascending (4th) part

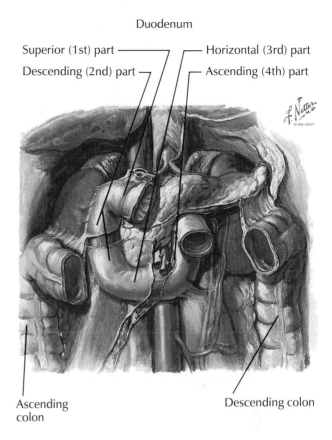

Ascending colon

Descending colon

PLATE 261

CUT through attachment of **falciform ligament** (*not shown*) to anterior abdominal wall until incision meets incision of right triangular ligament. Most of falciform ligament is to remain attached to liver.

NOTE that for next step, use of fingers is recommended.

BLUNT DISSECT deep to **bare area** of **diaphragm**.

RETRACT liver alternately superiorly and inferiorly to cut posterior layer of coronary ligament.

ELEVATE liver from posterior abdominal wall, and blunt dissect **inferior vena cava** free from liver. Note that **hepatic veins** must be cut as they enter inferior vena cava. Approach hepatic veins from superior aspect of liver.

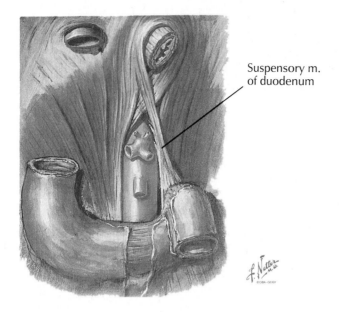

Suspensory m. of duodenum

PLATE 253

DIRECT attention to spleen.

BLUNT DISSECT deep to convex surface of spleen to free any adhesions.

CAUTION   During next step, preserve entrance of branches of proper hepatic artery, common hepatic duct, and portal vein into porta hepatis.

BLUNT DISSECT deep to **duodenum**.

IDENTIFY 2nd part of duodenum as it passes anterior to right kidney, 3rd part as it crosses inferior vena cava and aorta, and 4th part as it ascends to join jejunum.

LOCATE suspensory muscle of duodenum attached to duodenojejunal flexure from right crus of diaphragm. Note that identification of this structure as muscle is difficult because it contains only few muscle fibers.

CUT suspensory muscle of duodenum and adhesions that attach duodenojejunal flexure to posterior abdominal wall.

BLUNT DISSECT deep to **ascending colon** to free it from posterior abdominal wall.

LOCATE and CUT phrenicocolic ligament between left (splenic) colic flexure and diaphragm.

BLUNT DISSECT deep to **descending colon** with fingers to free it from posterior abdominal wall and left kidney.

CAUTION   During next step, preserve anterior and posterior vagal trunks.

BLUNT DISSECT around circumference of **esophagus** where it enters abdominal cavity through **esophageal hiatus**. Use fingers to free esophagus from all surrounding tissue.

PULL esophagus through its hiatus into abdomen.

RETRACT stomach, abdominal esophagus, liver, duodenum, and pancreas en bloc inferiorly to expose abdominal aorta above celiac trunk.

TAG each artery of **celiac trunk** for easier identification later.

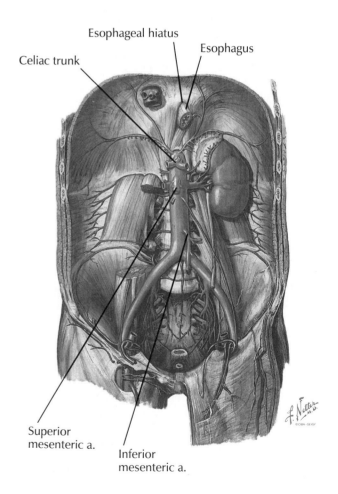

Esophageal hiatus

Esophagus

Celiac trunk

Superior mesenteric a.

Inferior mesenteric a.

PLATE 247

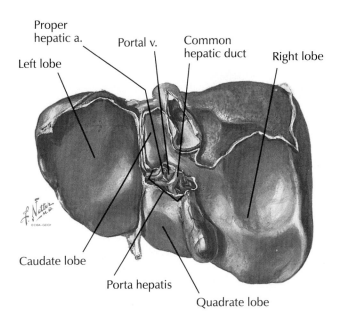

Proper
hepatic a.
Portal v.
Common
hepatic duct
Left lobe
Right lobe
Caudate lobe
Porta hepatis
Quadrate lobe

PLATE 270

CUT 3 branches of celiac trunk separately, distal to their origins, leaving celiac trunk attached to aorta.

CUT and TAG superior mesenteric artery proximal to origin of inferior pancreaticoduodenal artery.

CUT and TAG inferior mesenteric artery proximal to origin of left colic artery.

CUT and TAG superior rectal artery distal to rectosigmoid arteries, which branch from inferior mesenteric artery.

TIE sigmoid colon with 2 ligatures distal to last rectosigmoid artery.

CUT sigmoid colon between ligatures.

CAUTION During next step, preserve left ureter.

BLUNT DISSECT root of mesentery and sigmoid mesocolon free from posterior abdominal wall.

REMOVE freed abdominal viscera from abdominal cavity, placing viscera on tray in its usual anatomical arrangement, anterior aspect facing upward.

EXAMINE regions of liver again now that organ is mobile.

LOCATE caudate lobe, which was not visible until removal of viscera from abdomen.

BLUNT DISSECT liver tissue away to expose branches of biliary duct, hepatic artery, and portal vein. Use 1st forceps to protect ducts, arteries, and veins and 2nd forceps to remove hepatic tissue.

NOTE that branches of hepatic arteries accompany branches of portal vein and bile canaliculi. These 3 vessels enter **porta hepatis** to pass together in substance of liver, and are surrounded by sheath of connective tissue.

FOLLOW branching of **left hepatic artery** sufficiently to understand that it supplies caudate lobe and part of **quadrate lobe** as well as left lobe. Use 1st forceps to protect arteries and 2nd forceps to remove hepatic tissue.

REVIEW segmentation of liver in DISCUSSION **4.9**.

INCISE gallbladder from fundus to union of common hepatic duct with cystic duct (**Figure 18**).

EXAMINE smooth and honeycombed interior and **spiral part** of **cystic duct**.

Figure 18

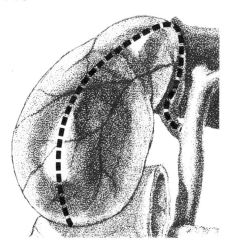

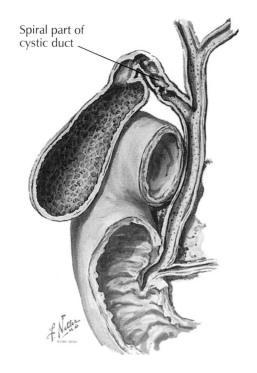

Spiral part of cystic duct

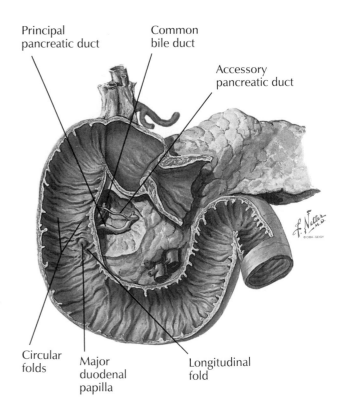

Principal pancreatic duct
Common bile duct
Accessory pancreatic duct

Circular folds
Major duodenal papilla
Longitudinal fold

PLATE 262

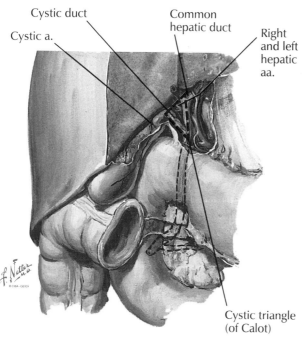

Cystic duct
Cystic a.
Common hepatic duct
Right and left hepatic aa.
Cystic triangle (of Calot)

PLATE 276

TRACE cystic artery to its origin, usually from right hepatic artery.

DEFINE boundaries of **cystic triangle** (of **Calot**) as liver, cystic duct, and common hepatic duct. Cystic artery is usually located within its boundaries.

OPEN 2nd part of duodenum.

IDENTIFY circular folds of mucosa and **longitudinal fold** of duodenum.

LOCATE major duodenal papilla in medial wall of 2nd part of duodenum in proximal end of longitudinal fold. Openings from **common bile duct** and **principal pancreatic duct** usually empty into hepatopancreatic ampulla located in major duodenal papilla. If accessory pancreatic duct is present, it is located superior and anterior to major duodenal papilla.

REARRANGE freed abdominal viscera on tray so that posterior aspect is facing upward. This should illustrate relationships of viscera and their vasculature to posterior abdominal wall.

TRACE formation of portal vein from posterior aspect.

DIRECT attention to pancreas.

CLEAN pancreatic ducts by preserving them with 1st forceps and removing pancreatic tissue with 2nd forceps.

FOLLOW principal pancreatic duct to its union with common bile duct. Note that main pancreatic duct extends from tail through body, neck, and head of pancreas and receives many small ductules.

LOOK for inconstant **accessory pancreatic duct** in head of pancreas.

EXAMINE hilus of spleen, noting extensive vascular supply and branching of **short gastric arteries** from splenic artery.

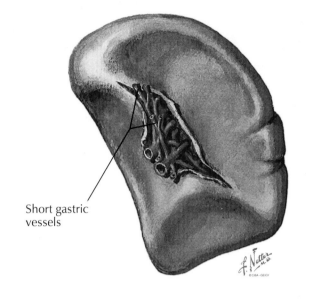

Short gastric
vessels

PLATE 279

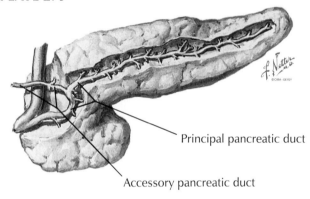

Principal pancreatic duct

Accessory pancreatic duct

PLATE 281

COMPLETE dissection of any arteries or autonomic plexuses that were inaccessible when viscera remained *in situ*.

EXAMINE relationship (beds) of various viscera with structures remaining in posterior abdominal wall.

DISSECTION 4.5
KIDNEY AND SUPRARENAL GLAND

Complete DISSECTION **4.4** Removal of Abdominal Viscera.

Read DISCUSSIONS **4.14** Kidneys and Ureters, **4.15** Suprarenal Glands, and **4.16** Diaphragm.

PLACE cadaver in supine position.

STUDY topographic relations of **kidneys** to removed viscera and structures in posterior abdominal wall (see DISCUSSION **4.14**).

CAUTION   During next step, preserve ureters, ovarian or testicular vessels, and branches of lumbar plexus.

REMOVE parietal peritoneum from posterior abdominal wall and abdominal surface of diaphragm with forceps and fingers.

IDENTIFY pararenal fat external to **renal fascia**, and identify **perirenal fat** surrounding kidney.

IDENTIFY right renal artery as it passes posterior to inferior vena cava, and identify **left renal artery**.

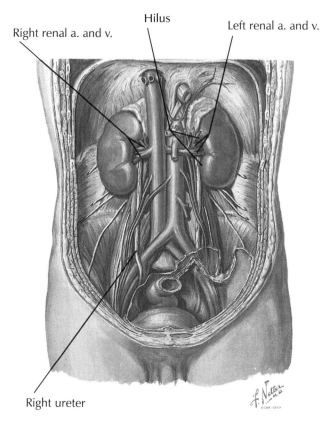

Right renal a. and v.   Hilus   Left renal a. and v.

Right ureter

PLATE 315

PLATE 328

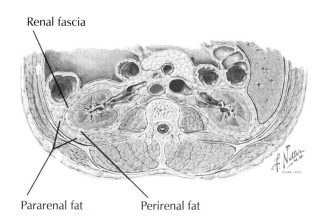

Renal fascia

Pararenal fat   Perirenal fat

IDENTIFY left renal vein as it passes anterior to aorta, and identify **right renal vein**. Note that renal veins enter **hilus** of **kidney** anterior to renal arteries.

IDENTIFY ureters as they pass from kidney over posterior abdominal wall into pelvis. Note that ureters leave hilus of kidney posterior to renal arteries.

LOOK for arteries to ureters from renal, testicular or ovarian, aortic, and common iliac sources.

CLEAN perirenal fat from hilus of kidney.

SECTION kidney along its lateral border with scalpel, extending incision medially toward hilus but preserving renal vessels and ureter.

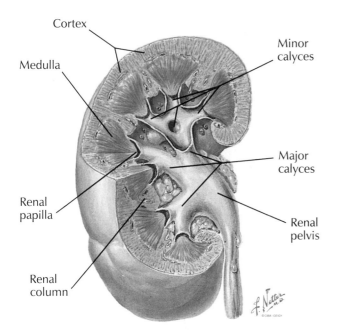

Cortex

Medulla

Minor calyces

Major calyces

Renal papilla

Renal pelvis

Renal column

PLATE 317

EXAMINE cortex and **medulla** of **kidney**.

IDENTIFY several **renal papilla**, **minor** and **major calyces**, and **renal pelvis**.

STUDY arterial distribution of kidneys.

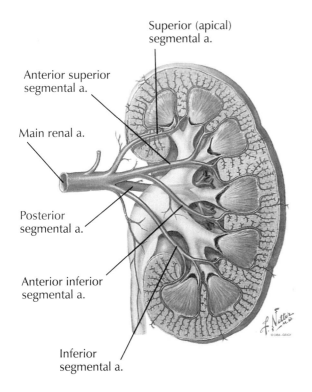

Superior (apical) segmental a.

Anterior superior segmental a.

Main renal a.

Posterior segmental a.

Anterior inferior segmental a.

Inferior segmental a.

PLATE 319

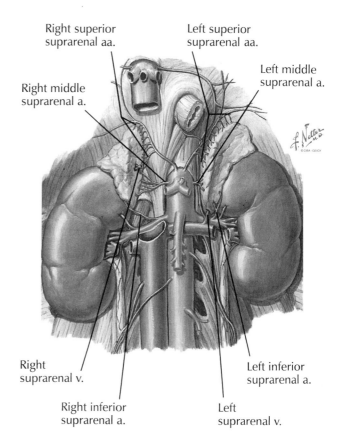

Right superior suprarenal aa.

Left superior suprarenal aa.

Right middle suprarenal a.

Left middle suprarenal a.

Right suprarenal v.

Left inferior suprarenal a.

Right inferior suprarenal a.

Left suprarenal v.

PLATE 318

STUDY topographic relations of **suprarenal glands** to kidneys, to removed viscera, and to structures in posterior abdominal wall (see DISCUSSION **4.15**).

LOCATE inferior suprarenal arteries, which originate from renal arteries; **middle suprarenal arteries**, which originate from aorta; and **superior suprarenal arteries**, which originate from inferior phrenic arteries. Note that origins of inferior phrenic arteries will be examined later in this dissection.

LOCATE right suprarenal vein, which drains into inferior vena cava, and **left suprarenal vein**, which drains into left renal vein.

SECTION suprarenal glands horizontally with scissors, preserving arteries and veins.

EXAMINE cortex and **medulla** of **suprarenal gland**.

REFLECT right kidney and suprarenal gland to left and left kidney and suprarenal gland to right as inspection of diaphragm and posterior abdominal wall continues.

73

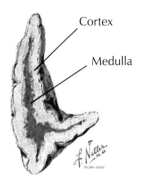

Cortex

Medulla

f. Netter
©CIBA-GEIGY

PLATE 329

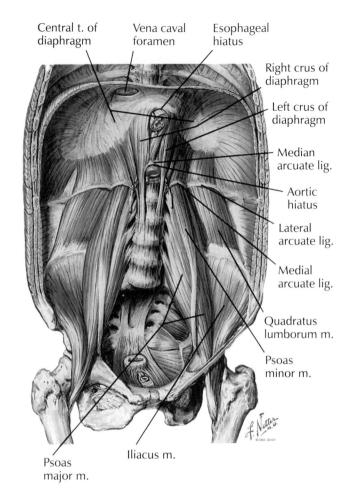

Central t. of diaphragm
Vena caval foramen
Esophageal hiatus
Right crus of diaphragm
Left crus of diaphragm
Median arcuate lig.
Aortic hiatus
Lateral arcuate lig.
Medial arcuate lig.
Quadratus lumborum m.
Psoas minor m.
Psoas major m.
Iliacus m.

f. Netter
©CIBA-GEIGY

PLATE 246

IDENTIFY central tendon and muscular part of abdominal surface of **diaphragm**.

OBSERVE vena caval foramen in central tendon.

IDENTIFY medial arcuate ligament arching anterior to psoas major muscle between transverse process to body of vertebra L2.

IDENTIFY lateral arcuate ligament arching anterior to **quadratus lumborum muscle** between rib 12 and transverse process of vertebra L2.

OBSERVE that **right crus** of **diaphragm** attaches to bodies of vertebrae L1–3 and is split by **esophageal hiatus.**

OBSERVE that **left crus** of **diaphragm** attaches to bodies of vertebrae L1, 2.

OBSERVE that **median arcuate ligament** connects medial borders of right and left crura to form **aortic hiatus.**

LOCATE right and **left phrenic nerves** (*not shown*) on inferior surface of diaphragm.

CAUTION Preserve subcostal, iliohypogastric, ilioinguinal, lateral femoral cutaneous, and genitofemoral nerves during inspection of muscles of posterior abdominal wall.

INSPECT origin of quadratus lumborum muscle from transverse processes of vertebrae L3–5 and iliac crest and its insertion to rib 12.

PRESERVE subcostal, iliohypogastric, and **ilioinguinal nerves,** which pass anterior to quadratus lumborum muscle after exiting lateral to **psoas major muscle.**

INSPECT origin of psoas major muscle from transverse processes and intervertebral discs of vertebrae L1–5.

PRESERVE genitofemoral nerve, which exits psoas major muscle on its anterior surface.

FOLLOW psoas major muscle as it passes deep to inguinal ligament lateral to external iliac artery.

LOOK for inconstant **psoas minor muscle,** which originates from bodies of vertebrae T12, L1 to insert to pecten pubis.

OBSERVE iliacus muscle and its investing fascia, attached to iliac fossa. Its tendon joins tendon of psoas major anteriorly, and they insert together to lesser trochanter of femur.

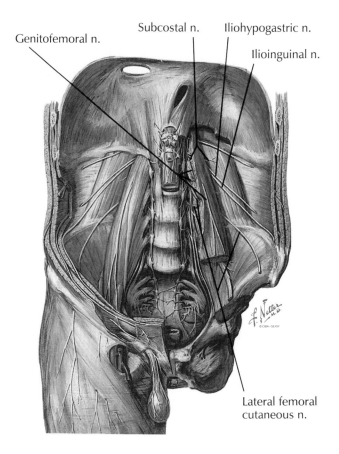

Genitofemoral n.

Subcostal n.

Iliohypogastric n.

Ilioinguinal n.

Lateral femoral cutaneous n.

PLATE 250

PRESERVE lateral femoral cutaneous nerve, which exits lateral side of psoas major muscle to pass anterior to iliacus muscle.

CAUTION   During following inspection, preserve aortic plexus and branches of aorta associated with ganglia.

FOLLOW abdominal aorta from aortic hiatus to its bifurcation anterior to body of vertebra L4.

NOTE that 3 unpaired branches (celiac, superior mesenteric, and inferior mesenteric) of aorta were studied in DISSECTIONS **4.2** and **4.3**.

EXAMINE 8 paired branches of abdominal aorta.

LOCATE **right inferior phrenic artery** from its origin from aorta between crura of diaphragm to its passage posterior to inferior vena cava, and locate **left inferior phrenic artery** from its similar origin to its passage posterior to removed esophagus.

IDENTIFY renal arteries. Note relation of superior mesenteric artery passing anterior to right renal artery.

FOLLOW (in male) **testicular arteries** from their origin from aorta just inferior to origin of superior mesenteric artery to where they cross ureter and to their exit through deep inguinal ring.

FOLLOW (in female) **ovarian arteries** from their origin from aorta just inferior to origin of superior mesenteric artery to where they cross ureter and common iliac arteries to their descent into pelvis.

IDENTIFY common iliac arteries between L4 and lumbosacral joints. Note that both common iliac arteries are crossed by ureters and left common iliac artery is crossed by superior rectal artery and vein.

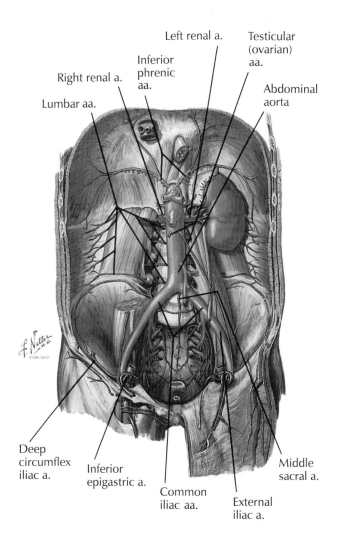

Right renal a.

Left renal a.

Inferior phrenic aa.

Testicular (ovarian) aa.

Lumbar aa.

Abdominal aorta

Deep circumflex iliac a.

Inferior epigastric a.

Common iliac aa.

External iliac a.

Middle sacral a.

PLATE 247

ELEVATE aorta just superior to its bifurcation and inspect 1 of 4 pairs of **lumbar arteries**, which originate from posterior surface of aorta.

LOOK for unpaired **middle sacral artery**, which passes anterior to body of vertebra L5 into pelvis.

FOLLOW external iliac artery as it passes medial to psoas major muscle to exit deep to medial part of inguinal ligament. Note that close to inguinal ligament it is crossed superiorly by ductus deferens (in male) or round ligament of uterus (in female).

LOCATE origin of **inferior epigastric artery** from external iliac artery.

LOCATE deep circumflex iliac artery branching from external iliac artery to pass along superior edge of iliac crest.

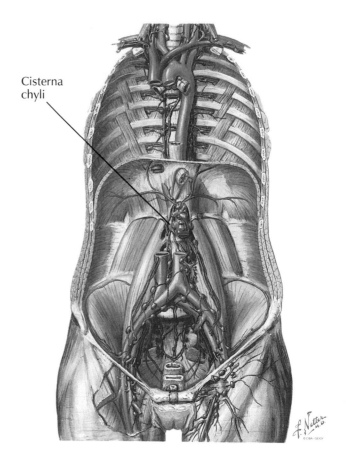

PLATE 249

LOCATE formation of inferior vena cava by union of **common iliac veins** anterior and to right of body of vertebra L5. Note that left common iliac vein is longer than right common iliac vein.

NOTE that common iliac veins and **external iliac veins** lie medial to common iliac and external iliac arteries.

LOCATE middle sacral vein, which drains into left common iliac vein.

ELEVATE distal inferior vena cava to expose **lumbar veins**. Note that 2 lower pairs of lumbar veins drain into inferior vena cava.

TRACE 2 upper pairs of lumbar veins, which pass through diaphragm to drain into azygos and hemiazygos veins.

FOLLOW (in male) **right testicular** and **right renal veins** to where they join inferior vena cava and **left testicular vein** to where it joins **left renal vein**.

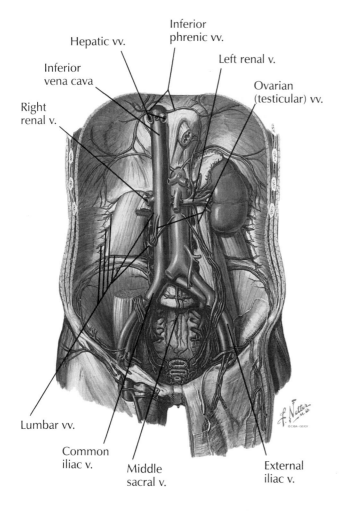

PLATE 248

FOLLOW (in female) **right ovarian** and **right renal veins** to where they join inferior vena cava and **left ovarian vein** to where it joins **left renal vein**.

TRACE inferior phrenic veins to where they drain into inferior vena cava.

EXAMINE cut ends of **hepatic veins**, which join inferior vena cava.

CAUTION During following steps, preserve cisterna chyli deep to aorta.

BLUNT DISSECT deep to aorta to free it from vertebral bodies.

RETRACT aorta to right, and cut lumbar arteries branching from it.

LOCATE cisterna chyli as it lies on vertebral column at level of T12, L1 (level of celiac trunk).

DISSECTION 4.6
POSTERIOR ABDOMINAL WALL

Complete DISSECTION **4.5** Kidney and Suprarenal Gland.

Read DISCUSSIONS **4.17** Posterior Abdominal Wall and **4.18** Lumbar Plexus.

PLACE cadaver in supine position.

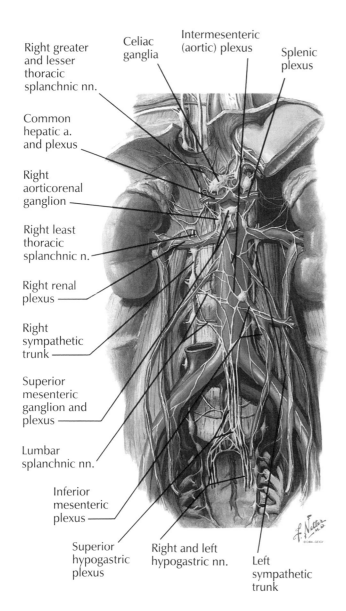

Right greater and lesser thoracic splanchnic nn.

Celiac ganglia

Intermesenteric (aortic) plexus

Splenic plexus

Common hepatic a. and plexus

Right aorticorenal ganglion

Right least thoracic splanchnic n.

Right renal plexus

Right sympathetic trunk

Superior mesenteric ganglion and plexus

Lumbar splanchnic nn.

Inferior mesenteric plexus

Superior hypogastric plexus

Right and left hypogastric nn.

Left sympathetic trunk

PLATE 304

OBSERVE remnants of **intermesenteric (aortic) plexus** on abdominal aorta, and follow this autonomic plexus along branches of aorta. Note that regional naming of these plexuses is determined by name of accompanying artery.

IDENTIFY celiac, aorticorenal, renal, superior mesenteric, and inferior mesenteric ganglia.

TRACE greater thoracic splanchnic nerve from celiac ganglion retrograde through diaphragm to its origin from T5–9. Note that left greater splanchnic nerve pierces <u>left</u> crus of diaphragm, and right greater splanchnic nerve pierces <u>right</u> crus.

TRACE lesser thoracic splanchnic nerve from aorticorenal ganglion retrograde to its origin from T10, 11. Note that lesser splanchnic nerve pierces diaphragm slightly posterior to greater thoracic splanchnic nerve.

TRACE least thoracic splanchnic nerve from renal ganglion retrograde to its origin from T12 to where it passes posterior to medial arcuate ligament.

NOTE that all these autonomic ganglia are very close and extremely interconnected and intertwined.

LOCATE superior hypogastric plexus descending over bifurcation of aorta. Note that **right** and **left hypogastric nerves** may be distinguishable passing along common iliac arteries.

LOOK for **lumbar splanchnic nerves** from L1, 2 ganglia joining inferior mesenteric ganglion directly from sympathetic trunk.

LOOK for lumbar splanchnic nerves from L3, 4 ganglia joining superior hypogastric plexus directly from sympathetic trunk.

RETRACT abdominal aorta and inferior vena cava to <u>right</u> as much as possible.

TRACE course of **left sympathetic trunk** as it passes on anterior lateral surfaces of bodies of lumbar vertebrae. Note that both sympathetic trunks pass deep to medial arcuate ligaments, medial to psoas major muscle and anterior to sacral promontory into pelvis.

NOTE that following dissection is to be done on <u>right</u> side only.

CAUTION   During next step, preserve genitofemoral nerve, which emerges from psoas major muscle to course inferiorly on anterior surface of psoas major muscle, and subcostal, iliohypogastric, and ilioinguinal nerves as they exit from lateral side of psoas major muscle.

REMOVE <u>right</u> psoas major and minor muscles to expose formation of **lumbar plexus.**

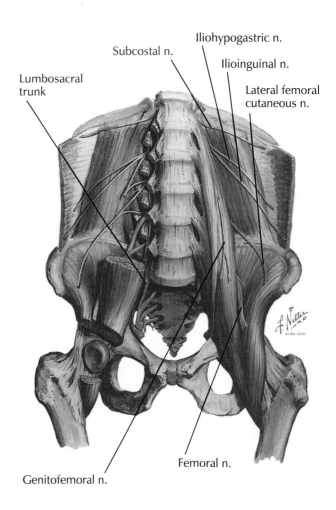

PLATE 466

DISSECT with forceps in one hand while branches of lumbar plexus are protected by forceps in other hand. Parts of psoas major muscle may be cut with scissors only after inspection has confirmed that no nerve branches are within.

TRACE genitofemoral nerve to its origin from ventral rami of spinal nerves L1, 2.

FOLLOW femoral branch (*not shown*) of genitofemoral nerve to where it passes deep to inguinal ligament. Note that **genital branch** of genitofemoral nerve was followed to cremaster muscle in DISSECTION **2.4.**

IDENTIFY subcostal nerve, and follow it proximally to its origin from ventral ramus of spinal nerve T12.

IDENTIFY iliohypogastric nerve, and follow it proximally to its origin from ventral ramus of spinal nerve L1.

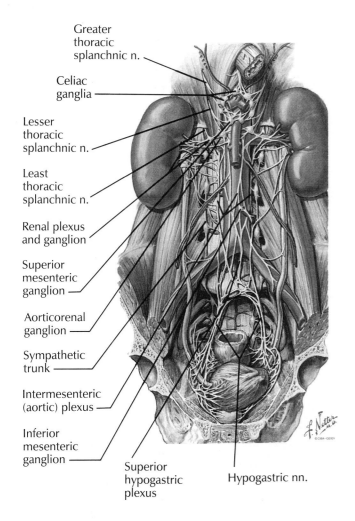

PLATE 326

79

FOLLOW iliohypogastric nerve distally between internal abdominal oblique and transversus abdominis muscles. Locate where its lateral cutaneous branch pierces muscle layers above iliac crest and its anterior cutaneous branch pierces them above superficial inguinal ring.

IDENTIFY ilioinguinal nerve, and follow it proximally to its origin from ventral ramus of spinal nerve L1.

FOLLOW ilioinguinal nerve's distal course, which is similar but inferior to course of iliohypogastric nerve, to its passage through superficial inguinal ring.

IDENTIFY lateral femoral cutaneous nerve as it exits deep to inguinal ligament near anterior superior iliac spine, and follow it retrograde to its origin from ventral rami of spinal nerves L2, 3.

FOLLOW lateral femoral cutaneous nerve distally to where it passes deep to inguinal ligament medial to anterior superior iliac spine.

IDENTIFY femoral nerve as it exits lateral to remaining fibers of psoas major muscle, and follow it retrograde to its origin from ventral rami of spinal nerves L2–4.

FOLLOW femoral nerve distally to where it passes deep to inguinal ligament lateral to external iliac artery.

IDENTIFY obturator nerve (*not shown*) as it exits deep and medial to remaining fibers of psoas major muscle, and follow it proximally to its origin from ventral rami of spinal nerves L2–4.

FOLLOW obturator nerve distally to where it passes deep to common iliac vessels and enters pelvis. Note that its complete path will be traced in DISSECTIONS **7.3** and **7.4**.

LOOK for branches from femoral nerve to iliacus muscle and for branches from ventral rami of L1–4 directly to psoas major and quadratus lumborum muscles.

LOCATE lumbosacral trunk from ventral rami of spinal nerves L4, 5 as it passes medial to obturator nerve.

NOTE that common variation is presence of inconstant **accessory obturator nerve** (*not shown*), which originates from ventral rami of spinal nerves L3, 4. It passes along medial border of psoas major muscle to exit anterior to pecten pubis.

Section 5

UPPER LIMB

DISSECTION 5.1

AXILLARY REGION

Complete DISSECTION **2.1** Pectoral Region.

Read DISCUSSIONS **5.1** Surface Anatomy, **5.2** Bones, **5.5** Axilla, **5.6** Brachial Plexus, and **5.11** Arteries.

COMPLETE removal of fat and fascia in axilla with forceps, fingers, and blunt-scissor dissection, taking care not to injure structures embedded in fat.

IDENTIFY intercostobrachial nerve as it crosses axilla from lateral cutaneous branch of 2nd intercostal nerve to join **medial brachial cutaneous nerve.**

IDENTIFY long thoracic nerve and **lateral thoracic artery** as they pass external to **serratus anterior muscle**.

TRACE lateral thoracic artery retrograde to axillary artery.

IDENTIFY following nerves, arteries, and veins, which pass through axilla into arm, by carefully cleaning deep fascia from upper part of arm.

LOCATE axillary vein (*not shown*) anterior medially and superficially placed in **axillary sheath** (*not shown*). Note that axillary vein may consist of 2 or more parallel and anastomosing vessels.

NOTE entrance of cephalic vein into axillary vein within deltopectoral triangle (*not labeled*).

BLUNT DISSECT tributaries free from their accompanying arterial branches.

REMOVE axillary vein and its tributaries to clear field of dissection.

IDENTIFY medial antebrachial cutaneous nerve and medial brachial cutaneous nerve situated medial to axillary vein.

IDENTIFY upper, middle (thoracodorsal), and **lower subscapular nerves** on anterior surface of subscapularis muscle.

CLEAN anterior surface of **latissimus dorsi, teres major,** and **subscapularis muscles**.

BLUNT DISSECT latissimus dorsi muscle free from ribs and serratus anterior muscle.

IDENTIFY axillary artery, and use it as point of reference for following identifications.

IDENTIFY ulnar nerve, which is medial to 3rd part of axillary artery and passes anterior to tendon of latissimus dorsi and medial to medial antebrachial cutaneous nerve.

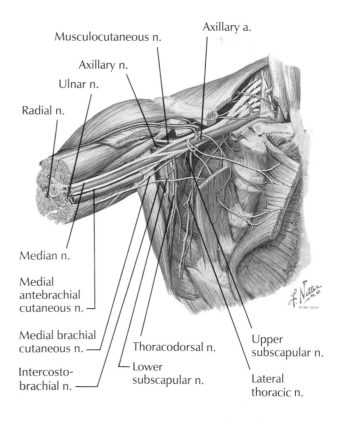

Musculocutaneous n.

Axillary a.

Axillary n.

Ulnar n.

Radial n.

Median n.

Medial antebrachial cutaneous n.

Medial brachial cutaneous n.

Intercosto-brachial n.

Thoracodorsal n.

Lower subscapular n.

Upper subscapular n.

Lateral thoracic n.

PLATE 404

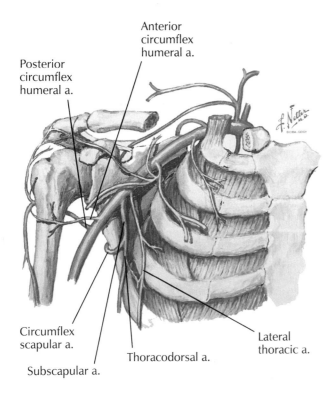

Posterior circumflex humeral a.

Anterior circumflex humeral a.

Circumflex scapular a.

Subscapular a.

Thoracodorsal a.

Lateral thoracic a.

PLATE 402

IDENTIFY median nerve anterior to axillary artery. Use M-shaped configuration for confirmation.

CLEAN coracobrachialis muscle and **short head** of **biceps brachii muscle.**

REFLECT coracobrachialis muscle laterally to expose **musculocutaneous nerve** as it enters coracobrachialis muscle.

ELEVATE axillary artery to expose **radial nerve.** Note that radial nerve accompanies **deep brachial artery.**

ELEVATE axillary artery to expose **axillary nerve.**

TRACE ulnar nerve proximally to its origin from **medial cord** (*not labeled*). Note branches of medial cord: medial antebrachial, medial brachial, medial pectoral, and medial contribution to median nerve.

TRACE median nerve proximally to its origin from medial cord and **lateral cord** (*not labeled*). Branch of median nerve from medial cord crosses anterior to axillary artery.

TRACE musculocutaneous nerve proximally to identify lateral cord. Note branches of lateral cord to lateral pectoral and median nerves.

TRACE radial nerve proximally to identify **posterior cord** (*not labeled*). Note subscapular branches of posterior cord: upper, middle, and lower. These nerves may arise from common trunk, or may appear to arise from axillary nerve.

IDENTIFY subscapular artery against posterior wall of axilla. It branches close to its source into circumflex scapular and thoracodorsal arteries.

IDENTIFY circumflex scapular artery passing between subscapularis and teres major muscles.

IDENTIFY thoracodorsal artery and nerve as they distribute to latissimus dorsi muscle.

IDENTIFY anterior circumflex humeral artery as it passes behind coracobrachialis muscle.

IDENTIFY posterior circumflex humeral artery as it passes between subscapularis and teres major muscles in company with axillary nerve. Anterior and posterior circumflex humeral arteries may arise separately or from common trunk. Posterior artery is usually larger.

DISSECTION 5.2
SCAPULAR REGION

Complete DISSECTION **1.1** Superficial Back.

Read DISCUSSIONS **5.6** Brachial Plexus, **5.7** Scapular Region, and **5.11** Arteries.

PLACE cadaver in prone position and a<u>b</u>duct arm until resistance is felt.

CLEAN posterior surface of **deltoid muscle**.

BLUNT DISSECT deep to scapular attachment of deltoid muscle with scissors or fingers to separate deltoid muscle from underlying **infraspinatus muscle**.

PLATE 399

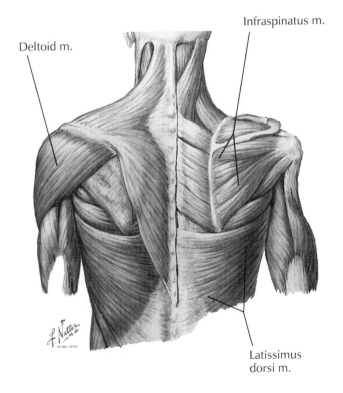

PLATE 407

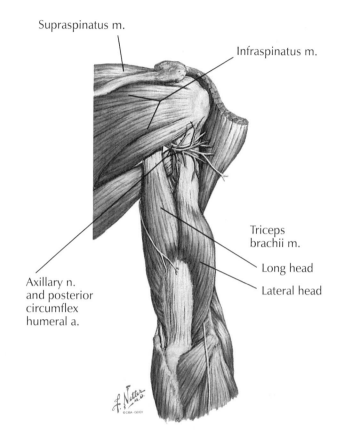

CUT deltoid muscle, using scalpel, along its scapular origin from medial end of spine, continuing around to anterior angle of acromion.

CAUTION   During next step, preserve axillary nerve and posterior circumflex humeral artery.

REFLECT deltoid muscle laterally toward its insertion to humerus.

IDENTIFY axillary nerve and **posterior circumflex humeral artery** on deep surface of deltoid muscle.

IDENTIFY nerve to **teres minor muscle**, which branches from inferior division of axillary nerve.

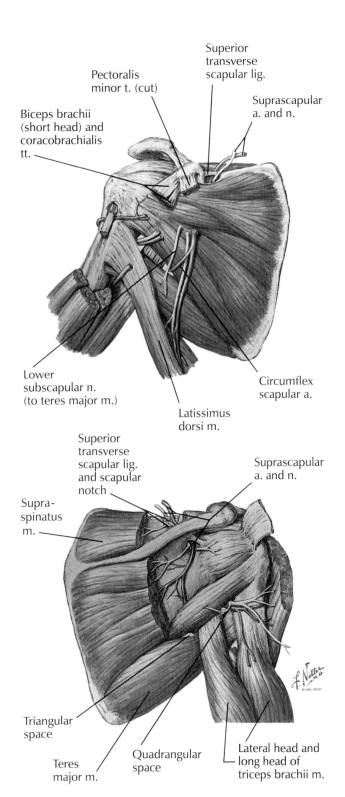

Pectoralis minor t. (cut)

Biceps brachii (short head) and coracobrachialis tt.

Superior transverse scapular lig.

Suprascapular a. and n.

Lower subscapular n. (to teres major m.)

Latissimus dorsi m.

Circumflex scapular a.

Superior transverse scapular lig. and scapular notch

Supra-spinatus m.

Suprascapular a. and n.

Triangular space

Teres major m.

Quadrangular space

Lateral head and long head of triceps brachii m.

PLATE 401

CLEAN infraspinatus and teres minor muscles.

DEFINE borders of **quadrangular space** as teres major and minor muscles and long head of triceps brachii muscle and humerus.

DEFINE borders of **triangular space** as long head of triceps brachii muscle and teres major and minor muscles.

LOOK for **circumflex scapular artery** deep to borders of triangular space.

CLEAN teres major muscle and **long head** of **triceps brachii muscle.**

CAUTION   During following steps, preserve suprascapular artery and nerve.

CLEAN supraspinatus muscle.

RETRACT superior border of supraspinatus muscle inferiorly to palpate bony surface deep to it.

LOCATE superior transverse ligament of scapula with fingers.

IDENTIFY suprascapular artery as it passes superior to transverse ligament, and clean area surrounding artery.

IDENTIFY suprascapular nerve as it passes beneath superior transverse ligament.

TRANSECT supraspinatus muscle medial to superior transverse ligament.

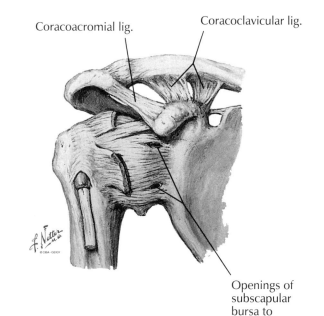

Coracoacromial lig.

Coracoclavicular lig.

Openings of subscapular bursa to shoulder joint

PLATE 398

REFLECT cut ends of supraspinatus muscle medially and laterally away from superior transverse ligament.

LOOK for branches of suprascapular nerve supplying supraspinatus muscle.

BLUNT DISSECT deep to muscle fibers and tendon of infraspinatus as it inserts to humerus.

TRANSECT infraspinatus muscle with scissors vertically, in line with posterior angle of acromion (*not labeled*).

REFLECT cut end of infraspinatus muscle medially, detaching fibers from scapula.

LOOK for branches of suprascapular nerve supplying infraspinatus muscle.

TURN cadaver to supine position.

INCISE skin of pectoral region (**Figure 3**), if DISSECTION **2.1** has not been completed.

CUT clavicular attachment of deltoid muscle as close to bone as possible.

REFLECT cut ends of deltoid muscle away from clavicle, leaving axillary nerve intact.

CLEAN coracoacromial ligament.

OPEN subacromial bursa. Observe that bursa may extend deep to deltoid muscle, where it is called **subdeltoid bursa.**

CLEAN coracoid attachments of **pectoralis minor** and **coracobrachialis muscles** and **short head** of **biceps brachii muscle.** Note that latter 2 muscles originate from common tendon.

LOCATE tendons of teres major and **latissimus dorsi** as they insert to humerus. Note that these tendons pass posterior to coracobrachialis muscle and short head of biceps brachii muscle and that tendon of latissimus dorsi attaches to humerus anterior to tendon of teres major.

LOCATE tendon of **pectoralis major** as it inserts to humerus. Note that this tendon passes anterior to both coracobrachialis muscle and short head of biceps brachii muscle.

DISSECTION 5.3
ARM

Complete DISSECTIONS **5.1** Axillary Region and **5.2** Scapular Region.

Read DISCUSSIONS **5.6** Brachial Plexus, **5.8** Arm, and **5.11** Arteries.

PLACE cadaver in supine position.

MARK location of cutaneous nerves and superficial veins on skin with felt-tip marker.

CAUTION   During skinning and following steps, preserve cephalic and basilic veins and cutaneous nerves.

INCISE skin of arm and forearm (**Figure 19**), adapting incision lines to rigor position of cadaver.

REMOVE skin and subcutaneous tissue of arm and forearm.

CAUTION   During next step, preserve medial and lateral pectoral nerves and thoracoacromial artery. Use fingers as guides to protect these structures by pulling up on pectoral muscles while cutting.

CUT tendon of **pectoralis major** 1 finger-width from its insertion to humerus, and cut tendon of **pectoralis minor** 1 finger-width from coracoid process.

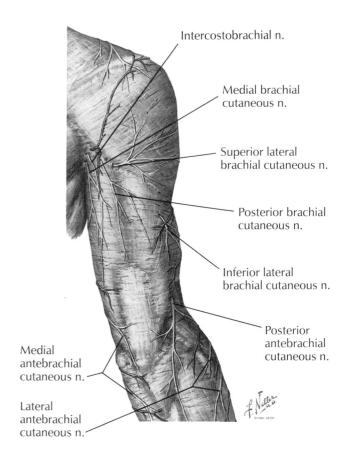

Supraclavicular nn.

Medial brachial cutaneous n.

Superior lateral brachial cutaneous n.

Cephalic v.

Inferior lateral brachial cutaneous n.

Posterior antebrachial cutaneous n.

Medial antebrachial cutaneous n.

Basilic v.

Intermediate cubital v.

Basilic v.

Intercostobrachial n.

Medial brachial cutaneous n.

Superior lateral brachial cutaneous n.

Posterior brachial cutaneous n.

Inferior lateral brachial cutaneous n.

Posterior antebrachial cutaneous n.

Medial antebrachial cutaneous n.

Lateral antebrachial cutaneous n.

PLATE 452

PLATE 452

88

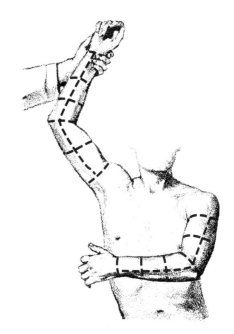

Figure 19

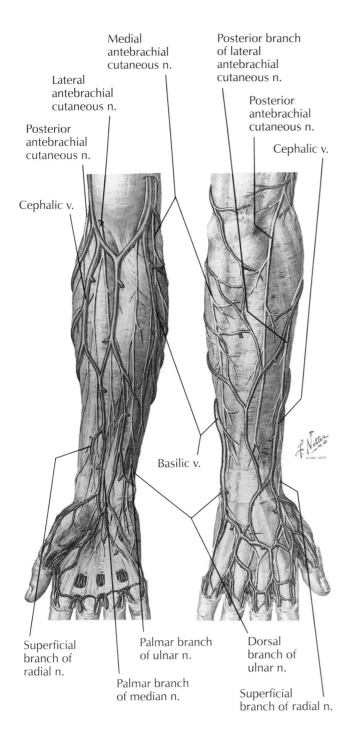

Medial antebrachial cutaneous n.

Lateral antebrachial cutaneous n.

Posterior antebrachial cutaneous n.

Cephalic v.

Posterior branch of lateral antebrachial cutaneous n.

Posterior antebrachial cutaneous n.

Cephalic v.

Basilic v.

Superficial branch of radial n.

Palmar branch of ulnar n.

Palmar branch of median n.

Dorsal branch of ulnar n.

Superficial branch of radial n.

PLATE 453

CUT and TAG "buttons" of pectoralis major and minor muscles attached to both medial and lateral pectoral nerves to use for later identification.

REMOVE pectoralis major and minor muscles, except for muscle "buttons."

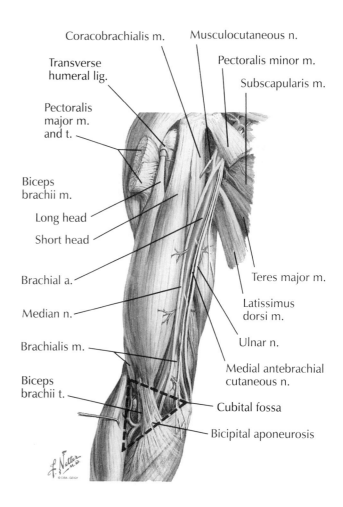

Coracobrachialis m.

Musculocutaneous n.

Transverse humeral lig.

Pectoralis minor m.

Subscapularis m.

Pectoralis major m. and t.

Biceps brachii m.

Long head

Short head

Brachial a.

Median n.

Brachialis m.

Biceps brachii t.

Teres major m.

Latissimus dorsi m.

Ulnar n.

Medial antebrachial cutaneous n.

Cubital fossa

Bicipital aponeurosis

PLATE 408

RETRACT brachial plexus and axillary artery laterally to complete cleaning tendons of **latissimus dorsi** and **teres major**.

CLEAN anterior surface of **subscapularis muscle** to complete exposure of subscapular nerves and vessels.

IDENTIFY serratus anterior muscle, and palpate its insertion to medial margin of anterior surface of scapula. Note that costal origins may have been removed if DISSECTION **2.1** preceded inspection of upper limb.

IDENTIFY long and **short heads** of **biceps brachii muscle** and **coracobrachialis muscle**.

IDENTIFY transverse humeral ligament.

DEFINE boundaries of **cubital fossa** as imaginary line between medial and lateral epicondyles of humerus and between brachioradialis and pronator teres muscles.

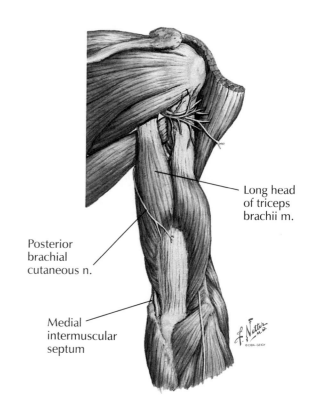

Posterior brachial cutaneous n.

Long head of triceps brachii m.

Medial intermuscular septum

PLATE 407

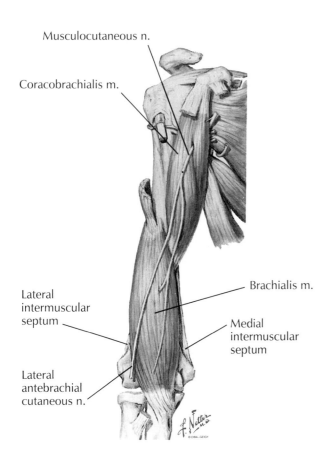

Musculocutaneous n.

Coracobrachialis m.

Brachialis m.

Lateral intermuscular septum

Medial intermuscular septum

Lateral antebrachial cutaneous n.

PLATE 406

IDENTIFY bicipital aponeurosis and tendon of **biceps brachii** within cubital fossa.

IDENTIFY brachial artery and **median nerve** passing anterior to coracobrachialis muscle.

IDENTIFY musculocutaneous nerve entering coracobrachialis muscle.

ELEVATE biceps brachii muscle to expose **brachialis muscle**.

LOCATE musculocutaneous nerve passing between biceps brachii and brachialis muscles and its branches to both those muscles.

LOOK for **lateral antebrachial cutaneous nerve** piercing brachial fascia lateral to biceps brachii muscle above elbow.

LOOK for passage of **medial antebrachial cutaneous nerve** between median and ulnar nerves.

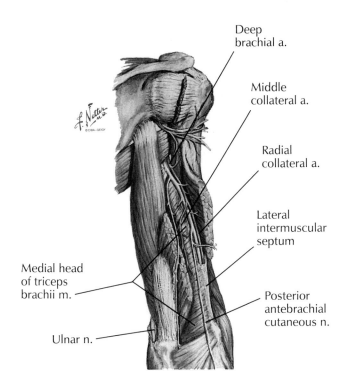

Deep
brachial a.

Middle
collateral a.

Radial
collateral a.

Lateral
intermuscular
septum

Medial head
of triceps
brachii m.

Posterior
antebrachial
cutaneous n.

Ulnar n.

PLATE 407

IDENTIFY medial head of **triceps brachii muscle**
by its attachment to posterior surface of medial
and lateral intermuscular septa.

CAUTION   During next step, preserve branches
of radial nerve and deep brachial artery.

TRANSECT long head of triceps brachii muscle 3
finger-widths inferior to passage of axillary nerve.

TRANSECT lateral head of triceps brachii muscle
along course of radial groove, protecting radial
nerve and deep brachial artery.

LOOK for **ascending branch** (*not labeled*) of
deep brachial artery, which is deep to deltoid
muscle, and for **middle collateral artery**, which
is descending branch of deep brachial artery.

PLATE 409

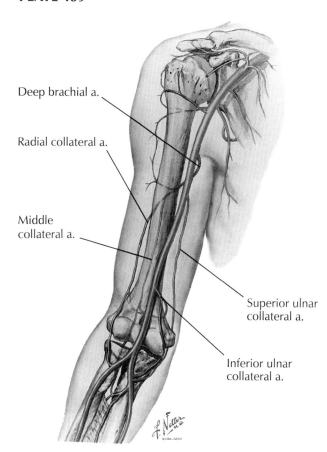

Deep brachial a.

Radial collateral a.

Middle
collateral a.

Superior ulnar
collateral a.

Inferior ulnar
collateral a.

TRACE brachial artery. Note that median nerve
crosses it midarm from lateral to medial.

LOCATE origin of **deep brachial artery** from
medial side of brachial artery, and follow its
passage between medial and lateral heads of
triceps brachii muscle. Note that name changes to
radial collateral artery when it approaches elbow.

IDENTIFY radial nerve, which accompanies deep
brachial artery.

ADDUCT upper limb to expose its posterior
surface by crossing it over thorax obliquely
(**Figure 19**).

IDENTIFY lateral and **long heads** of **triceps
brachii muscle**, and separate heads to expose
radial nerve and deep brachial artery.

IDENTIFY medial and **lateral intermuscular septa**
by attachments of distal brachialis muscle to their
anterior surfaces.

LOOK for origins of branches of radial nerve before radial nerve passes into radial groove.

TRACE posterior brachial cutaneous nerve from its passage inferior to tendons of latissimus dorsi and teres major to medial side of long head of triceps brachii muscle.

LOCATE nerve to **long head** of **triceps brachii muscle** (*not labeled*) from radial nerve.

IDENTIFY ulnar nerve as it passes superficial to medial head of triceps brachii muscle.

LOOK for origins of branches of radial nerve as it spirals around humerus.

LOCATE origin of **nerves** to **lateral head** of **triceps brachii muscle** (*not labeled*) from radial nerve.

TRACE nerve to **medial head** of **triceps brachii muscle** (*not labeled*) from radial nerve as it accompanies ulnar nerve. Note that it may also be called ulnar collateral nerve.

IDENTIFY posterior antebrachial cutaneous nerve as it becomes superficial below inferior border of lateral head of triceps brachii muscle.

TRACE radial nerve distally to where it pierces lateral intermuscular septum.

REPLACE upper limb in supine position.

TRACE brachial artery to where it passes deep to bicipital aponeurosis.

REMOVE brachial vein (*not shown*) and **basilic vein** to expose branches of brachial artery.

TRACE superior ulnar collateral artery from its origin from brachial artery near insertion of coracobrachialis muscle to where it pierces medial intermuscular septum. Note that it accompanies ulnar nerve.

TRACE inferior ulnar collateral artery from its origin above bicipital aponeurosis to its division into anterior and posterior branches.

DISSECTION 5.4
POSTERIOR FOREARM

Complete DISSECTION **5.3** Arm.

Read DISCUSSIONS **5.6** Brachial Plexus, **5.9** Forearm, and **5.11** Arteries.

DEFINE attachments of **anconeus muscle** between lateral epicondyle of humerus and lateral border of olecranon process of ulna. Anconeus muscle will appear to be continuous with medial head of triceps brachii muscle.

CUT muscle fibers of anconeus that insert to olecranon. Use blunt scissors to feel bone, and then cut fibers from bone.

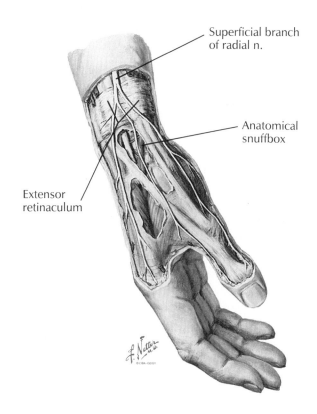

Superficial branch of radial n.

Anatomical snuffbox

Extensor retinaculum

PLATE 440

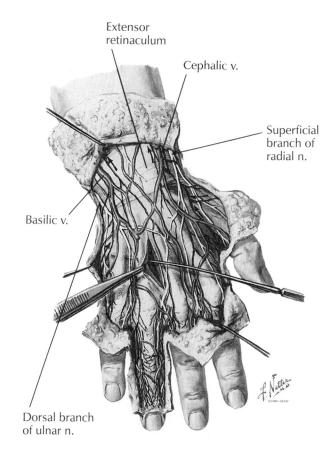

Extensor retinaculum

Cephalic v.

Superficial branch of radial n.

Basilic v.

Dorsal branch of ulnar n.

PLATE 441

REFLECT anconeus muscle toward lateral epicondyle to expose nerve to **anconeus muscle** from **radial nerve** (*not shown*).

DIRECT attention to dorsal surface of hand.

MARK location of superficial veins and cutaneous nerves on dorsal surface of hand with felt-tip marker.

CAUTION During next step, preserve superficial veins and cutaneous nerves of hand.

SKIN dorsal surface of hand. Note that skin is loose from underlying deep fascia.

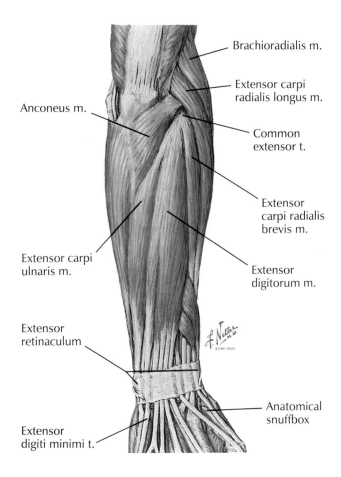

Brachioradialis m.

Extensor carpi
radialis longus m.

Anconeus m.

Common
extensor t.

Extensor
carpi radialis
brevis m.

Extensor carpi
ulnaris m.

Extensor
digitorum m.

Extensor
retinaculum

Anatomical
snuffbox

Extensor
digiti minimi t.

PLATE 418

DEFINE superior and inferior borders of **extensor retinaculum** so that remaining deep antebrachial fascia may be removed from forearm muscles during following steps.

REVIEW contents of compartments of extensor retinaculum. Each compartment will be opened as dissection progresses.

CONFIRM attachments of extensor retinaculum to distal radius and styloid process of ulna.

CAUTION   During following steps, preserve superficial radial nerve and dorsal branch of ulnar nerve.

REMOVE cephalic and **basilic veins.**

CLEAN superficial muscles and tendons on posterior surface of forearm and dorsal surface of hand.

BLUNT DISSECT with fingers and scissors to separate muscles and tendons from each other.

LOCATE origins of **brachioradialis** and **extensor carpi radialis longus muscles** from supracondylar ridge of humerus. Note that extensor carpi radialis longus muscle originates distal to brachioradialis muscle.

IDENTIFY superficial branch of **radial nerve** as it exits from deep to brachioradialis muscle and courses superficial to anatomical snuffbox and to lateral side of dorsal surface of hand.

PLATE 419

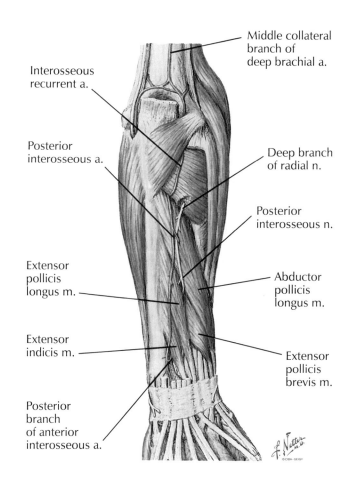

Interosseous
recurrent a.

Middle collateral
branch of
deep brachial a.

Posterior
interosseous a.

Deep branch
of radial n.

Posterior
interosseous n.

Extensor
pollicis
longus m.

Abductor
pollicis
longus m.

Extensor
indicis m.

Extensor
pollicis
brevis m.

Posterior
branch
of anterior
interosseous a.

TRACE brachioradialis muscle to its insertion to styloid process of radius.

TRACE tendon of extensor carpi radialis longus proximal to extensor retinaculum where it is crossed superficially by outcropping muscles. Continue tracing tendon distal to extensor retinaculum to its insertion to base of metacarpal bone 2.

ELEVATE brachioradialis muscle to expose course of superficial radial nerve and radial artery.

LOCATE common extensor tendon, which attaches to lateral epicondyle of humerus.

IDENTIFY extensor carpi radialis brevis muscle, which lies deep to extensor carpi radialis longus muscle.

TRACE tendon of extensor carpi radialis brevis proximal to extensor retinaculum where it is crossed superficially by outcropping muscles. Continue tracing tendon distal to extensor retinaculum to its insertion to base of metacarpal bone 3.

IDENTIFY extensor digitorum muscle, and follow it to its formation of 4 tendons proximal to extensor retinaculum.

BLUNT DISSECT tendons of extensor digitorum to separate and determine extent of **intertendinous connections** on dorsal surface of hand.

TRACE tendons of extensor digitorum to their insertions to **dorsal expansions (extensor hoods)** of index through little fingers. Note that each extensor expansion divides into 3 bands over proximal phalanx. **Central band** (*not labeled*) attaches to base of middle phalanx, and **collateral bands** (*not labeled*) continue distally to base of distal phalanx.

IDENTIFY tendon of **extensor digiti minimi**, which joins tendon of extensor digitorum on radial side of little finger. Note that belly of extensor digiti minimi muscle is in common with belly of extensor digitorum muscle.

IDENTIFY extensor carpi ulnaris muscle and its humeral head, which originates from common extensor tendon.

RETRACT proximal part of extensor carpi ulnaris muscle medially to determine attachment of its ulnar head to middle part of posterior surface of ulna.

TRACE tendon of extensor carpi ulnaris distally through extensor retinaculum to base of metacarpal bone 5.

IDENTIFY dorsal cutaneous branch of **ulnar nerve** as it emerges from deep to flexor carpi ulnaris muscle (DISSECTION **5.5**) and onto medial side of dorsal surface of hand.

MAKE 3 vertical cuts in extensor retinaculum with scissors over tendons of extensor carpi ulnaris, extensor digiti minimi, and extensor digitorum.

RETRACT laterally tendons and muscle bellies of extensor carpi ulnaris, extensor digiti minimi, and extensor digitorum.

LOCATE branches of **deep radial nerve** on deep surface of these muscles.

IDENTIFY posterior interosseous nerve (continuation of deep radial nerve) and **posterior interosseous artery** between retracted muscles and outcropping muscles.

CAUTION During following steps, preserve branches of posterior interosseous nerve and artery.

CUT muscle bellies of extensor carpi ulnaris, extensor digiti minimi, and extensor digitorum distal to entrance of nerves.

REFLECT both cut ends of extensor carpi ulnaris, extensor digiti minimi, and extensor digitorum muscles superiorly and inferiorly to expose supinator and outcropping muscles.

BLUNT DISSECT origins of extensor digitorum and extensor carpi radialis brevis muscles apart with scissors to expose origin of humeral head of supinator muscle from common extensor tendon.

LOCATE ulnar head of supinator muscle inferior to radial notch of ulna.

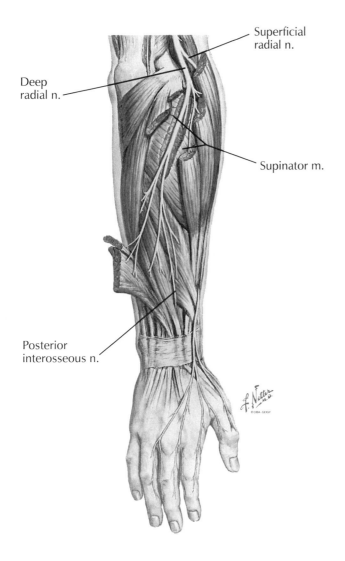

Deep
radial n.

Superficial
radial n.

Supinator m.

Posterior
interosseous n.

PLATE 451

LOCATE origin of **extensor pollicis brevis muscle** from interosseous membrane and radius distal to attachment of abductor pollicis longus muscle.

TRACE tendon of extensor pollicis brevis to insertion to base of proximal phalanx of thumb.

NOTE that abductor pollicis longus and extensor pollicis brevis muscles cross superficially to tendons of extensor carpi radialis longus and brevis.

LOCATE origin of **extensor pollicis longus muscle** from interosseous membrane and ulna distal to attachment of abductor pollicis longus muscle.

TRACE tendon of extensor pollicis longus to insertion to base of distal phalanx of thumb. Note that its tendon passes medial to dorsal tubercle of radius.

LOCATE origin of **extensor indicis muscle** from interosseous membrane and ulna distal to attachment of extensor pollicis longus muscle.

TRACE tendon of extensor indicis to union with tendon of extensor digitorum on radial side of index finger.

IDENTIFY branches of **posterior interosseous nerve** to extensor indicis, extensor pollicis longus, extensor pollicis brevis, and abductor pollicis longus muscles.

ELEVATE brachioradialis muscle again to expose branches of superficial radial nerve, which lie deep to proximal part of muscle.

TRACE branches of radial nerve to extensor carpi radialis longus and brevis muscles and to lateral part of brachialis muscle.

LOCATE origin of **interosseous recurrent artery** near inferior border of supinator muscle, and trace it superiorly as it continues posterior to lateral epicondyle to anastomose with **middle collateral artery** from deep brachial artery.

CUT extensor retinaculum for each compartment containing tendons of extensor indicis, extensor pollicis longus, extensor pollicis brevis, and abductor pollicis longus to expose arterial supply to dorsal surface of wrist and hand.

FOLLOW supinator muscle as it wraps around proximal radius.

TRACE passage of deep branch of radial nerve through supinator muscle.

BLUNT DISSECT to separate each of following muscles.

LOCATE origin of **abductor pollicis longus muscle** from interosseous membrane and radius and ulna.

TRACE tendon of abductor pollicis longus to its insertion to base of metacarpal bone 1.

SEPARATE extensor indicis and extensor pollicis longus muscles to expose interosseous membrane.

LOOK for **posterior branch** of **anterior interosseous artery** piercing interosseous membrane proximal to wrist.

DEFINE borders of **anatomical snuffbox** as tendons of abductor pollicis longus and extensor pollicis brevis and longus.

IDENTIFY radial artery deep to these tendons.

LOCATE dorsal carpal artery (*not labeled*) and **1st dorsal metacarpal artery** as branches from radial artery, which originate just proximal to passage of radial artery through 1st dorsal interosseus muscle.

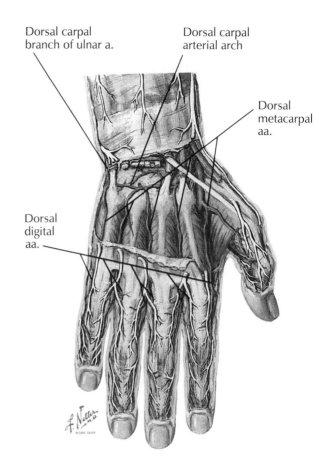

Dorsal carpal branch of ulnar a.

Dorsal carpal arterial arch

Dorsal metacarpal aa.

Dorsal digital aa.

PLATE 442

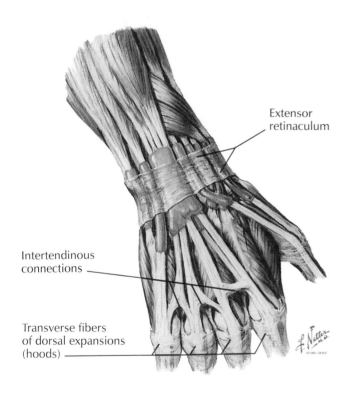

Extensor retinaculum

Intertendinous connections

Transverse fibers of dorsal expansions (hoods)

PLATE 443

CONTINUE with following steps only if time permits.

TRACE dorsal carpal branch of **radial artery** as it passes posterior to wrist to anastomose with **dorsal carpal branch** of **ulnar artery** and **posterior branch** of **anterior interosseous artery** to form **dorsal carpal arch**.

LOCATE dorsal metacarpal arteries, which branch from dorsal carpal arch.

LOCATE dorsal digital arteries, which branch from dorsal metacarpal arteries. Note that 2 dorsal digital arteries arise from each dorsal metacarpal artery to supply facing sides of adjacent fingers.

SUPERFICIAL ANTERIOR FOREARM AND HAND

Complete DISSECTION **5.3** Arm.

Read DISCUSSIONS **5.6** Brachial Plexus, **5.9** Forearm, **5.10** Hand, and **5.11** Arteries.

MARK location of palmar cutaneous branch of median and ulnar nerves and palmaris brevis muscle on palm of hand with felt-tip marker.

CAUTION During following steps, preserve palmar cutaneous branch of median nerve. It branches from median nerve just proximal to palmar carpal ligament, and passes in subcutaneous tissue over thenar eminence.

PLATE 432

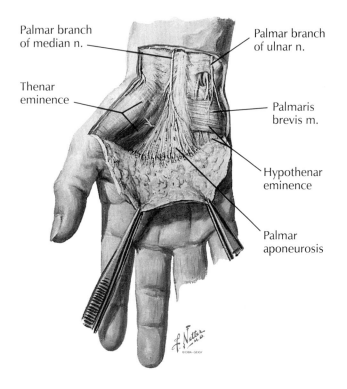

PLATE 420

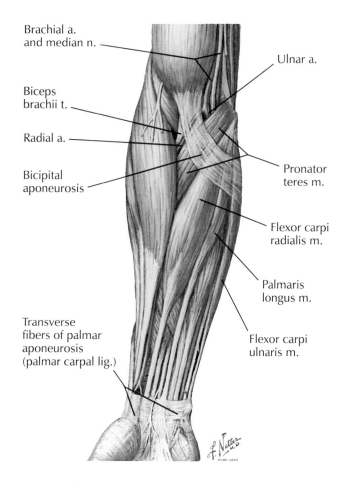

CAUTION Preserve palmaris brevis muscle and palmar cutaneous branch of ulnar nerve located in subcutaneous tissue of hypothenar eminence.

SKIN palm of hand. Note that skin tightly adheres to underlying deep fascia.

IDENTIFY palmar branch of **median nerve, palmaris brevis muscle**, and **palmar branch** of **ulnar nerve.**

CLEAN **palmar aponeurosis** with forceps and scissors.

DIRECT attention to cubital fossa and muscles that originate from medial epicondyle of humerus by common flexor tendon.

BLUNT DISSECT bicipital aponeurosis free from brachial artery and median nerve.

REMOVE bicipital aponeurosis with scissors to expose relationship of **median nerve** medial to **brachial artery**, which is medial to tendon of **biceps brachii**.

IDENTIFY pronator teres, flexor carpi radialis, palmaris longus, and **flexor carpi ulnaris muscles.**

CLEAN origin of **radial** and **ulnar arteries.** Note that radial artery crosses superficial to tendon of biceps brachii and ulnar artery passes deep to pronator teres muscle.

LOCATE radial recurrent artery ascending between brachialis and brachioradialis muscles.

LOCATE anterior ulnar recurrent artery ascending between pronator teres and brachialis muscles.

LOCATE posterior ulnar recurrent artery ascending deep to pronator teres muscle.

TRACE median nerve as it passes through humeral and ulnar heads of pronator teres muscle.

RETRACT pronator teres muscle, brachial artery, and median nerve as far medially as possible and brachioradialis muscle as far laterally as possible.

LOCATE insertion of tendon of biceps brachii to **tuberosity** of **radius** (*not shown*).

LOCATE insertion of tendon of brachialis to **tuberosity** of **ulna** (*not shown*).

DIRECT attention to wrist.

DEFINE superior and inferior borders of **palmar carpal ligament** so that remaining deep antebrachial fascia may be removed from muscles as dissection progresses.

CONFIRM attachment of palmar carpal ligament to styloid processes of ulna and radius.

SEPARATE remaining superficial muscles and tendons on anterior surface of forearm.

CAUTION During next step, preserve superficial palmar arterial arch and accompanying branches of median nerve.

BLUNT DISSECT deep to **fibrous bands** that extend from palmar aponeurosis to base of index through little fingers.

CAUTION During next step, preserve ulnar nerve and artery deep to medial palmar carpal ligament.

CUT fibrous bands of palmar aponeurosis from fingers, and progressively free palmar aponeurosis with palmar carpal ligament attached to it. Blunt dissect and use only very small scissor snips.

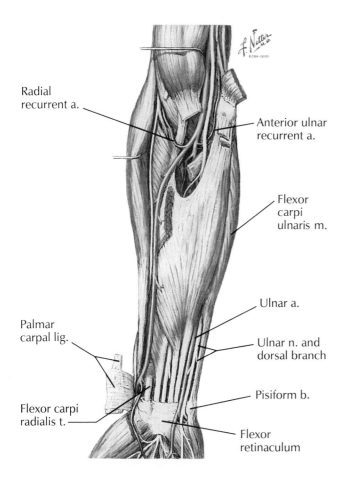

Radial recurrent a.

Anterior ulnar recurrent a.

Flexor carpi ulnaris m.

Ulnar a.

Ulnar n. and dorsal branch

Palmar carpal lig.

Pisiform b.

Flexor carpi radialis t.

Flexor retinaculum

PLATE 421

REFLECT palmar aponeurosis proximally with tendon of palmaris longus attached to it.

IDENTIFY ulnar nerve and **artery** superficial to flexor retinaculum between pisiform bone and hook of hamate bone.

TRACE tendon of **flexor carpi radialis** to its passage deep to thenar muscles. Note that its insertion will be inspected in DISSECTION **5.7**.

TRACE tendon of **flexor carpi ulnaris** to pisiform bone. In DISSECTION **5.7**, pisohamate and hamatometacarpal ligaments (*not labeled*) will be identified as continuations of tendon of flexor carpi ulnaris to base of metacarpal bone 5.

TRANSECT pronator teres muscle 3 finger-widths proximal to its radial insertion, and continue incision at same level across belly of flexor carpi radialis muscle.

PLATE 432

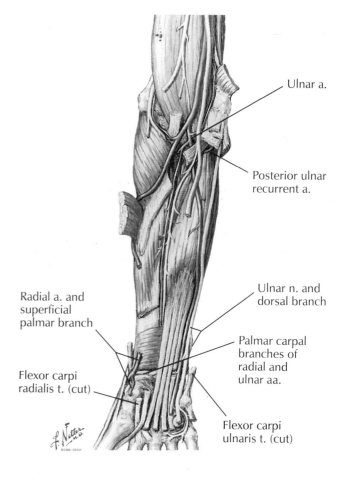

Ulnar a.

Posterior ulnar recurrent a.

Radial a. and superficial palmar branch

Ulnar n. and dorsal branch

Palmar carpal branches of radial and ulnar aa.

Flexor carpi radialis t. (cut)

Flexor carpi ulnaris t. (cut)

PLATE 422

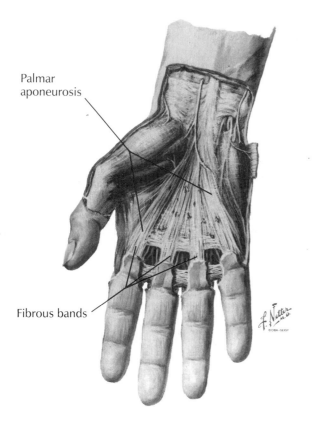

Palmar aponeurosis

Fibrous bands

LOCATE branches of median nerve deep to proximal bellies of pronator teres, flexor carpi radialis, and palmaris longus muscles.

RETRACT flexor carpi ulnaris muscle medially to expose course of ulnar nerve and artery.

LOCATE branches of ulnar nerve deep to proximal belly of flexor carpi ulnaris muscle.

REFLECT proximal cut ends of pronator teres, flexor carpi radialis, and palmaris longus muscles as far superiorly as possible.

LOCATE origin of flexor digitorum superficialis muscle from common flexor tendon.

CONFIRM additional origin of flexor digitorum superficialis muscle from ulnar tuberosity, oblique line of radius, and fibrous arch between ulna and radius.

CAUTION   During following steps, preserve contents of carpal tunnel.

BLUNT DISSECT deep to **flexor retinaculum**.

CONFIRM attachment of flexor retinaculum laterally to scaphoid and trapezium bones and medially to pisiform bone and hook of hamate bone.

CUT middle of flexor retinaculum vertically with scissors. Note that ulnar artery and nerve do <u>not</u> pass deep to flexor retinaculum.

ELEVATE 4 tendons of flexor digitorum superficialis out of carpal tunnel. Note that median nerve is superficial to tendons of middle and ring fingers, which pass superficial to tendons of index and little fingers.

LOCATE origin of **superficial palmar branch** of **radial artery** within or near borders of anatomical snuffbox. It will pass through thenar eminence to contribute to **superficial palmar arch** by joining ulnar artery.

LOCATE origin of **palmar carpal branch** of **radial artery** over distal radius. It passes deep to flexor tendons, and joins palmar carpal branch of ulnar artery to form **palmar carpal arch**.

DISSECTION 5.6
DEEP ANTERIOR FOREARM AND HAND

Complete DISSECTION **5.5** Superficial Anterior Forearm and Hand.

Read DISCUSSIONS **5.6** Brachial Plexus, **5.9** Forearm, **5.10** Hand, and **5.11** Arteries.

LOCATE median nerve in **carpal tunnel**.

PLATE 422

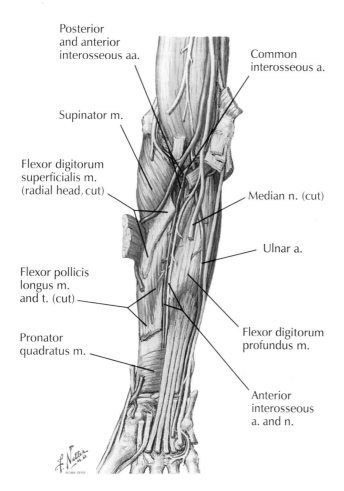

Posterior and anterior interosseous aa.

Common interosseous a.

Supinator m.

Flexor digitorum superficialis m. (radial head, cut)

Median n. (cut)

Flexor pollicis longus m. and t. (cut)

Ulnar a.

Pronator quadratus m.

Flexor digitorum profundus m.

Anterior interosseous a. and n.

TRACE median nerve proximally where it usually adheres to deep surface of **flexor digitorum superficialis muscle**.

BLUNT DISSECT median nerve free of flexor digitorum superficialis muscle. Note that medial retraction of flexor digitorum superficialis muscle may assist dissection.

TRANSECT flexor digitorum superficialis muscle midway in arm.

REFLECT proximal cut ends of flexor digitorum superficialis, palmaris longus, and pronator teres muscles to expose deep muscles. Note that neurovascular supply will be cut for reflection.

IDENTIFY flexor digitorum profundus muscle medially and **flexor pollicis longus muscle** laterally.

IDENTIFY ulnar artery passing superficial to flexor digitorum profundus muscle.

LOCATE origin of flexor digitorum profundus muscle from ulna and interosseous membrane.

LOCATE origin of flexor pollicis longus muscle from radius and interosseous membrane.

DIRECT attention to cubital fossa.

LOCATE origin of **common interosseous artery** from ulnar artery.

IDENTIFY interosseous recurrent artery (*not labeled*) as branch of common interosseous artery, and trace its passage superficial to supinator muscle.

TRACE common interosseous artery to its branching into **anterior** and **posterior interosseous arteries**. Follow posterior interosseous artery to **interosseous membrane** (*not shown*).

LOCATE median nerve in cubital fossa.

SEPARATE flexor digitorum profundus and flexor pollicis longus muscles vertically with fingers to expose anterior interosseous nerve and artery.

IDENTIFY origin of **anterior interosseous nerve** from median nerve.

LOCATE branches of anterior interosseous nerve to flexor digitorum profundus and flexor pollicis longus muscles.

BLUNT DISSECT flexor digitorum profundus and flexor pollicis longus muscles free from interosseous membrane, radius, and ulna.

TRANSECT flexor digitorum profundus and flexor pollicis longus muscles midway in arm.

REFLECT flexor digitorum profundus and flexor pollicis longus muscles distally to expose interosseous membrane. Note that neurovascular supply will be cut for reflection.

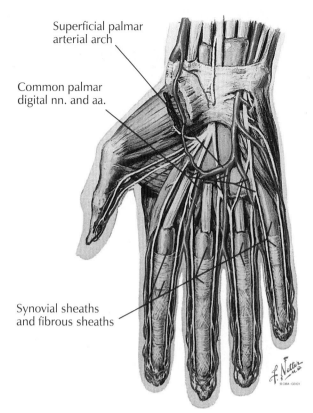

Superficial palmar arterial arch

Common palmar digital nn. and aa.

Synovial sheaths and fibrous sheaths

PLATE 439

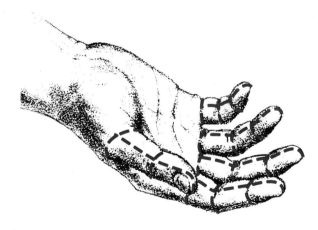

Figure 20

IDENTIFY pronator quadratus muscle on distal radius and ulna.

TRACE anterior interosseous nerve and artery to proximal border of pronator quadratus muscle where they pierce interosseous membrane.

DIRECT attention to hand.

CAUTION During next steps, preserve deep transverse metacarpal ligaments.

INCISE skin of fingers (**Figure 20**).

REMOVE skin from fingers as close to fingertips as possible.

IDENTIFY deep transverse metacarpal ligaments (*not shown*) between heads of metacarpal bones.

IDENTIFY superficial palmar arch and origins of **common palmar digital arteries**.

CUT common palmar digital arteries, ulnar artery, and superficial palmar branch of radial artery from their contributions to superficial palmar arch.

REMOVE superficial palmar arch.

IDENTIFY annular and **cruciate ligaments** of **fibrous tendon sheaths** of 1 finger.

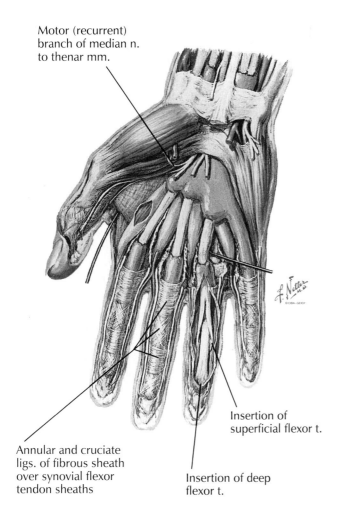

Motor (recurrent) branch of median n. to thenar mm.

Insertion of superficial flexor t.

Annular and cruciate ligs. of fibrous sheath over synovial flexor tendon sheaths

Insertion of deep flexor t.

PLATE 433

CAUTION During next step, do <u>not</u> damage tendons enclosed in fibrous sheaths.

OPEN fibrous sheaths of index through little fingers lengthwise with scissors. Cutting deep transverse metacarpal ligaments may facilitate this step.

CUT synovial sheath lengthwise over each tendon.

ELEVATE tendons of flexor digitorum superficialis and flexor digitorum profundus from tendon sheaths.

LOCATE insertions of flexor digitorum superficialis muscle to base of middle phalanges and insertions of flexor digitorum profundus muscle to base of distal phalanges.

LOCATE vincula between tendons and floor of tendon sheaths.

IDENTIFY lumbrical muscles and their origins from tendons of flexor digitorum profundus and insertions to extensor expansions. Note that lumbrical muscles pass metacarpophalangeal joints on radial side.

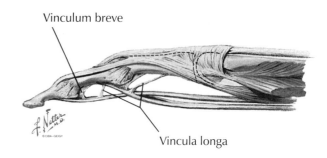

Vinculum breve

Vincula longa

PLATE 437

LOCATE branches of median nerve to radial lumbrical muscles 1, 2.

LOCATE branches of ulnar nerve to ulnar lumbrical muscles 3, 4.

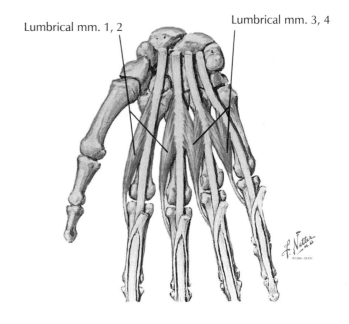

Lumbrical mm. 1, 2

Lumbrical mm. 3, 4

PLATE 436

IDENTIFY abductor digiti minimi muscle on ulnar side of hypothenar eminence. Locate its origin from pisiform bone and its insertion to base of proximal phalanx of little finger.

IDENTIFY flexor digiti minimi brevis muscle lateral to abductor digiti minimi muscle. Locate its origin from hook of hamate bone and medial flexor retinaculum, and locate its insertion to base of proximal phalanx of little finger.

TRACE deep ulnar nerve between abductor digiti minimi and flexor digiti minimi brevis muscles to locate branches to abductor digiti minimi, flexor digiti minimi brevis, and opponens digiti minimi muscles.

TRANSECT abductor digiti minimi and flexor digiti minimi brevis muscles to expose **opponens digiti minimi muscle**. Locate its insertion to length of shaft of metacarpal bone 5 and its common origin with flexor digiti minimi brevis muscle from hook of hamate bone and flexor retinaculum. Note that fibers may blend.

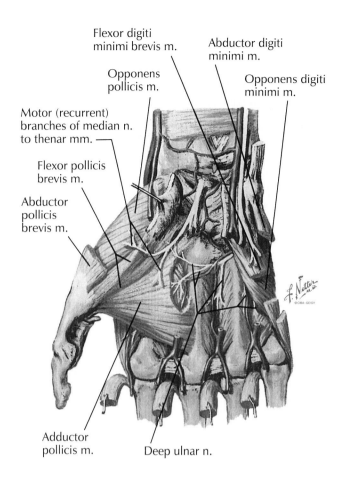

Flexor digiti minimi brevis m.
Abductor digiti minimi m.
Opponens pollicis m.
Opponens digiti minimi m.
Motor (recurrent) branches of median n. to thenar mm.
Flexor pollicis brevis m.
Abductor pollicis brevis m.
Adductor pollicis m.
Deep ulnar n.

PLATE 438

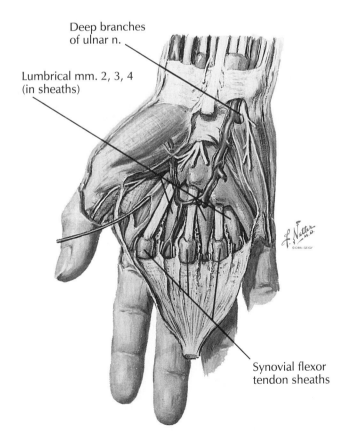

Deep branches of ulnar n.
Lumbrical mm. 2, 3, 4 (in sheaths)
Synovial flexor tendon sheaths

PLATE 433

IDENTIFY abductor pollicis brevis muscle, and locate its origin from trapezium bone and flexor retinaculum and its insertion to lateral side of base of proximal phalanx of thumb.

CAUTION During next step, locate and protect tendon of abductor pollicis longus on lateral side of thenar eminence.

CUT abductor pollicis brevis muscle from its attachment to trapezium bone.

REFLECT abductor pollicis brevis muscle superiorly to expose flexor pollicis brevis and opponens pollicis muscles.

IDENTIFY superficial head of **flexor pollicis brevis muscle**, and locate its common origin with abductor pollicis brevis muscle from trapezium bone and its insertion to base of proximal phalanx of thumb medial to insertion of abductor pollicis brevis muscle.

LOOK for motor branches of recurrent median nerve to thenar muscles.

CUT recurrent median nerve where it enters thenar eminence.

CUT superficial head of flexor pollicis brevis muscle from its attachment to trapezium bone.

REFLECT superficial head of flexor pollicis brevis muscle to expose tendon of flexor pollicis longus.

RETRACT tendon of flexor pollicis longus laterally to expose deep head of **flexor pollicis brevis muscle**, locating its origin from trapezoid bone and its insertion to base of proximal phalanx of thumb in common with its superficial head.

IDENTIFY opponens pollicis muscle, and locate its origin from trapezium bone and flexor retinaculum to its insertion to length of shaft of metacarpal bone 1.

REFLECT 9 tendons within carpal tunnel as far distally as possible, preserving median nerve by reflecting it laterally, to expose deep muscles of palm and deep palmar arch.

IDENTIFY adductor pollicis muscle. Note that this muscle has 2 heads of origin, oblique and transverse.

LOCATE origin of oblique head of adductor pollicis muscle from capitate bone and bases of metacarpal bones 2, 3.

LOCATE insertion of oblique head of adductor pollicis muscle to medial side of base of proximal phalanx of thumb.

LOCATE origin of transverse head of adductor pollicis muscle from length of metacarpal bone 3 and its insertion in common with its oblique head to medial side of base of proximal phalanx of thumb.

LOCATE branches of deep ulnar nerve supplying adductor pollicis muscle.

CUT transverse head of adductor pollicis muscle from its metacarpal attachment.

REFLECT adductor pollicis muscle toward thumb to expose palmar interosseus muscles.

LOCATE contribution from radial artery to **deep palmar arch** originating deep to oblique head of adductor pollicis muscle.

FOLLOW deep palmar arch to contribution from **deep palmar branch** of **ulnar artery** originating deep to flexor digiti minimi brevis muscle.

IDENTIFY passage of **princeps pollicis artery** in interosseous space 1 along metacarpal bone 1.

IDENTIFY passage of **radialis indicis artery** in interosseous space 1 along lateral side of index finger.

CUT origins of princeps pollicis, radialis indicis, and **palmar metacarpal arteries** from deep palmar arch.

NOTE that deep branch of ulnar nerve accompanies ulnar side of deep palmar arch.

REMOVE deep palmar arch.

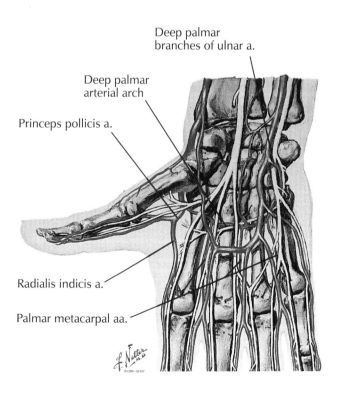

Deep palmar branches of ulnar a.

Deep palmar arterial arch

Princeps pollicis a.

Radialis indicis a.

Palmar metacarpal aa.

PLATE 439

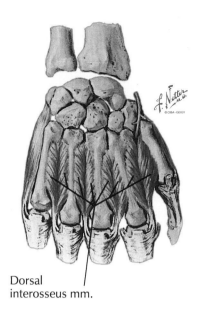

Dorsal
interosseus mm.

PLATE 438

IDENTIFY 1 of 3 **palmar interosseus muscles**, and locate its origin from metacarpal bone and its insertion to base of proximal phalanx and extensor expansion. Note unipennate form of palmar interosseus muscles.

BLUNT DISSECT deep to palmar interosseus muscles to separate them from 4 bipennate **dorsal interosseus muscles**.

DIRECT attention to dorsal surface of hand.

LOCATE origins of dorsal interosseus muscles from adjacent metacarpal bones and their insertions to extensor expansions and base of proximal phalanges.

DIRECT attention to palm of hand.

LOOK for branches of deep ulnar nerves to both palmar and dorsal interosseus muscles.

PLATE 438

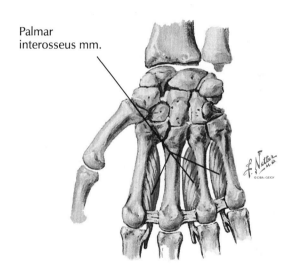

Palmar
interosseus mm.

JOINTS OF UPPER LIMB

Complete DISSECTIONS **5.1** Axillary Region, **5.2** Scapular Region, **5.3** Arm, **5.4** Posterior Forearm, **5.5** Superficial Anterior Forearm and Hand, and **5.6** Deep Anterior Forearm and Hand.

Read DISCUSSIONS **5.2** Bones, **5.3** Joints and Ligaments, and **5.4** Movements and Muscle Actions.

NOTE that shoulder, elbow, and wrist dissections are to be done unilaterally to preserve other limb for review.

TURN cadaver to either supine or prone position, as needed, to expose capsules of joints.

Shoulder

CLEAN capsule of **sternoclavicular joint** if DISSECTION **8.2** has <u>not</u> been completed.

OPEN sternoclavicular joint around entire circumference with scalpel if DISSECTION **8.2** has <u>not</u> been completed.

IDENTIFY articular disc between manubrium and clavicle and rib 1 if DISSECTION **8.2** has <u>not</u> been completed.

PALPATE acromion and **coracoid process** of **scapula** and **greater tubercle** of **humerus**.

CAUTION   During next step, preserve tendinous insertions of rotator cuff muscles and tendons of long heads of biceps and triceps brachii.

REMOVE all other muscles, arteries, veins, and nerves from shoulder with scalpel and scissors.

OPEN acromioclavicular joint with scalpel.

IDENTIFY inconstant **articular disc** (*not shown*), which separates joint cavity.

IDENTIFY coracoclavicular (trapezoid and **conoid) ligaments**.

SEVER coracoclavicular ligaments from inferior surface of clavicle with scalpel.

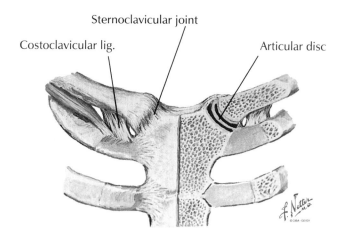

Costoclavicular lig. Sternoclavicular joint Articular disc

PLATE 395

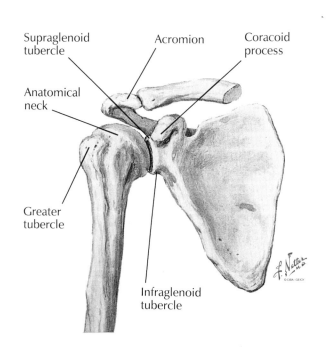

Supraglenoid tubercle Acromion Coracoid process

Anatomical neck

Greater tubercle

Infraglenoid tubercle

PLATE 396

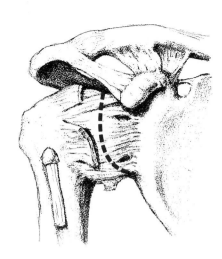

Figure 21

SEVER coracoacromial ligament with scissors or scalpel.

SEVER tendon of supraspinatus as it inserts to greater tubercle of humerus, and separate it from superior part of **glenohumeral capsule**.

SEPARATE tendons of infraspinatus and teres minor from posterior part of glenohumeral capsule.

SEVER tendon of subscapularis from lesser tubercle, and separate it from anterior part of glenohumeral capsule.

LOOK for **subscapular bursa** deep to subscapularis muscle.

INSPECT superior capsule to define **coracohumeral ligament**.

LOOK for communication between subscapular bursa and synovial cavity of shoulder joint located around middle glenohumeral ligament.

LOCATE transverse ligament of **humerus** attaching between greater and lesser tubercles over tendon of long head of biceps brachii and intertubercular groove.

LOOK for **intertubercular synovial sheath** extending inferior to transverse ligament of humerus.

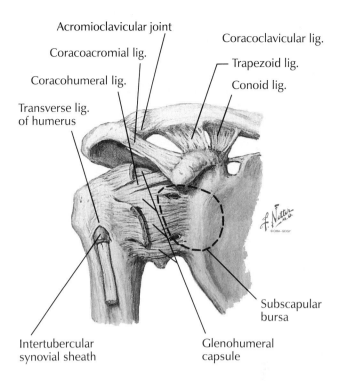

Acromioclavicular joint
Coracoacromial lig.
Coracohumeral lig.
Transverse lig. of humerus
Coracoclavicular lig.
Trapezoid lig.
Conoid lig.
Subscapular bursa
Intertubercular synovial sheath
Glenohumeral capsule

PLATE 398

INCISE entire circumference of glenohumeral capsule, beginning cut inferior to transverse ligament (**Figure 21**).

INSPECT anterior capsule to define **superior, middle**, and **inferior glenohumeral ligaments**.

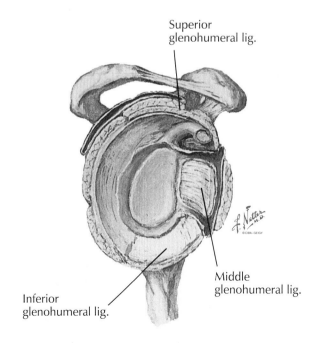

Superior glenohumeral lig.
Inferior glenohumeral lig.
Middle glenohumeral lig.

PLATE 398

NOTE that capsule is attached from **margin** of **glenoid fossa** to **anatomical neck** of **humerus**.

IDENTIFY **glenoid labrum**, **articular cartilage** of **head** of **humerus**, and **glenoid cavity**.

TRACE tendon of long head of biceps brachii to its origin from **supraglenoid tubercle**.

TRACE tendon of long head of triceps brachii to its origin from **infraglenoid tubercle**.

Elbow

PALPATE olecranon of **ulna** and **medial** and **lateral epicondyles** of **humerus**.

REMOVE muscles, arteries, veins, and nerves from elbow with scalpel and scissors.

CAUTION During next step, preserve ulnar and radial collateral ligaments.

CLEAN capsule of **elbow joint**.

IDENTIFY anterior part of **ulnar collateral ligament** between medial epicondyle of humerus and coronoid process of ulna.

IDENTIFY posterior part of **ulnar collateral ligament** between medial epicondyle of humerus and olecranon of ulna and oblique part between olecranon and coronoid process of ulna.

IDENTIFY **radial collateral ligament** between lateral epicondyle and neck of radius and as its contribution to annular ligament.

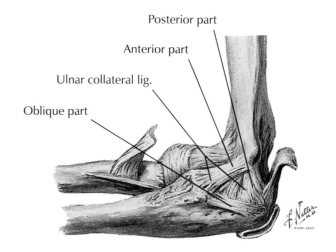

Posterior part
Anterior part
Ulnar collateral lig.
Oblique part

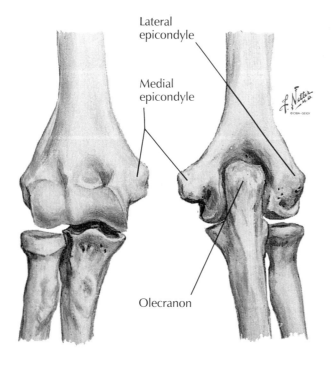

Lateral epicondyle
Medial epicondyle
Olecranon

PLATE 411

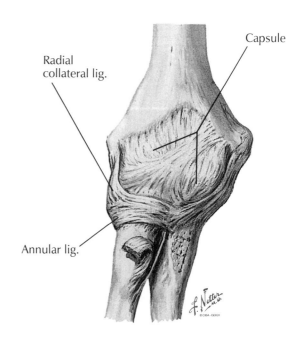

Capsule
Radial collateral lig.
Annular lig.

PLATE 412

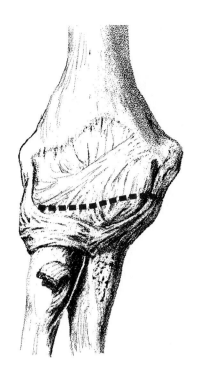

Figure 22

IDENTIFY annular ligament as it passes around head of radius, attaching to anterior and posterior margins of radial notch of ulna.

INCISE anterior capsule of elbow joint (**Figure 22**).

INSPECT articular cartilage on articular surfaces of distal humerus and proximal radius and ulna.

Wrist

PALPATE styloid processes of **radius** and **ulna**.

IDENTIFY individual carpal bones on skeleton.

IDENTIFY bifid tendon of flexor carpi radialis as it inserts to bases of metacarpal bones 2, 3.

IDENTIFY pisohamate and hamatometacarpal ligaments as continuations of tendon of flexor carpi ulnaris between pisiform bone and hook of hamate bone and base of metacarpal bone 5.

REMOVE all muscles, arteries, veins, and nerves from wrist and hand with scalpel and scissors.

CLEAN palmar and dorsal **capsule** of **wrist joint**.

DEFINE radiocarpal and **ulnocarpal ligaments**, naming individual components by attachments to carpal bones. Note that palmar ligaments are more substantial than dorsal ligaments.

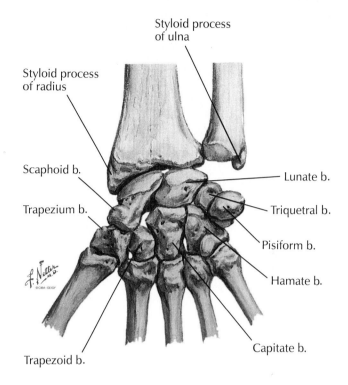

PLATE 426

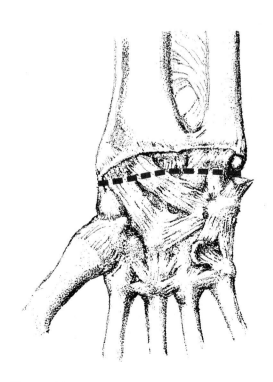

Figure 23

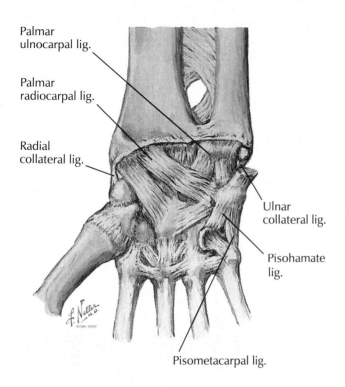

Palmar
ulnocarpal lig.

Palmar
radiocarpal lig.

Radial
collateral lig.

Ulnar
collateral lig.

Pisohamate
lig.

Pisometacarpal lig.

PLATE 428

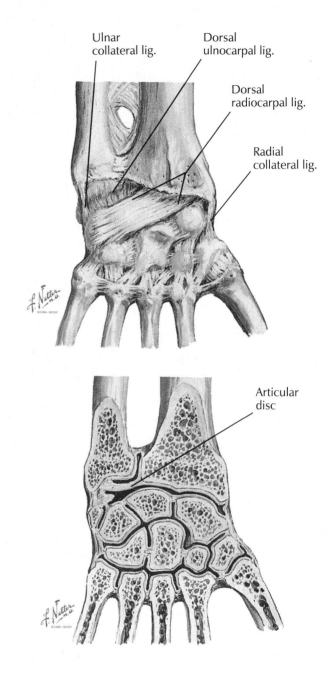

Ulnar
collateral lig.

Dorsal
ulnocarpal lig.

Dorsal
radiocarpal lig.

Radial
collateral lig.

Articular
disc

PLATE 429

IDENTIFY radial and **ulnar collateral ligaments** of wrist.

OPEN anterior surface of capsule of wrist joint (**Figure 23**). Hyperextend hand at wrist before making horizontal incision.

EXAMINE articular disc between distal ends of radius and ulna.

INSPECT articular cartilage on distal articular surfaces of radius, ulna, and carpal bones.

Section 6
LOWER LIMB

DISSECTION 6.1
GLUTEAL REGION

Complete DISSECTION **1.1** Superficial Back.

Read DISCUSSIONS **6.1** Surface Anatomy, **6.2** Bones, **6.6** Gluteal Region, **6.10** Sacral Plexus, and **6.11** Arteries.

TRANSECT cadaver through intervertebral disc level L2, 3 to facilitate turning lower limb in following dissections.

PLACE cadaver in prone position.

MARK location of cutaneous nerves and superficial veins on skin of posterior thigh with felt-tip marker.

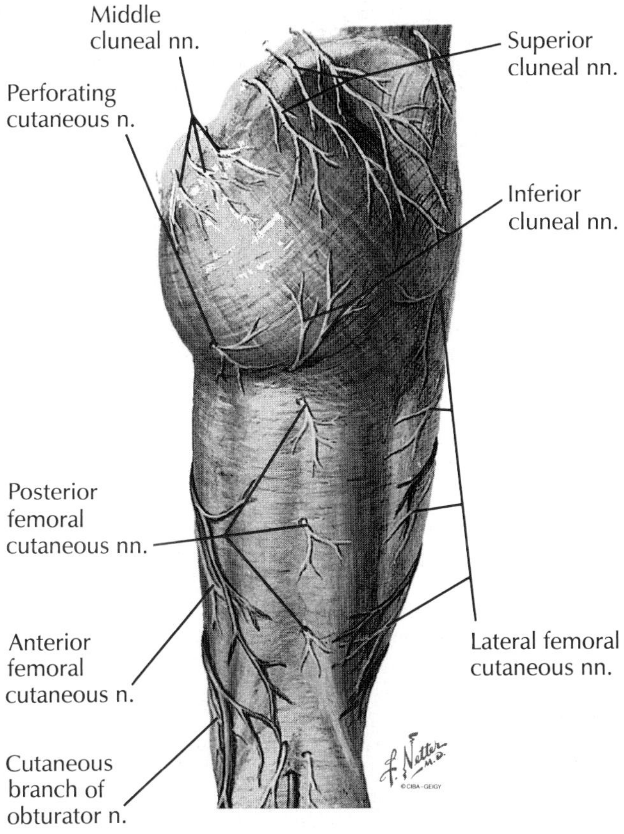

CAUTION During following steps, preserve cutaneous nerves on posterior thigh and iliotibial tract on lateral thigh.

INCISE skin of gluteal and posterior thigh regions (**Figure 24**). Note that distal incision is 1 hand-width inferior to tibial plateau (*not labeled*).

REMOVE skin and subcutaneous tissue from gluteal region and posterior surface of thigh. Fascia lata encloses thigh muscles as "support stocking" of deep fascia. Superficial tissue may be removed to this plane.

IDENTIFY lateral cutaneous branch of **iliohypogastric nerve**, which pierces deep fascia over lateral 1/3 of iliac crest.

Middle cluneal nn.

Superior cluneal nn.

Perforating cutaneous n.

Inferior cluneal nn.

Posterior femoral cutaneous nn.

Anterior femoral cutaneous n.

Lateral femoral cutaneous nn.

Cutaneous branch of obturator n.

PLATE 513

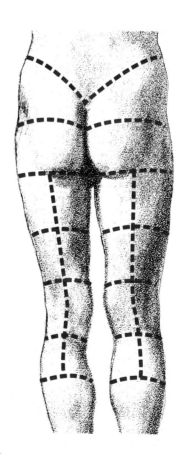

Figure 24

115

IDENTIFY superior cluneal nerves (dorsal primary rami of lumbar spinal levels 1–3), which pierce deep fascia over medial 2/3 of iliac crest. Note that these nerves may not have been preserved.

IDENTIFY middle cluneal nerves (dorsal primary rami of sacral spinal level 1–3), which pierce **gluteus maximus muscle** between posterior superior iliac spine and tip of coccyx.

IDENTIFY inferior cluneal nerves (branches of posterior femoral cutaneous nerves), which wind superiorly around inferior border of gluteus maximus muscle.

LOOK for representative branches of posterior femoral cutaneous nerve piercing fascia lata on posterior surface of thigh.

IDENTIFY gluteus maximus muscle.

DEFINE inferior and superior borders of gluteus maximus muscle by blunt dissection, and clean anterior and posterior borders of **iliotibial tract**.

LOCATE origin of iliotibial tract from anterior iliac crest and its insertion to Gerdy's tubercle on lateral condyle of tibia.

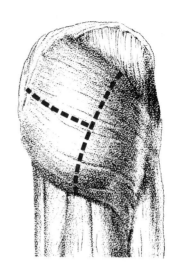

Figure 25

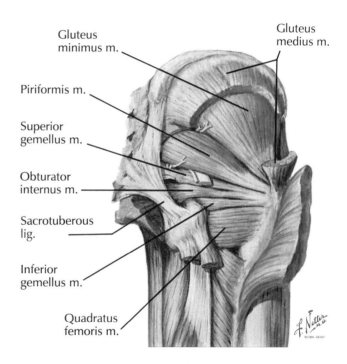

Gluteus minimus m.

Piriformis m.

Superior gemellus m.

Obturator internus m.

Sacrotuberous lig.

Inferior gemellus m.

Quadratus femoris m.

Gluteus medius m.

PLATE 465 detail

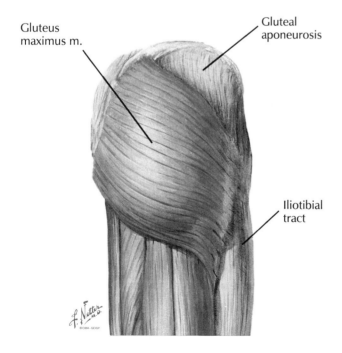

Gluteus maximus m.

Gluteal aponeurosis

Iliotibial tract

PLATE 465 detail

BLUNT DISSECT deep to gluteus maximus muscle, using fingers, to locate **inferior gluteal nerve** and **artery** and **superior gluteal artery**.

TRANSECT gluteus maximus muscle (**Figure 25**) with vertical incision lateral to gluteal nerves and arteries.

REFLECT lateral part of gluteus maximus muscle laterally to expose insertion of deeper fibers to gluteal tuberosity.

CAUTION During next step, preserve inferior gluteal nerve and artery and superior gluteal artery.

TRANSECT medial half of gluteus maximus muscle horizontally between superior and inferior gluteal vessels to lateral border of sacrotuberous ligament (**Figure 25**).

BLUNT DISSECT deep part of gluteus maximus muscle free from its origin from sacrotuberous ligament.

REFLECT 2 medial parts of gluteus maximus muscle medially and away from each other to expose underlying structures. Note that neurovascular elements may be cut to complete reflection.

REMOVE inferior gluteal vein and its tributaries.

CLEAN sacrotuberous ligament.

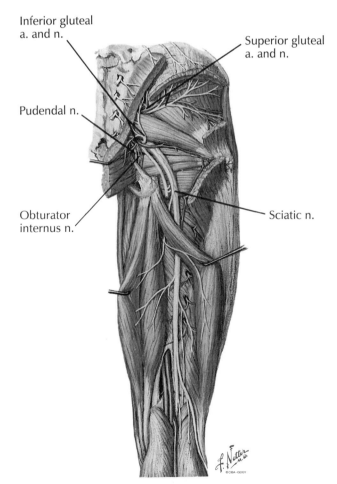

Inferior gluteal a. and n.

Superior gluteal a. and n.

Pudendal n.

Obturator internus n.

Sciatic n.

PLATE 472

IDENTIFY piriformis muscle by passage of inferior gluteal nerve and artery into greater sciatic foramen inferior to it and superior gluteal nerve and artery superior to it.

TRACE superior gluteal nerve deep to gluteus medius muscle.

REMOVE gluteal aponeurosis (fascia lata over part of gluteus medius muscle not covered by gluteus maximus muscle).

IDENTIFY gluteus medius muscle, and define its inferior border.

BLUNT DISSECT, with fingers, deep to inferior border of gluteus medius muscle to determine fascia plane between gluteus medius and gluteus minimus muscles and location of superior and inferior branches of superior gluteal nerve.

CAUTION During next step, protect origin of gluteus minimus muscle.

CUT gluteus medius muscle along its attachment to iliac crest and external wing of ilium.

REFLECT gluteus medius muscle toward its insertion to greater trochanter of femur.

LOCATE superior gluteal nerve on deep surface of gluteus medius muscle.

IDENTIFY gluteus minimus muscle located deep to gluteus medius muscle.

IDENTIFY sciatic nerve. Common peroneal nerve may <u>not</u> be enclosed with tibial nerve as complete sciatic nerve. In that case, common peroneal nerve pierces piriformis muscle. Note that sciatic nerve has no branches in gluteal region.

IDENTIFY posterior femoral cutaneous nerve passing inferior to piriformis muscle and medial to sciatic nerve.

CAUTION During following inspection of muscles, preserve neurovascular structures passing superficial to muscles.

CLEAN tendon of **obturator internus**. Note that tendon may be difficult to clean because **superior** and **inferior gemellus muscles** attach to it as they insert to greater trochanter of femur.

RETRACT sciatic nerve medially to aid following inspection.

DETERMINE origins of superior gemellus muscle from ischial spine and inferior gemellus muscle from ischial tuberosity.

CLEAN quadratus femoris muscle, and determine both its origin from ischial tuberosity and its insertion to intertrochanteric crest.

IDENTIFY nerve to **quadratus femoris** (*not shown*) located between sciatic and posterior femoral cutaneous nerves and exiting greater sciatic foramen to pass deep to superior gemellus muscle.

TRACE branches of nerve to quadratus femoris to its named muscle and to inferior gemellus muscle.

TRANSECT quadratus femoris muscle to expose tendon of **obturator externus** (*not shown*), which will be studied in DISSECTION **6.2**.

RETRACT sciatic nerve laterally to aid following inspection.

IDENTIFY obturator internus nerve located between posterior femoral cutaneous nerve and sacrotuberous ligament and above superior gemellus muscle.

TRACE branches of obturator internus nerve to its named muscle and to superior gemellus muscle.

IDENTIFY internal pudendal artery (*not shown*) medial to obturator internus nerve.

IDENTIFY pudendal nerve medial to internal pudendal artery.

NOTE that pudendal nerve and internal pudendal artery pass around posterior surface of ischial spine to enter lesser sciatic foramen.

DISSECTION 6.2
ANTERIOR AND MEDIAL THIGH

Complete DISSECTION **6.1** Gluteal Region.

Read DISCUSSIONS **4.18** Lumbar Plexus, **6.5** Fasciae, **6.7** Thigh, and **6.11** Arteries.

PLACE cadaver in supine position.

MARK location of cutaneous nerves and superficial veins on skin of anterior thigh with felt-tip marker.

CAUTION During following steps, preserve cutaneous nerves and great saphenous vein on anterior thigh.

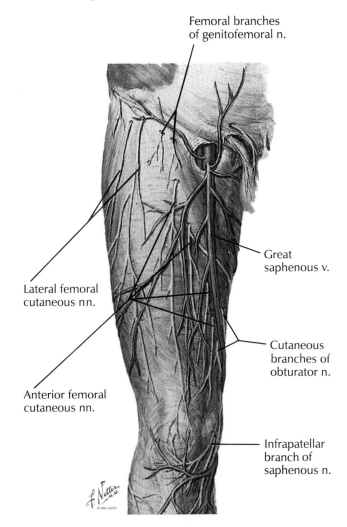

Femoral branches of genitofemoral n.

Lateral femoral cutaneous nn.

Anterior femoral cutaneous nn.

Great saphenous v.

Cutaneous branches of obturator n.

Infrapatellar branch of saphenous n.

PLATE 512 detail

INCISE skin of anterior thigh (**Figure 26**).

REMOVE skin and subcutaneous tissue from anterior surface of thigh. Fascia lata will enclose thigh muscles as "support stocking" of deep fascia. Superficial tissue may be removed to this plane.

IDENTIFY branches of **lateral femoral cutaneous nerve** as they pierce fascia lata inferior to lateral 1/3 of inguinal ligament.

IDENTIFY femoral branch of **genitofemoral nerve** (*not labeled*) as it pierces fascia lata near or emerges through **fossa ovalis (saphenous opening)**.

REIDENTIFY cutaneous branch of **ilioinguinal nerve** as it emerges through superficial inguinal ring. Note that this branch was originally identified in DISSECTION **2.4**.

IDENTIFY anterior femoral cutaneous nerves as they pierce fascia lata along course of great saphenous vein and below inguinal ligament on middle of anterior surface of thigh.

IDENTIFY cutaneous branch of **obturator nerve** as it pierces fascia lata 1 to 2 hand-widths inferior to pubic bone on medial surface of thigh.

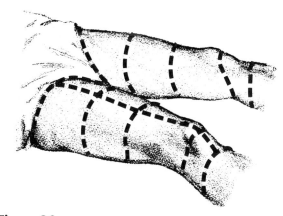

Figure 26

IDENTIFY infrapatellar branch of **saphenous nerve** as it pierces fascia lata medial to patella.

LOCATE great saphenous vein by blunt dissection posterior to medial knee.

TRACE great saphenous vein to where it enters **fossa ovalis** (**saphenous opening**).

IDENTIFY cribriform fascia in saphenous opening.

LOOK for **superficial epigastric**, **superficial circumflex iliac**, and **superficial external pudendal veins** as tributaries to great saphenous vein.

LOCATE superficial inguinal lymph nodes, but do not preserve them.

CAUTION During next step, preserve contents of femoral triangle.

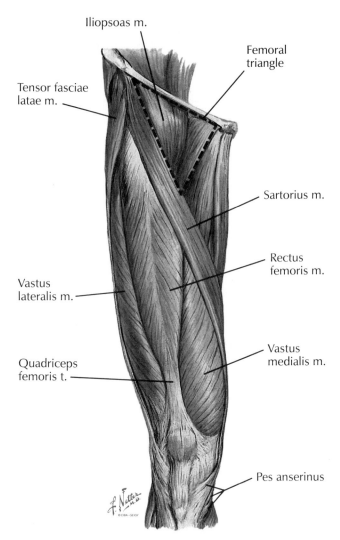

Iliopsoas m.

Femoral triangle

Tensor fasciae latae m.

Sartorius m.

Rectus femoris m.

Vastus lateralis m.

Quadriceps femoris t.

Vastus medialis m.

Pes anserinus

PLATE 462

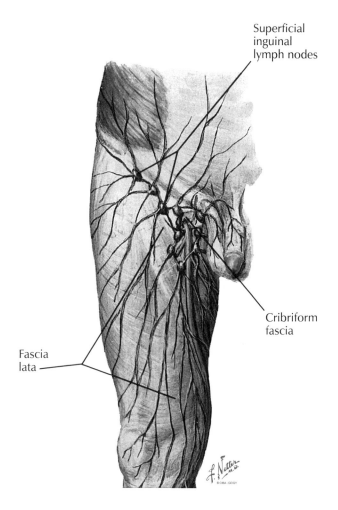

Superficial inguinal lymph nodes

Cribriform fascia

Fascia lata

PLATE 514 detail

REMOVE fascia lata from muscles of anterior and medial thigh.

IDENTIFY tensor fasciae latae muscle, its origin from anterior iliac crest and anterior superior iliac spine, and its insertion to iliotibial tract.

BLUNT DISSECT deep to tensor fasciae latae muscle to locate branch of **superior gluteal nerve** (*not shown*) to tensor fasciae latae muscle.

CUT along anterior and posterior borders of **iliotibial tract**, leaving gluteus maximus and tensor fasciae latae muscles attached to it.

PRESERVE attachments of iliotibial tract to anterior iliac crest and to Gerdy's tubercle on lateral condyle of tibia.

DEFINE boundaries of **femoral triangle** as inguinal ligament, sartorius muscle, and adductor longus muscle.

CAUTION During next step, preserve femoral sheath with femoral artery and vein enclosed and branches of femoral nerve.

CLEAN floor of femoral triangle.

IDENTIFY sartorius muscle, its origin from anterior superior iliac spine, and its insertion to medial proximal tibia by **pes anserinus**.

TRACE branches of **femoral nerve** to sartorius muscle.

BLUNT DISSECT deep to sartorius muscle to preserve fascial roof of adductor canal and structures within adductor canal.

TRANSECT sartorius muscle midway between its origin and insertion.

PLATE 470

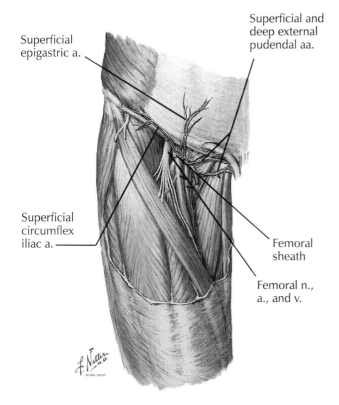

Superficial epigastric a.

Superficial and deep external pudendal aa.

Superficial circumflex iliac a.

Femoral sheath

Femoral n., a., and v.

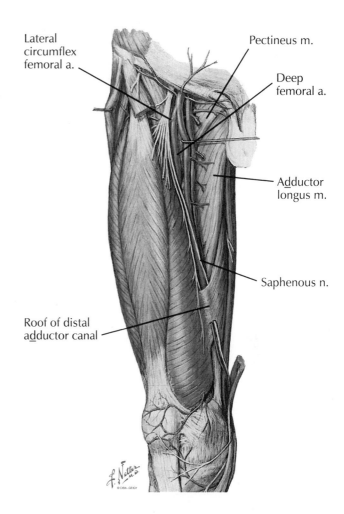

Lateral circumflex femoral a.

Pectineus m.

Deep femoral a.

Adductor longus m.

Saphenous n.

Roof of distal adductor canal

PLATE 470

REFLECT both cut ends of sartorius muscle away from anterior surface of thigh, cutting any vessels that enter sartorius muscle on its deep surface.

RETRACT tensor fasciae latae muscle laterally.

IDENTIFY rectus femoris muscle and its origin from anterior inferior iliac spine by its straight tendon and from rim of acetabulum by its reflected tendon.

RETRACT iliotibial tract laterally to clean **vastus lateralis muscle**.

LOCATE lateral intermuscular septum (*not shown*) extending from iliotibial tract posterior to vastus lateralis muscle.

IDENTIFY vastus medialis muscle, and separate rectus femoris muscle from it with fingers.

TRACE distal vastus lateralis and medialis muscles to where they join rectus femoris muscle to form tendon of **quadriceps femoris**.

TRACE branches of femoral nerve to deep surface of rectus femoris muscle.

TRANSECT belly of rectus femoris muscle halfway.

REFLECT both ends of rectus femoris muscle to expose **vastus intermedius muscle**.

RETRACT contents of femoral triangle medially or laterally to aid following muscle identifications.

PLATE 471

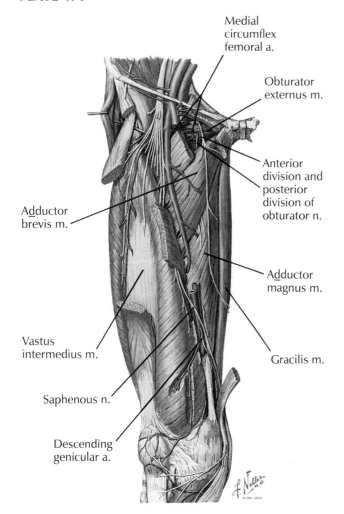

Medial circumflex femoral a.

Obturator externus m.

Anterior division and posterior division of obturator n.

Adductor brevis m.

Adductor magnus m.

Vastus intermedius m.

Gracilis m.

Saphenous n.

Descending genicular a.

LOCATE insertion of iliopsoas muscle to lesser trochanter. Note that origin of and nerves to psoas major and minor muscles were examined in DISSECTIONS **4.5** and **4.6**. Origin of iliacus muscle will be examined in DISSECTIONS **7.3** and **7.4**.

IDENTIFY pectineus muscle, and palpate its insertion to pectineal line of femur.

TRACE branch of femoral nerve to pectineus muscle.

CLEAN fat from **femoral canal** (*not labeled*) medial to **femoral vein**.

OPEN femoral sheath with vertical incision.

IDENTIFY femoral artery and vein.

LOCATE origins of **superficial** and **deep external pudendal**, **superficial epigastric**, and **superficial circumflex iliac arteries** as they branch from femoral artery.

LOCATE origin of **deep femoral artery** as it branches from lateral side of femoral artery.

LOCATE origin of **medial circumflex femoral artery** (*not shown*) from deep femoral artery, passing between **iliopsoas** and **pectineus muscles**.

LOCATE origin of **lateral circumflex femoral artery** from deep femoral artery passing superficial to tendon of iliopsoas.

TRACE femoral artery and vein and **saphenous nerve** as they descend in **adductor canal**.

CAUTION During next step, preserve contents of adductor hiatus.

CLEAN anterior surfaces of adductor longus and adductor magnus muscles.

LOCATE adductor hiatus in tendinous attachment of adductor magnus to linea aspera.

LOCATE descending genicular artery branching from femoral artery and dividing into **saphenous branch**, which accompanies saphenous nerve, and **articular branch**, which pierces vastus medialis muscle before serving medial side of knee. Note that fibers of vastus medialis muscle are to be dissected to trace articular artery.

DIRECT attention to muscles of medial thigh.

IDENTIFY gracilis muscle, and palpate its origin from inferior pubic ramus and its insertion by pes anserinus.

IDENTIFY adductor longus muscle.

TRACE deep femoral artery as it passes posterior to adductor longus muscle.

CAUTION   During next step, preserve anterior division of obturator nerve.

ELEVATE adductor longus and pectineus muscles, and blunt dissect posterior to them to expose **adductor brevis muscle**.

LOCATE branch of obturator nerve to adductor longus muscle on its deep surface.

LOCATE perforating branches of deep femoral artery piercing adductor muscles.

CUT pectineus muscle along pectineal line of pubic bone.

REFLECT pectineus muscle to expose **anterior division** of **obturator nerve** and adductor brevis muscle and **obturator externus muscle**.

LOCATE obturator nerve as it exits obturator canal. Note that anterior division passes anterior to adductor brevis muscle and posterior division passes deep to adductor brevis muscle.

TRACE branches of anterior obturator nerve to adductor brevis and gracilis muscles.

LOCATE posterior division of **obturator nerve** passing deep to adductor brevis muscle.

TRANSECT adductor longus muscle 1 hand-width from pubic bone.

REFLECT both cut ends to expose **adductor magnus muscle**.

TRANSECT adductor brevis muscle between its origin and insertion.

REFLECT adductor brevis muscle to expose proximal fibers of adductor magnus muscle.

LOCATE branches of posterior division of obturator nerve to proximal part of adductor magnus muscle.

CUT pubic attachment of adductor magnus muscle.

REFLECT superior fibers of adductor magnus muscle to expose obturator externus muscle.

LOOK for branch of posterior division of obturator nerve to obturator externus muscle.

NOTE that insertions of adductor muscles will be inspected in DISSECTION **6.3**.

POSTERIOR THIGH

Complete DISSECTION **6.1** Gluteal Region.

Read DISCUSSIONS **6.5** Fasciae, **6.7** Thigh, **6.10** Sacral Plexus, and **6.11** Arteries.

PLACE cadaver in prone position.

SEPARATE hamstring muscles with fingers.

PLATE 465

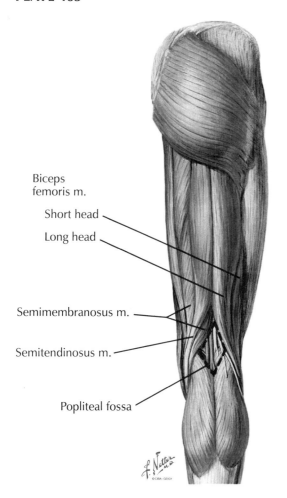

Biceps femoris m.

Short head

Long head

Semimembranosus m.

Semitendinosus m.

Popliteal fossa

IDENTIFY semitendinosus and **semimembranosus muscles** and **long head** of **biceps femoris muscle**.

LOCATE common tendon from ischial tuberosity for long head of biceps femoris muscle and semitendinosus muscle.

LOCATE short head of biceps femoris muscle arising from distal part of linea aspera and lateral supracondylar ridge.

TRACE tendon of biceps femoris to head of fibula.

TRACE tendon of semitendinosus to pes anserinus. Note tendon is round.

TRACE flat tendon of semimembranosus to medial condyle of tibia.

LOCATE nerves to semitendinosus and semimembranosus muscles and long head of biceps femoris muscle from tibial (medial) side of **sciatic nerve**. Note that these nerves usually branch quite high on sciatic nerve.

LOCATE nerve to short head of biceps femoris muscle from peroneal (lateral) side of sciatic nerve.

RETRACT hamstring muscles and sciatic nerve medially or laterally to expose insertion of **adductor magnus muscle** to linea aspera.

LOCATE nerve to ischiocondylar part of adductor magnus muscle from tibial (medial) side of sciatic nerve. Note that proximal fibers of adductor magnus muscle receive branches from posterior division of obturator nerve.

TRACE medial circumflex femoral artery between proximal adductor magnus and quadratus femoris muscles.

LOCATE perforating arteries as they pierce adductor magnus muscle.

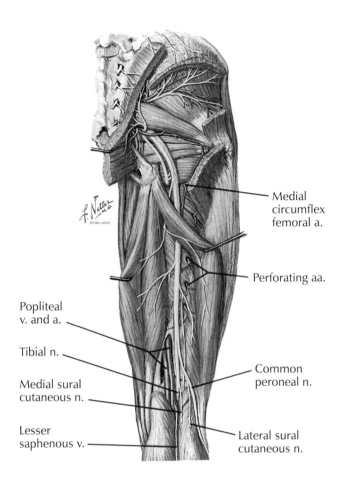

Medial circumflex femoral a.

Perforating aa.

Popliteal v. and a.

Tibial n.

Medial sural cutaneous n.

Lesser saphenous v.

Common peroneal n.

Lateral sural cutaneous n.

PLATE 472

DEFINE boundaries of **popliteal fossa** as semimembranosus and biceps femoris muscles and medial and lateral heads of gastrocnemius muscle.

TRACE lesser saphenous vein in company with **medial sural cutaneous nerve** into popliteal fossa to its drainage into **popliteal vein**.

REMOVE popliteal vein and its tributaries.

TRACE lateral sural cutaneous nerve in relation to popliteal border of biceps femoris muscle to **common peroneal nerve** in popliteal fossa.

LOOK for articular branches of common peroneal nerve in popliteal fossa.

TRACE tibial nerve as it passes popliteal fossa vertically.

SEPARATE 2 heads of **gastrocnemius muscle** to expose tibial nerve.

IDENTIFY popliteal artery.

IDENTIFY medial superior genicular artery, which branches from popliteal artery and passes superior to medial condyle of femur, anterior to semitendinosus and semimembranosus muscles.

PLATE 486

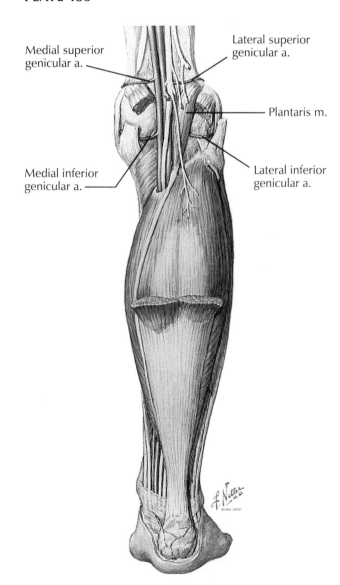

Medial superior genicular a.

Lateral superior genicular a.

Plantaris m.

Medial inferior genicular a.

Lateral inferior genicular a.

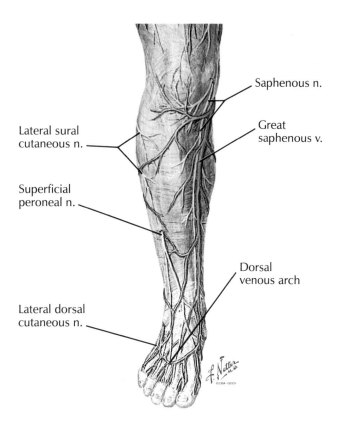

Lateral sural cutaneous n.

Saphenous n.

Great saphenous v.

Superficial peroneal n.

Dorsal venous arch

Lateral dorsal cutaneous n.

PLATE 512 detail

IDENTIFY lateral superior genicular artery, which branches from popliteal artery and passes superior to lateral condyle of femur, anterior to biceps femoris muscle.

IDENTIFY medial inferior genicular artery, which branches from popliteal artery and passes inferior to medial condyle of tibia, deep to medial head of gastrocnemius muscle.

IDENTIFY lateral inferior genicular artery, which branches from popliteal artery and winds around lateral condyle of tibia, superior to head of fibula, deep to lateral head of gastrocnemius muscle.

IDENTIFY **middle genicular artery** (*not shown*), which branches from popliteal artery and pierces oblique popliteal ligament (reflected tendon of semimembranosus) to enter knee.

CLEAN attachment of **plantaris muscle** to lateral condyle of femur.

CLEAN fat from popliteal fossa.

LOCATE branch of tibial nerve to plantaris muscle.

DIRECT attention to leg.

MARK location of cutaneous nerves and superficial veins on skin of leg with felt-tip marker.

CAUTION   During next step, preserve cutaneous nerves and great and lesser saphenous veins.

INCISE skin of leg and foot (**Figure 27**).

TURN lower limb as needed to complete incisions.

CAUTION   During skinning, preserve dorsal venous arch and origin of lesser saphenous vein from lateral side of arch.

REMOVE skin and subcutaneous tissue from entire circumference of leg and from dorsal surface of foot. Leave skin on toes.

PLATE 513 detail

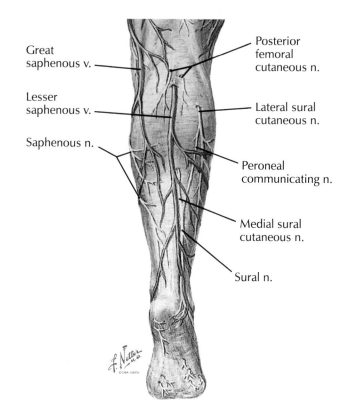

Great saphenous v.

Lesser saphenous v.

Saphenous n.

Posterior femoral cutaneous n.

Lateral sural cutaneous n.

Peroneal communicating n.

Medial sural cutaneous n.

Sural n.

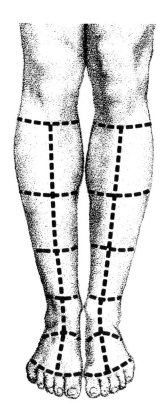

Figure 27

PLACE cadaver in prone position.

TRACE lesser saphenous vein as it passes posterior to lateral malleolus and on lateral surface of leg to enter popliteal fossa.

LOOK for cutaneous nerves of posterior leg.

IDENTIFY **medial** and **lateral sural cutaneous nerves** as they emerge near or from popliteal fossa.

IDENTIFY **peroneal communicating nerve**, which is branch of lateral sural cutaneous nerve that connects to medial sural cutaneous nerve.

IDENTIFY **sural nerve**, which is formed by union of peroneal communicating and medial sural cutaneous nerves and extends posterior to lateral malleolus.

IDENTIFY **lateral dorsal cutaneous nerve** (name of sural nerve changes as it serves lateral surface of foot) as it passes from lateral malleolus to lateral surface of little toe.

TURN cadaver to supine position.

LOOK for cutaneous nerves of anterior leg and dorsal surface of foot.

IDENTIFY **saphenous nerve**, which pierces crural fascia inferior to medial surface of knee. It accompanies great saphenous vein.

IDENTIFY cutaneous branches of **superficial peroneal nerve** as they pierce anterior lateral crural fascia halfway between knee and ankle. Note medial and intermediate dorsal branches.

DISSECTION 6.4
ANTERIOR LEG

Complete DISSECTIONS **6.2** Anterior and Medial Thigh and **6.3** Posterior Thigh.

Read DISCUSSIONS **6.8** Leg, **6.10** Sacral Plexus, and **6.11** Arteries.

PLACE cadaver in supine position.

INCISE skin of toes (**Figure 28**).

REMOVE skin, subcutaneous tissue, and superficial veins of toes.

CLEAN dorsal surface of foot, and remove dorsal venous arch.

DEFINE boundaries of **superior extensor retinaculum** between distal fibula and tibia just superior to malleoli.

Figure 28

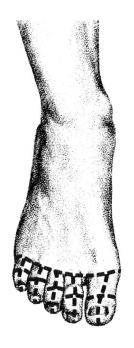

DEFINE boundaries of **inferior extensor retinaculum** and its division into superior band, which attaches to medial malleolus, and inferior band, which extends around medial side of foot to attach to plantar aponeurosis.

DEFINE boundaries of **superior** and **inferior peroneal retinacula** between lateral malleolus and calcaneus.

NOTE that muscles of leg are studied and dissected better by considering contents of lateral, anterior, and posterior compartments separately. Posterior compartment will be examined in DISSECTION **6.5**.

Lateral Compartment

TURN lower limb as needed to complete dissection.

IDENTIFY peroneus longus muscle on lateral side of leg, and locate its origin from proximal 2/3 of fibula.

TRACE tendon of peroneus longus to superior peroneal retinaculum.

RETRACT peroneus longus muscle laterally to expose **peroneus brevis muscle** and its origin from distal 2/3 of fibula.

NOTE that tendon of peroneus brevis passes anterior to tendon of peroneus longus under superior and inferior peroneal retinacula.

CUT superior and inferior peroneal retinacula, and free tendons of peroneus longus and brevis.

TRACE peroneus brevis muscle to its insertion on base of metatarsal bone 5. Note that insertion of peroneus longus muscle will be examined in DISSECTION **6.6**.

LOCATE common peroneal nerve as it exits popliteal fossa medial to tendon of biceps femoris.

TRACE common peroneal nerve to posterior border of peroneus longus muscle where it passes deep to muscle.

BLUNT DISSECT between proximal peroneus longus and brevis muscles to determine division of common peroneal nerve into **superficial** and **deep peroneal nerves**.

TRANSECT peroneus longus muscle just proximal to division of common peroneal nerve.

LOOK for **recurrent articular branch** to **knee** from common peroneal nerve.

TRACE superficial peroneal nerve between peroneus longus and brevis muscles. Note its terminal cutaneous branches as well as its muscular branches to both peroneus longus and brevis muscles.

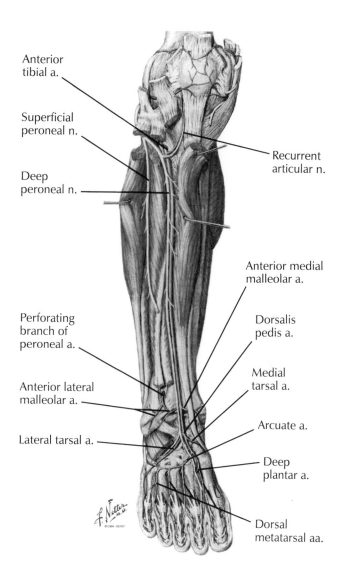

Anterior tibial a.

Superficial peroneal n.

Deep peroneal n.

Recurrent articular n.

Anterior medial malleolar a.

Perforating branch of peroneal a.

Dorsalis pedis a.

Medial tarsal a.

Anterior lateral malleolar a.

Arcuate a.

Lateral tarsal a.

Deep plantar a.

Dorsal metatarsal aa.

PLATE 489

TRACE deep peroneal nerve to its entry through proximal extensor digitorum longus muscle. Note that it pierces **anterior intermuscular septum** (*not shown*) to reach extensor digitorum longus muscle.

Anterior Compartment

SEPARATE extensor digitorum longus and **tibialis anterior muscles** to superior extensor retinaculum.

CUT superior and inferior extensor retinacula vertically with scissors to free tendons.

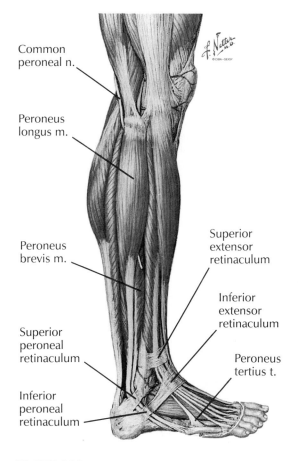

Common peroneal n.

Peroneus longus m.

Peroneus brevis m.

Superior peroneal retinaculum

Inferior peroneal retinaculum

Superior extensor retinaculum

Inferior extensor retinaculum

Peroneus tertius t.

PLATE 490

129

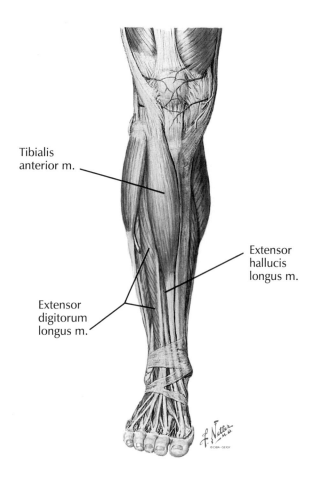

Tibialis anterior m.

Extensor hallucis longus m.

Extensor digitorum longus m.

PLATE 488

TRACE tendons of extensor digitorum longus to their insertions to 2nd through little toes. Note that central band of **extensor expansion** attaches to base of middle phalanx, and collateral bands attach to base of distal phalanx.

IDENTIFY peroneus tertius muscle, and follow its tendon to base of metatarsal bone 5.

TRACE tendon of tibialis anterior to its insertion to medial cuneiform bone and base of metatarsal bone 1. Note that tendon of tibialis anterior passes through superior band of inferior extensor retinaculum, not deep to it.

RETRACT extensor digitorum longus muscle laterally and tibialis anterior muscle medially to expose **extensor hallucis longus muscle**.

TRACE tendon of extensor hallucis longus to its insertion to distal phalanx of big toe.

IDENTIFY extensor digitorum brevis muscle on dorsal surface of foot deep to tendons of extensor digitorum longus and peroneus tertius.

TRACE tendons of extensor digitorum brevis to their insertions to lateral side of tendons of extensor digitorum longus to big through 4th toes. Note that tendon of extensor digitorum brevis to big toe may attach directly to proximal phalanx and is then called **extensor hallucis brevis muscle**.

CAUTION During next step, preserve anterior tibial artery and deep peroneal nerve.

REFLECT tibialis anterior muscle medially and extensor digitorum longus muscle laterally, and clean space between them.

TRACE deep peroneal nerve from where it pierces proximal extensor digitorum longus muscle to where it crosses ankle.

PLATE 498

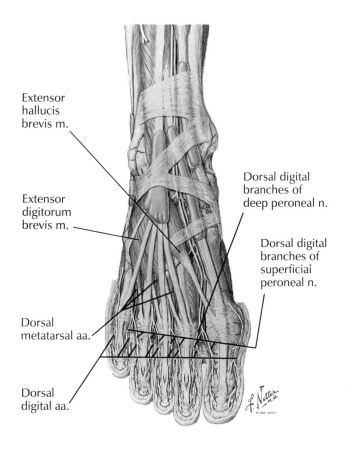

Extensor hallucis brevis m.

Extensor digitorum brevis m.

Dorsal metatarsal aa.

Dorsal digital aa.

Dorsal digital branches of deep peroneal n.

Dorsal digital branches of superficial peroneal n.

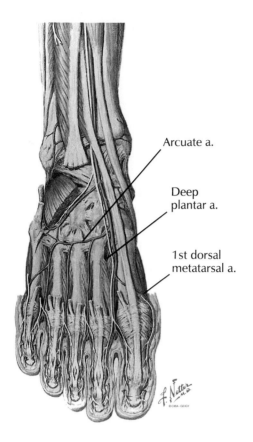

Arcuate a.

Deep
plantar a.

1st dorsal
metatarsal a.

PLATE 499

LOOK for branches of deep peroneal nerve to muscles of anterior compartment.

TRACE lateral branch of deep peroneal nerve deep to extensor digitorum brevis muscle.

TRACE medial branch of deep peroneal nerve to its cutaneous termination as **dorsal digital nerves** to cleft between big and 2nd toes.

LOCATE anterior tibial artery proximally in leg between extensor digitorum longus and tibialis anterior muscles and distally between extensor hallucis longus and tibialis anterior muscles. Note that anterior tibial artery becomes superficial at level of ankle between tendons of extensor hallucis longus and extensor digitorum longus.

LOCATE origin of **anterior tibial recurrent artery** from proximal anterior tibial artery, and follow its passage superiorly through proximal tibialis anterior muscle.

LOOK for **anterior lateral malleolar arteries** proximal to ankle, passing deep to tendons of extensor digitorum longus and peroneus tertius.

LOOK for **anterior medial malleolar arteries** proximal to ankle, passing deep to tendons of extensor hallucis longus and tibialis anterior.

LOOK for **perforating branch** of **peroneal artery** piercing interosseous membrane 3 finger-widths above lateral malleolus. Reflect extensor digitorum longus muscle laterally to facilitate inspection.

TRACE dorsalis pedis artery from its origin from anterior tibial artery to its division into deep plantar artery and 1st dorsal metatarsal artery.

CAUTION During next step, preserve branches of dorsalis pedis artery.

BLUNT DISSECT deep to extensor digitorum brevis muscle.

TRANSECT belly of extensor digitorum brevis muscle, and reflect cut ends.

RETRACT tendons of extensor digitorum longus laterally.

LOCATE origin of **lateral tarsal branches** from dorsalis pedis artery, and follow them as they pass laterally deep to extensor digitorum brevis muscle. Note that lateral tarsal artery accompanies lateral branch of deep peroneal nerve.

LOCATE origin of **medial tarsal branches**, which pass medially from dorsalis pedis artery over tarsal bones.

LOCATE arcuate artery, which passes laterally over bases of metatarsal bones.

LOCATE dorsal metatarsal arteries, which arise from arcuate artery to serve interosseous spaces 2–4. Note that **2 dorsal digital arteries** arise from each dorsal metatarsal artery.

LOCATE deep plantar artery as it passes deep through interosseous space 1.

LOCATE 1st dorsal metatarsal artery passing to medial side of big toe.

DISSECTION 6.5
POSTERIOR LEG

Complete DISSECTIONS **6.2** Anterior and Medial Thigh and **6.3** Posterior Thigh.

Read DISSECTIONS **6.8** Leg, **6.10** Sacral Plexus, and **6.11** Arteries.

PLACE cadaver in prone position.

NOTE that muscles of posterior leg are studied and dissected better by considering contents of superficial and deep posterior compartments separately.

Superficial Posterior Compartment

REMOVE crural fascia (*not shown*) of posterior leg, including superficial nerves and veins.

IDENTIFY gastrocnemius muscle and its insertion to tuberosity of calcaneus by calcaneal tendon.

BLUNT DISSECT deep to gastrocnemius muscle to separate tendon of **plantaris** from gastrocnemius muscle.

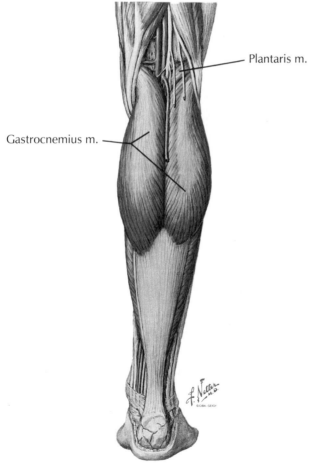

Plantaris m.

Gastrocnemius m.

PLATE 485

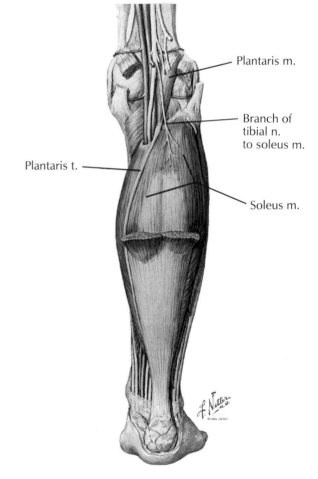

Plantaris m.

Branch of tibial n. to soleus m.

Plantaris t.

Soleus m.

PLATE 486

CAUTION During next step, preserve belly of plantaris muscle.

TRANSECT medial and lateral heads of gastrocnemius muscle 1 finger-width distal to their origins from respective medial and lateral femoral condyles.

LOCATE branches of tibial nerve to gastrocnemius muscle.

LOCATE branches of popliteal artery to gastrocnemius muscle.

CUT nerve and arterial branches to gastrocnemius muscle, leaving segment of vessel and nerve for future reference.

REFLECT gastrocnemius muscle toward calcaneal tendon.

REIDENTIFY plantaris muscle and its origin from lateral supracondylar ridge of femur.

TRANSECT belly of plantaris muscle.

REFLECT inferior part of plantaris muscle and its tendon toward calcaneal tendon.

IDENTIFY soleus muscle and its origin from soleal line of tibia, upper fibula, and fibrous arch between bones.

LOCATE branches of tibial nerve to soleus muscle.

BLUNT DISSECT deep to soleus muscle to free tibial nerve and posterior tibial artery.

CUT soleus muscle free, first from its tibial origin and then from its fibular origin.

REFLECT soleus muscle toward calcaneal tendon, cutting nerves and arteries on its deep surface to facilitate dissection.

Deep Posterior Compartment

CAUTION During next step, preserve tibial nerve and popliteal artery.

IDENTIFY popliteus muscle in inferior part of popliteal fossa. Note that popliteus muscle exits posterior capsule of knee inferior to **arcuate ligament** (*not labeled*).

TRACE branch of tibial nerve to popliteus muscle as nerve winds around inferior border of muscle.

TRACE popliteal artery to where it branches into **anterior** and **posterior tibial arteries**.

LOOK for origin of **posterior tibial recurrent branch** of anterior tibial artery. It ascends deep to popliteus muscle.

CLEAN fat from space anterior to calcaneal tendon.

PLATE 487

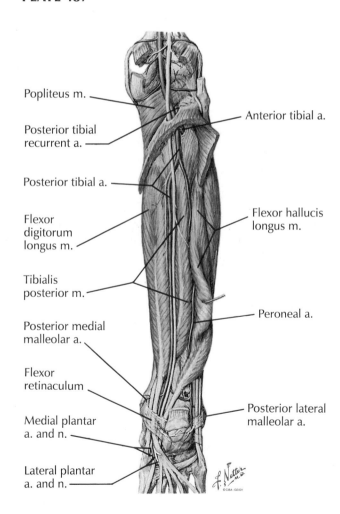

Popliteus m.

Posterior tibial recurrent a.

Posterior tibial a.

Flexor digitorum longus m.

Tibialis posterior m.

Posterior medial malleolar a.

Flexor retinaculum

Medial plantar a. and n.

Lateral plantar a. and n.

Anterior tibial a.

Flexor hallucis longus m.

Peroneal a.

Posterior lateral malleolar a.

J. Netter

133

DEFINE boundaries of **flexor retinaculum** from medial malleolus to medial surface of calcaneus.

IDENTIFY flexor hallucis longus muscle and its origin from lower 2/3 of fibula.

IDENTIFY flexor digitorum longus muscle and its origin from medial tibia.

TRACE tendons of these 2 muscles deep to flexor retinaculum.

TRACE posterior tibial artery and tibial nerve between tendons of flexor hallucis longus and flexor digitorum longus. Note branches to both these muscles from artery.

LOCATE origin of **peroneal artery** from posterior tibial artery 2 finger-widths below division of popliteal artery into anterior and posterior tibial arteries.

RETRACT belly of flexor hallucis longus muscle laterally and belly of flexor digitorum longus muscle medially with fingers.

IDENTIFY tibialis posterior muscle and its origin from tibia, fibula, and interosseous membrane.

LOCATE branches of posterior tibial artery and tibial nerve to tibialis posterior muscle.

TRACE tendon of tibialis posterior deep to flexor retinaculum where it is located anterior to tendon of flexor digitorum longus.

TRACE peroneal artery between flexor hallucis longus and tibialis posterior muscles. Note branches to both these muscles from artery.

LOCATE origin of **posterior lateral malleolar branch** from peroneal artery.

LOCATE origins of **medial calcaneal** and **posterior medial malleolar branches** from posterior tibial artery.

CUT flexor retinaculum to expose structures that pass deep to it. Clean this area by removing segments of retinaculum that wrap around each tendon.

LOCATE medial and **lateral plantar nerves** and arteries as they originate deep to flexor retinaculum. These nerves and arteries will be examined in DISSECTION **6.6**.

FOOT

Complete DISSECTIONS **6.4** Anterior Leg and **6.5** Posterior Leg.

Read DISCUSSIONS **6.9** Foot, **6.10** Sacral Plexus, and **6.11** Arteries.

PLACE cadaver in either prone or supine position. Elevate foot to facilitate dissection.

REMOVE skin and subcutaneous tissue from plantar surface of foot.

REMOVE respective medial and lateral deep plantar fasciae from muscles to big and little toes.

CLEAN plantar aponeurosis from calcaneus to digital bands attaching to **fibrous sheaths** of toes.

CAUTION   During next step, preserve medial plantar nerve and superficial branch of lateral plantar nerve.

BLUNT DISSECT deep to plantar aponeurosis with closed scissors to free aponeurosis for removal.

CUT digital bands as close to toes as possible without damaging structures near base of toes.

REFLECT plantar aponeurosis toward calcaneus until attachment to its deep surface of flexor digitorum brevis muscle is encountered.

TRANSECT plantar aponeurosis at this point, and discard it.

NOTE that plantar muscles of foot are studied and dissected better by considering them in layers.

1st Layer

IDENTIFY abductor hallucis muscle and its origin from medial side of calcaneus.

TRACE tendon of abductor hallucis to its insertion to base of proximal phalanx of big toe.

IDENTIFY abductor digiti minimi muscle and its origin from inferior lateral side of calcaneus.

TRACE tendon of abductor digiti minimi to its insertion to base of proximal phalanx of little toe.

IDENTIFY flexor digitorum brevis muscle and its origin from deep surface of plantar aponeurosis and middle portion of calcaneus.

PLATE 500

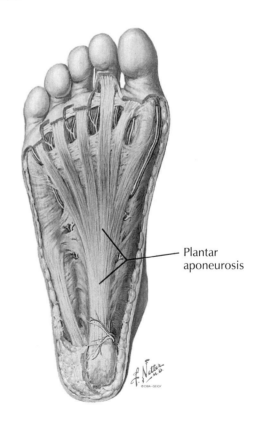

Plantar aponeurosis

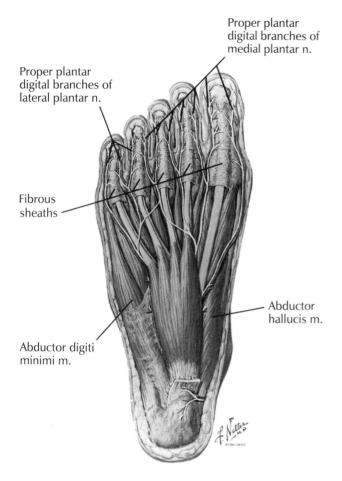

Proper plantar
digital branches of
medial plantar n.

Proper plantar
digital branches of
lateral plantar n.

Fibrous
sheaths

Abductor digiti
minimi m.

Abductor
hallucis m.

PLATE 501

IDENTIFY superficial branch of **lateral plantar nerve** as it surfaces on lateral side of flexor digitorum brevis muscle.

TRACE superficial branch of lateral plantar nerve to its division into proper plantar digital branch to little toe and 1 common plantar digital nerve, which divides into 2 proper plantar digital nerves for cleft between 4th and little toes.

CAUTION   During next step, preserve structures deep to abductor hallucis and flexor digitorum brevis muscles.

BLUNT DISSECT deep to abductor hallucis brevis and flexor digitorum brevis muscles with closed scissors to establish plane for transection of muscles.

TRANSECT abductor hallucis muscle as close to calcaneal attachments as possible.

PLATE 502

Fibrous
sheaths

Lumbrical
mm.

Flexor
hallucis
brevis m.

Flexor
hallucis
longus t.

Flexor
digitorum
longus t.

Medial plantar
a. and n.

Superficial
branch
of lateral
plantar n.

TRACE 4 tendons of flexor digitorum brevis to proximal border of fibrous sheaths for 2nd through little toes. Insertions of these tendons will be examined during dissection of 2nd plantar layer.

IDENTIFY medial and **lateral plantar nerves** on medial side of foot before their passage deep to abductor hallucis muscle.

TRACE medial plantar nerve from between abductor hallucis and flexor digitorum brevis muscles to its division into proper plantar digital branch to big toe and 3 **common plantar digital nerves**.

LOOK for only 2 of **proper plantar digital nerves** that arise from these common plantar digital nerves.

TRANSECT flexor digitorum brevis muscle as close to calcaneal attachments as possible.

LOCATE branches to abductor digiti minimi muscle from superficial lateral plantar nerve.

REFLECT abductor hallucis and flexor digitorum brevis muscles toward toes. Note following 3 steps.

LOCATE branches of medial plantar nerve to abductor hallucis and flexor digitorum brevis muscles.

IDENTIFY branches of **medial plantar artery** that accompany medial plantar nerve branches.

CUT medial plantar nerve and arterial branches to continue reflection of tendons of abductor hallucis and flexor digitorum longus.

2nd Layer

LOCATE muscular branches from medial plantar nerve to flexor hallucis brevis of 3rd layer, and **lumbrical muscle 1** (most medial) of 2nd layer.

IDENTIFY lateral plantar nerve and **artery** as they travel laterally across foot between quadratus plantae muscle of 2nd layer and reflected flexor digitorum brevis muscle of 1st layer.

TRACE tendon of **flexor digitorum longus** to its division into 4 tendons, which enter digital fibrous sheaths of 2nd through little toes. Note that these tendons pass deep to tendons of flexor digitorum brevis.

IDENTIFY quadratus plantae muscle, its origin from calcaneus, and its insertion to tendons of flexor digitorum longus.

LOCATE muscular branches from lateral plantar nerve supplying quadratus plantae muscle.

IDENTIFY 4 lumbrical muscles and origins of unipennate lumbrical muscle 1 and bipennate lumbrical muscles 2–4 originating from adjacent tendons of flexor digitorum longus.

IDENTIFY insertions of lumbrical muscles to extensor expansions of 2nd through little toes.

INCISE fibrous sheaths of 2nd through little toes lengthwise, protecting tendons of flexor digitorum longus and brevis.

LIFT tendons of flexor digitorum longus and brevis out of fibrous sheaths.

LOCATE tendons of flexor digitorum brevis as they insert to bases of middle phalanges and tendons of flexor digitorum longus to bases of distal phalanges.

TRACE tendon of **flexor hallucis longus** as it crosses deep to tendon of flexor digitorum longus.

INCISE fibrous sheath of big toe lengthwise, protecting tendon of flexor hallucis longus.

TRACE tendon of flexor hallucis longus to attachment to distal phalanx of big toe.

LOCATE division of lateral plantar nerve into superficial and deep branches.

LOCATE branches from **superficial branch** of **lateral plantar nerve** to flexor digiti minimi brevis and interosseus muscles of interosseous space 4.

NOTE that branches of lateral plantar artery accompany branches of lateral plantar nerve.

CUT attachments of quadratus plantae muscle to calcaneus.

CUT tendon of flexor digitorum longus before it crosses inferior to tendon of flexor hallucis longus.

REFLECT quadratus plantae muscle and tendons of flexor digitorum longus toward toes.

LOOK for branches to 3 lateral lumbrical muscles from deep branch of lateral plantar nerve.

CUT nerve branches from lateral and medial plantar nerves to complete reflection of quadratus plantae muscle and tendons of flexor digitorum longus.

NOTE that 3rd and 4th layers may be dissected on opposite foot if preservation of deep arterial plantar arch and deep branches of lateral plantar nerve is difficult.

PLATE 503

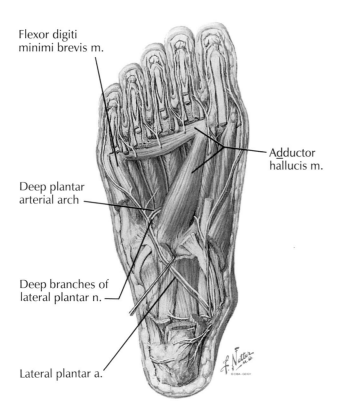

Flexor digiti minimi brevis m.

Adductor hallucis m.

Deep plantar arterial arch

Deep branches of lateral plantar n.

Lateral plantar a.

3rd Layer

IDENTIFY 2 heads of **flexor hallucis brevis muscle**, 1 of which lies on each side of tendon of flexor hallucis longus.

IDENTIFY 2 heads of **adductor hallucis muscle**. Note that both heads insert with lateral head of flexor hallucis brevis muscle to base of proximal phalanx of big toe.

IDENTIFY **flexor digiti minimi brevis muscle** located medial to abductor digiti minimi muscle.

DETACH flexor hallucis brevis muscle from its origin on lateral cuneiform bone and cuboid bone.

DETACH oblique head of adductor hallucis muscle from its origin on bases of metatarsal bones 2–4.

REFLECT medial head of flexor hallucis brevis muscle and oblique head of adductor hallucis muscle toward big toe.

TRACE lateral plantar artery down to origin of **deep plantar arch**. Use passage of lateral plantar artery as guide for cleaning away remnants of reflected muscles.

TRACE deep plantar arch to its anastomosis with **deep plantar artery** from dorsalis pedis artery. Note that deep plantar artery from dorsalis pedis artery pierces interosseous space 1.

LOCATE 4 **plantar metatarsal arteries**, which arise from deep plantar arch. They pass deep to transverse head of adductor hallucis muscle.

LOOK for branches of **deep branch** of **lateral plantar nerve** to adductor hallucis muscle.

DETACH transverse head of adductor hallucis muscle from capsule of metatarsophalangeal joints 3–5.

REFLECT transverse head of adductor hallucis muscle toward big toe.

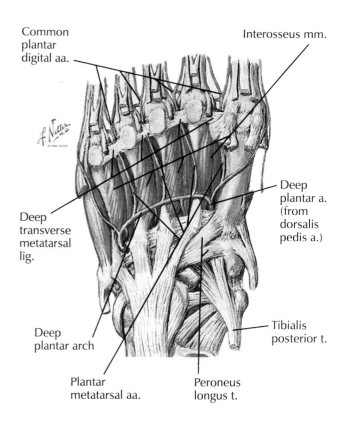

Common plantar digital aa.

Interosseus mm.

Deep transverse metatarsal lig.

Deep plantar a. (from dorsalis pedis a.)

Deep plantar arch

Plantar metatarsal aa.

Peroneus longus t.

Tibialis posterior t.

PLATE 504

LOCATE common plantar digital arteries, which arise from plantar metatarsal arteries deep to transverse head of adductor hallucis muscle.

4th Layer

CAUTION   During next steps, preserve tendons of previously reflected muscles.

CUT deep transverse metatarsal ligaments to facilitate manipulation of metatarsal bones.

IDENTIFY 3 plantar interosseus muscles in interosseous spaces 2–4. Note that they are unipennate.

IDENTIFY 4 dorsal interosseus muscles in interosseous spaces 1–4. Note that they are bipennate.

LOCATE branches of deep branch of lateral plantar nerve supplying interosseus muscles.

TRACE tendon of **tibialis posterior** to its insertion to tuberosity of navicular bone and its spreading attachments intermediate and lateral to cuneiform bones, cuboid bone, and base of metatarsal bone 4.

TRACE tendon of **peroneus longus** across plantar surface of foot to its insertion to medial cuneiform bone and base of metatarsal bone 1. Transect abductor digiti minimi muscle to observe tendon of peroneus longus deep to it. Continue following tendon by removing fascia that surrounds it to its insertion to medial side of foot. Note that tendon of peroneus longus passes deep to long plantar ligament.

DISSECTION 6.7

JOINTS OF LOWER LIMB

Complete DISSECTIONS **6.1** Gluteal Region, **6.2** Anterior and Medial Thigh, **6.3** Posterior Thigh, **6.4** Anterior Leg, **6.5** Posterior Leg, and **6.6** Foot.

Read DISCUSSIONS **6.2** Bones, **6.3** Joints and Ligaments, and **6.4** Movements and Muscle Actions.

NOTE that hip dissection is to be bilateral, in preparation for DISSECTIONS **7.1** and **7.2**. Knee and ankle dissections are to be done unilaterally to preserve other limb for review.

Hip Joint

PLACE cadaver in either supine or prone position, as needed, to expose capsules of joints.

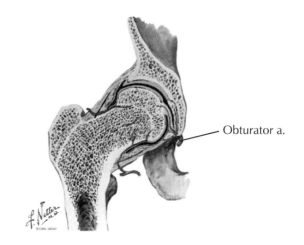

PLATE 474

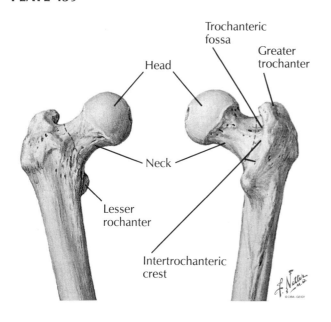

PLATE 459

PALPATE following bony landmarks cited in directions before removing indicated muscles, nerves, and vessels.

NOTE that sartorius muscle passes superficial to **neck** of **femur**, and femoral artery at its location (deep to inguinal ligament) passes superficial to **head** of **femur**.

SEVER gracilis muscle from its origin to **inferior pubic ramus**, and remove proximal part of muscle from hip.

SEVER tendon of sartorius from its origin to **anterior superior iliac spine**, and remove proximal part of muscle from hip.

CAUTION During next step, preserve origin of obturator externus muscle.

SEVER adductor longus and brevis muscles from their origins to **ischiopubic ramus**, and remove remaining parts of all adductor muscles.

SEVER tensor fasciae latae muscle from its origin to **iliac crest**, and reflect iliotibial tract with attached gluteus maximus and tensor fasciae latae muscles inferiorly. Note that vastus lateralis muscle must be freed from iliotibial tract.

TRANSECT femoral artery, vein, and nerve as they exit from beneath inguinal ligament.

SEVER tendon of gluteus medius from its insertion to posterior surface of **greater trochanter** of **femur**, and remove muscle.

SEVER tendon of gluteus minimus from its insertion to anterior surface of greater trochanter of femur, and reflect muscle posteriorly.

SEVER straight tendon of rectus femoris from its origin to **anterior inferior iliac spine** and reflected tendon from its origin to **posterior superior acetabulum**, and remove proximal part of muscle.

FREE obturator externus muscle at its origin from **obturator membrane**.

SEVER obturator artery as it exits **obturator canal** and **lateral** and **medial circumflex femoral arteries** as they branch from deep femoral artery.

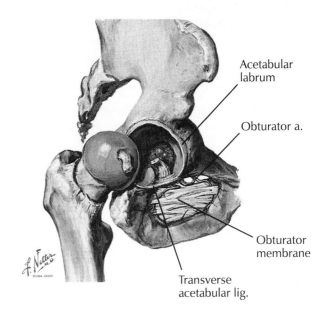

Acetabular labrum

Obturator a.

Obturator membrane

Transverse acetabular lig.

PLATE 458

CAUTION During next step, preserve iliopectineal bursa deep to iliopsoas muscle.

SEVER tendon of iliopsoas from its insertion to **lesser trochanter** of **femur**, and reflect iliopsoas muscle superiorly.

LOOK for **iliopectineal bursa** deep to iliopsoas muscle and superficial to anterior surface of capsule of hip joint.

SEVER tendon of piriformis from its insertion to greater trochanter of femur, and reflect piriformis muscle medially.

SEVER sciatic and posterior femoral cutaneous nerves as they exit greater sciatic foramen, and reflect distal cut ends inferiorly.

LOOK for articular branch to hip joint from nerve to quadratus femoris.

CAUTION During next step, preserve bursa deep to quadratus femoris muscle, and joint capsule deep to bursa.

SEVER quadratus femoris muscle from its insertion to **intertrochanteric crest** of **femur**, and reflect quadratus femoris muscle medially.

PLATE 458

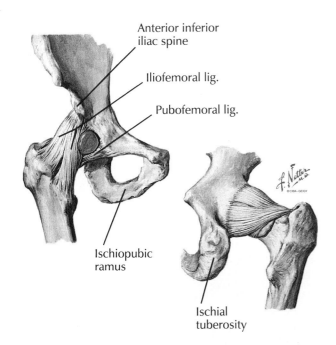

Anterior inferior iliac spine

Iliofemoral lig.

Pubofemoral lig.

Ischiopubic ramus

Ischial tuberosity

SEVER tendon of obturator internus from its insertion to **trochanteric fossa** of **femur**, and reflect obturator internus muscle with attached tendons of superior gemellus and inferior gemellus medially.

LOOK for bursa deep to obturator internus muscle and anterior to posterior surface of capsule of hip joint.

OBSERVE passage of tendon of obturator externus inferior to capsule of hip joint.

SEVER tendon of obturator externus from its insertion to trochanteric fossa of femur, and remove obturator externus muscle.

SEVER tendons of long head of biceps femoris, semitendinosus, and semimembranosus from their origins to ischial tuberosity, and reflect muscles inferiorly.

IDENTIFY inverted Y-shaped **iliofemoral ligament** attaching between anterior inferior iliac spine and intertrochanteric line of femur.

IDENTIFY **pubofemoral ligament** attaching between superior pubic ramus and inferior intertrochanteric line of femur.

MANIPULATE femur to determine which movements produce tautness in which ligaments.

SEVER ligaments of capsule of hip joint around entire circumference of capsule with scalpel.

OPEN hip joint and rupture **round ligament** of **femur** by force of dislocation and with scalpel (**Figure 29**).

OBSERVE acetabular labrum and **articular cartilage** on head of femur.

IDENTIFY **transverse acetabular ligament** between 2 ends of **lunate surface**.

LOOK for **artery** to **round ligament** of **femur** from anterior branch of obturator artery.

Knee

PALPATE patella, **lateral** and **medial epicondyles** and **condyles** of **femur**, **lateral** and **medial condyles** of **tibia**, **tuberosity** of **tibia**, and **head** of **fibula**.

SEVER iliotibial tract from its insertion to Gerdy's tubercle, and remove iliotibial tract.

CAUTION   During next step, preserve bursa deep to biceps femoris muscle.

SEVER short head of biceps femoris muscle at its origin from linea aspera and tendon of biceps femoris from its insertion to head of fibula, and remove muscle.

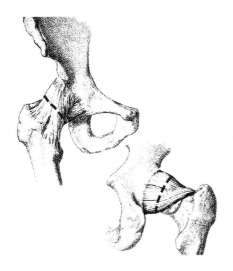

Figure 29

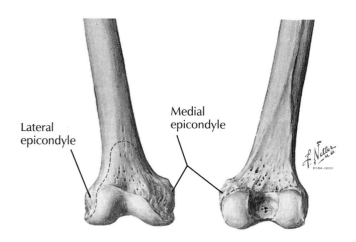

Lateral epicondyle

Medial epicondyle

PLATE 459 detail

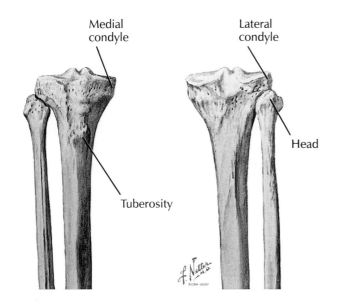

Medial condyle   Lateral condyle

Head

Tuberosity

PLATE 482 detail

LOOK for bursa deep to tendon of biceps femoris and superficial to fibular collateral ligament.

CAUTION   During following steps, preserve anserine bursa deep to pes anserinus.

REMOVE saphenous artery and nerve.

SEVER tendons of semitendinosus, gracilis, and sartorius as they insert to form pes anserinus and attach to anterior surface of medial condyle of tibia; remove these muscles.

LOOK for **anserine bursa** deep to pes anserinus and superficial to tibial collateral ligament.

CAUTION   During following steps, preserve bursa deep to semimembranosus muscle.

SEVER tendon of semimembranosus from its insertion to posterior surface of medial condyle of tibia, and remove muscle.

NOTE tendinous expansion of semimembranosus, which forms identifiable **oblique popliteal ligament** on posterior capsule of knee.

LOOK for bursa deep to tendon of semi-membranosus and superficial to tibial collateral ligament.

CAUTION   During following steps, preserve bursae deep to both heads of gastrocnemius muscle.

REMOVE remnants of gastrocnemius muscle from medial and lateral epicondyles of femur.

LOOK for bursae deep to medial and lateral heads of gastrocnemius muscle and superficial to posterior capsule of knee.

IDENTIFY tendon of **quadriceps femoris, patella,** and **patellar ligament**.

FOLLOW attachment of **medial** and **lateral retinacula** from distal vastus medialis and lateralis muscles to patella and medial and lateral condyles of tibia.

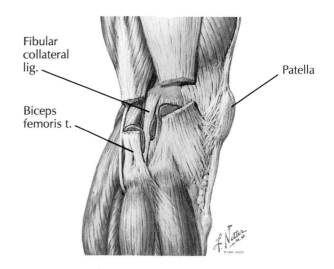

Fibular collateral lig.

Patella

Biceps femoris t.

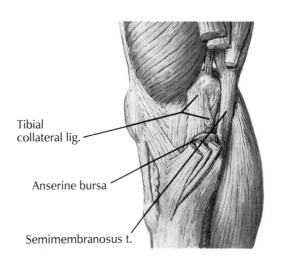

Tibial collateral lig.

Anserine bursa

Semimembranosus t.

PLATE 476

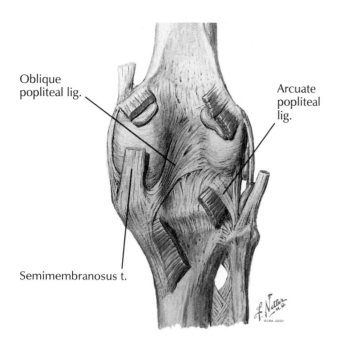

Oblique popliteal lig.

Arcuate popliteal lig.

Semimembranosus t.

PLATE 480

INCISE tendon of quadriceps femoris <u>vertically</u> 3 or 4 finger-widths superiorly from superior margin of patella.

LOOK for **suprapatellar bursa** deep to tendon of quadriceps femoris and superficial to distal anterior shaft of femur by retracting medial and lateral margins of incision.

REMOVE all branches of popliteal artery and veins and tibial and common peroneal nerves from popliteal fossa.

CAUTION   During next step, preserve ligaments of knee capsule.

CLEAN knee capsule by removing fat.

IDENTIFY fibular and **tibial collateral ligaments**.

IDENTIFY arcuate popliteal ligament between lateral condyle of femur and head of fibula.

NOTE that tendon of popliteus exits posterior capsule inferior to arcuate ligament.

TRANSECT quadriceps femoris muscle <u>horizontally</u> 1 hand-width superior to patella.

CUT horizontal fibers of vastus medialis muscle free from tendon of quadriceps femoris, and reflect distal cut end of quadriceps femoris muscle inferiorly to expose anterior capsule of knee.

IDENTIFY origin of **articularis genus muscle** deep to vastus intermedius muscle from distal femur.

INCISE attachment of anterior capsule to distal femur, and reflect capsule inferiorly.

FLEX knee to expose joint interior and **infrapatellar synovial fold**.

INSPECT extent and reflections of synovial membranes. Note that suprapatellar bursa is continuous with synovial sac of knee joint.

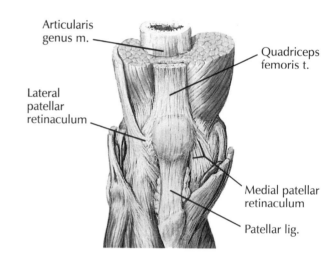

Articularis genus m.

Quadriceps femoris t.

Lateral patellar retinaculum

Medial patellar retinaculum

Patellar lig.

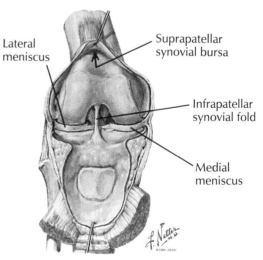

Lateral meniscus

Suprapatellar synovial bursa

Infrapatellar synovial fold

Medial meniscus

PLATE 477

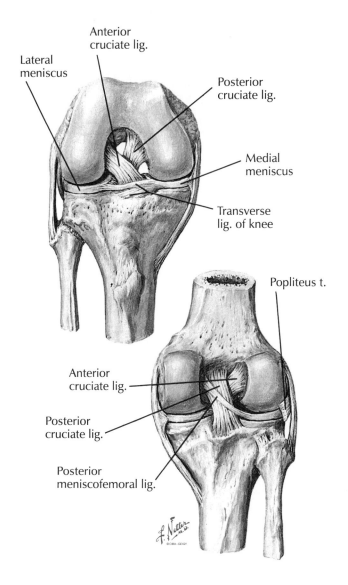

Lateral meniscus

Anterior cruciate lig.

Posterior cruciate lig.

Medial meniscus

Transverse lig. of knee

Popliteus t.

Anterior cruciate lig.

Posterior cruciate lig.

Posterior meniscofemoral lig.

PLATE 479

REMOVE infrapatellar synovial fold and fat.

OBSERVE articular cartilage (*not labeled*) on medial and lateral condyles and patellar surface of femur, posterior surface of patella, and superior surfaces of medial and lateral condyles of tibia.

OBSERVE attachment of oval-shaped **medial meniscus** to knee capsule and tibial collateral ligament.

OBSERVE that there is no attachment of circular-shaped **lateral meniscus** to knee capsule and fibular collateral ligament.

OBSERVE attachment of **anterior cruciate ligament** to anterior intercondylar fossa of tibia.

OBSERVE that **transverse ligament** of knee extends from anterior edge of lateral meniscus to anterior edge of medial meniscus.

EXTEND knee.

PRESERVE tibial and fibular collateral ligaments as dissection continues.

RETURN to examination of posterior knee.

INCISE posterior capsule of knee, initially placing scalpel on lateral condyle of femur to incise capsule vertically for approximately 2 finger-widths (**Figure 30**). Continue this scalpel incision horizontally 1 finger-width laterally. Then cut capsule with scissors horizontally along its entire posterior width.

EXAMINE interior of knee joint.

OBSERVE attachment of **posterior cruciate ligament** to **posterior intercondylar fossa** of **tibia**.

LOOK for **posterior meniscofemoral ligament** (part of posterior cruciate ligament) extending from medial condyle of femur to posterior surface of lateral meniscus.

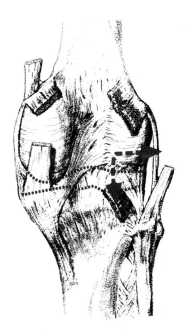

Figure 30

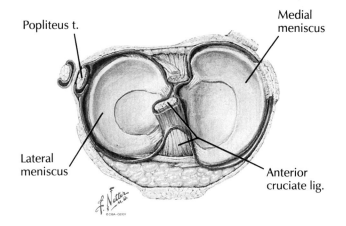

Popliteus t.

Medial meniscus

Lateral meniscus

Anterior cruciate lig.

PLATE 478

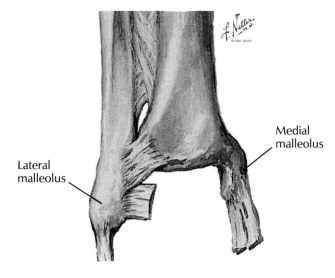

Lateral malleolus

Medial malleolus

PLATE 483 detail

OBSERVE posterior attachment of **anterior cruciate ligament** to medial surface of lateral condyle of femur.

OBSERVE origin of **popliteus muscle** within cavity of knee joint from lateral condyle of femur.

RETURN knee to flexion and look through opening in anterior surface of capsule.

TRACE posterior cruciate ligament to its anterior attachment to lateral surface of medial condyle of femur.

Ankle

PALPATE medial and **lateral malleoli, sustentaculum tali,** and **tuberosities** of **navicular bone** and **metatarsal bone 5.**

SEVER calcaneal tendon as it attaches to calcaneus, and remove triceps surae muscles.

CUT and **REMOVE** peroneal artery with calcaneal tendon.

REFLECT cut ends of tendons of flexor digitorum longus with attached muscles toward toes.

SEVER tendon of flexor hallucis longus from just proximal to distal phalanx of big toe, and reflect proximal cut end of tendon superiorly above **talocrural joint.**

REMOVE a**b**ductor hallucis muscle, medial and lateral heads of flexor hallucis brevis muscle, and transverse and oblique heads of a**dd**uctor hallucis muscle.

REMOVE a**b**ductor digiti minimi and flexor digiti minimi brevis muscles.

SEVER tendon of tibialis posterior from just distal to sustentaculum tali, and reflect proximal cut end of tendon of tibialis posterior superiorly above talocrural joint.

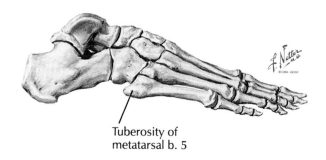

Tuberosity of metatarsal b. 5

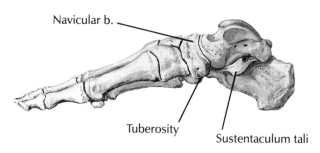

Navicular b.

Tuberosity

Sustentaculum tali

PLATE 493

146

REMOVE medial and lateral plantar nerves and arteries from plantar surface of foot, and remove posterior tibial artery from region of ankle.

SEVER tendon of peroneus brevis from its insertion to base of metatarsal bone 5, and reflect peroneus brevis muscle superiorly 1 hand-width above talocrural joint.

SEVER tendon of peroneus longus from just proximal to talocrural joint, and reflect peroneus longus muscle superiorly above talocrural joint.

SEVER tendons of extensor digitorum longus, peroneus tertius, and extensor hallucis from just proximal to extensor expansions, and reflect these muscles superiorly above talocrural joint.

REMOVE cut ends and tendon of extensor digitorum brevis from dorsal surface of foot.

SEVER tendon of tibialis anterior just proximal to talocrural joint, and reflect proximal cut end of tendon of tibialis anterior superiorly.

CUT anterior tibial artery proximal to origin of dorsalis pedis artery, and remove branches of dorsalis pedis artery from dorsal surface of foot.

CUT deep peroneal nerve at same level, and remove its branches from dorsal surface of foot.

CAUTION   During following steps, preserve capsule of ankle joint.

CLEAN dorsal surface of bones and ligaments of foot.

CLEAN capsule of ankle joint.

IDENTIFY posterior and **anterior tibiofibular ligaments**.

DEFINE component parts of **deltoid ligament** as follows.

OBSERVE that **posterior tibiotalar ligament** attaches from medial malleolus to posterior process of talus.

OBSERVE that **tibiocalcaneal ligament** attaches from medial malleolus to sustentaculum tali.

PLATE 495

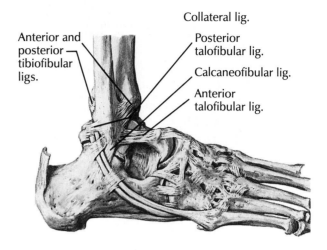

Collateral lig.

Anterior and posterior tibiofibular ligs.

Posterior talofibular lig.

Calcaneofibular lig.

Anterior talofibular lig.

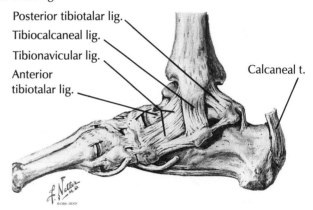

Deltoid lig.

Posterior tibiotalar lig.

Tibiocalcaneal lig.

Tibionavicular lig.

Anterior tibiotalar lig.

Calcaneal t.

f. Netter
©CIBA-GEIGY

OBSERVE that **tibionavicular ligament** attaches from medial malleolus to navicular bone.

OBSERVE that **anterior tibiotalar ligament** attaches from medial malleolus to head of talus.

DEFINE component parts of **lateral collateral ligament** as follows.

OBSERVE that **posterior talofibular ligament** attaches from lateral malleolus to posterior process of talus.

OBSERVE that **calcaneofibular ligament** attaches from lateral malleolus to tubercle on midlateral surface of calcaneus.

OBSERVE that **anterior talofibular ligament** attaches from lateral malleolus to neck of talus.

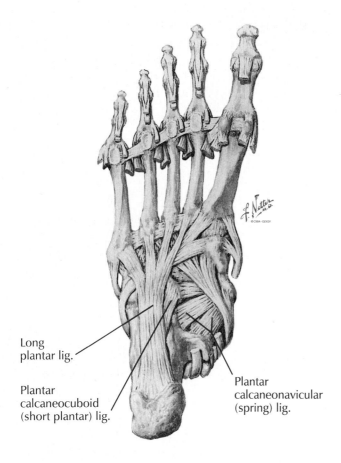

Long
plantar lig.

Plantar
calcaneocuboid
(short plantar) lig.

Plantar
calcaneonavicular
(spring) lig.

PLATE 496

CLEAN plantar surface of foot to define boundaries of 3 major ligaments.

OBSERVE that **long plantar ligament** attaches from anterior of tuberosity of calcaneus to posterior of tuberosity of cuboid bone and to bases of metatarsal bones 2–5. Note that long plantar ligament passes superficial to tendon of peroneus longus.

OBSERVE that **plantar calcaneocuboid (short plantar) ligament** is deep to long plantar ligament and attaches from tuberosity of calcaneus to cuboid bone proximal to groove for peroneus longus muscle.

OBSERVE that **plantar calcaneonavicular (spring) ligament** attaches from tuberosity of calcaneus to navicular bone.

OPEN talocrural joint partially by cutting components of lateral collateral ligament.

INSPECT articular cartilage (*not labeled*) on articular surfaces of talus by using deltoid ligament as hinge during separation of talus from tibia and fibula.

IMMOBILIZE talus with one hand, and produce eversion by pulling on tendon of peroneus longus.

PRODUCE inversion by pulling on tendons of tibialis anterior and posterior.

IDENTIFY posterior talocalcaneal ligament between posterior process of talus and calcaneus and **medial talocalcaneal ligament** between posterior process of talus and sustentaculum tali.

OPEN subtalar joint posteriorly by cutting posterior and medial talocalcaneal ligaments and slipping scalpel between talus and calcaneus to cut interosseous talocalcaneal ligament.

REMOVE talus, and inspect articular cartilage on calcaneus, which articulates with talus and cuboid bone. Inspect articular cartilage on talus, which articulates with calcaneus and navicular bone.

LOOK for internal **calcaneocuboid ligament** (*not shown*).

PLATE 494

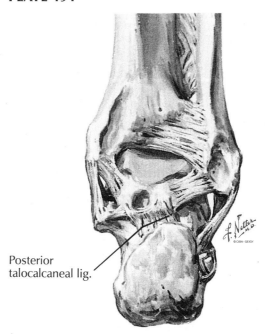

Posterior
talocalcaneal lig.

Section 7

PELVIS AND PERINEUM

DISSECTIONS

DISSECTION 7.1
FEMALE PERINEUM

Complete DISSECTIONS **4.6** Posterior Abdominal Wall, **6.1** Gluteal Region, and **6.7** Joints of Lower Limb.

Read DISCUSSIONS **6.2** Bones (Pelvic Girdle), **7.1** Pelvic Diaphragm, **7.2** Urogenital Diaphragm, **7.3** Ischiorectal Fossa, **7.4** Female External Genitalia, and **7.9** Arteries.

NOTE that following directions assume that <u>both</u> hip joints have been disarticulated.

PLACE cadaver with perineum facing up.

REMEMBER that directions are given as though cadaver were in anatomical position.

NOTE that bony pelvis with intact ligaments should be placed beside and in same position as cadaver.

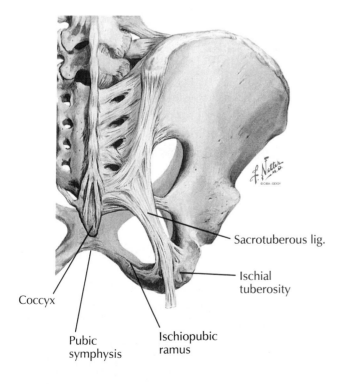

Coccyx

Pubic symphysis

Ischiopubic ramus

Sacrotuberous lig.

Ischial tuberosity

PLATE 335

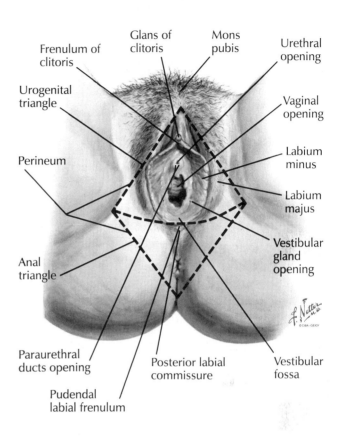

Frenulum of clitoris

Glans of clitoris

Mons pubis

Urethral opening

Urogenital triangle

Vaginal opening

Perineum

Labium minus

Labium majus

Anal triangle

Vestibular gland opening

Paraurethral ducts opening

Posterior labial commissure

Vestibular fossa

Pudendal labial frenulum

PLATE 354

PALPATE following bony landmarks: inferior border of **pubic symphysis, coccyx, ischial tuberosity, ischiopubic ramus**, and **sacrotuberous ligament**. Note that sacrotuberous ligament may have been cut on 1 side during gluteal dissection.

DEFINE boundaries of **perineum** as diamond-shaped space divided into **urogenital triangle** and **anal triangle**.

IDENTIFY mons pubis as fatty deposit anterior to pubic symphysis.

FOLLOW labia majora posteriorly to **posterior labial commissure**.

SPREAD labia majora with fingers, and identify **labia minora** bordering **vestibule**.

IDENTIFY external openings of **urethra** and **vagina** between labia minora.

LOOK for openings of **paraurethral ducts** on each side of urethral opening and for openings of ducts of **vestibular glands** on each side of vaginal opening.

FOLLOW labia minora posteriorly to their union as **pudendal frenulum** of **labia**, anteriorly to their union posterior to clitoris as **frenulum** of **clitoris**, and to their union anterior to clitoris as **prepuce** of **clitoris**.

LOCATE vestibular fossa posterior to vaginal opening and anterior to pudendal frenulum of labia.

IDENTIFY glans of **clitoris**.

IDENTIFY anus.

INCISE skin (**Figure 31**). Note that circular area of skin around anus will be dissected later. Skin of labia minora will not be removed.

REMOVE skin and discard it. Note that to understand varying descriptions of fascial layers, time should be afforded to careful dissection.

Figure 31

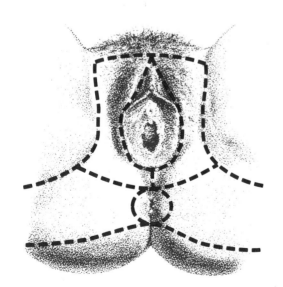

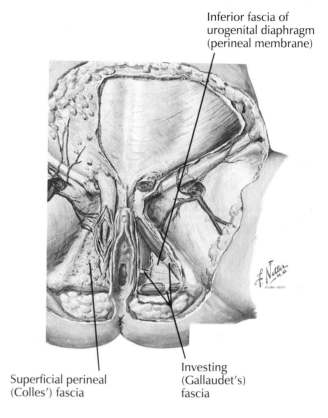

Superficial perineal (Colles') fascia

Inferior fascia of urogenital diaphragm (perineal membrane)

Investing (Gallaudet's) fascia

PLATE 355

EXAMINE superficial fatty subcutaneous tissue covering both urogenital and anal triangles.

REMOVE as much superficial fatty subcutaneous tissue as possible with forceps and paper towels. Make an effort <u>not</u> to cut this tissue away to preserve deep membranous subcutaneous tissue, called **superficial perineal (Colles') fascia**.

IDENTIFY Colles' fascia, which attaches to posterior border of urogenital triangle and laterally to ischiopubic rami.

BLUNT DISSECT deep to Colles' fascia to expose contents of **superficial perineal space (pouch)**.

IDENTIFY perineal artery and **superficial** and **deep branches** of **perineal nerve**.

CAUTION During next step, preserve posterior labial arteries and other branches of perineal artery, superficial branches of perineal nerve, and superficial transverse perineal muscle.

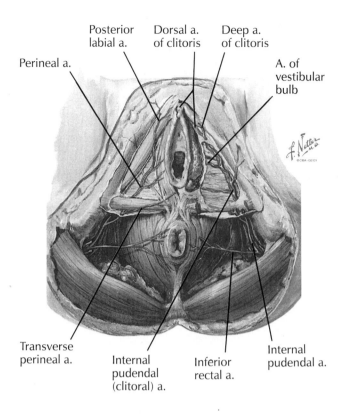

Perineal a. | Posterior labial a. | Dorsal a. of clitoris | Deep a. of clitoris | A. of vestibular bulb

Transverse perineal a. | Internal pudendal (clitoral) a. | Inferior rectal a. | Internal pudendal a.

PLATE 379

REMOVE Colles' fascia with forceps.

DEFINE boundaries of superficial perineal space between removed Colles' fascia and exposed **inferior fascia** of **urogenital diaphragm (perineal membrane)**.

IDENTIFY ischiocavernosus, bulbospongiosus, and **superficial transverse perineal muscles** and their **investing (Gallaudet's) fascia**.

IDENTIFY central tendon of **perineum**. Note that superficial transverse perineal and bulbospongiosus muscles attach to it.

IDENTIFY posterior labial arteries and **nerves** at most anterior part of urogenital triangle.

TRACE posterior labial arteries and nerves to their origins from perineal artery and superficial branch of perineal nerve, which are found inferior (superficial) to superficial transverse perineal muscle at posterior margin of urogenital triangle.

IDENTIFY deep branches of perineal nerve and artery as they pass through urogenital triangle. Note their entrance into urogenital triangle deep to superficial transverse perineal muscle.

IDENTIFY transverse perineal artery as it travels along surface of superficial transverse perineal muscle. Note that it branches from perineal artery.

TRANSECT superficial transverse perineal muscle, and reflect cut ends medially and laterally. Note that transverse perineal artery will be cut during this step.

CAUTION During next step, preserve bulbospongiosus muscle.

REMOVE labia minora with scalpel.

BLUNT DISSECT around borders of ischiocavernosus muscle enveloping **crus of clitoris**. Note that ischiocavernosus and bulbospongiosus muscles cannot be successfully dissected free of erectile tissue in female.

BLUNT DISSECT around borders of bulbospongiosus muscle to determine extent of **vestibular bulb** contained within.

EXAMINE corpus (body) of **clitoris**, and trace its roots back to crura of clitoris.

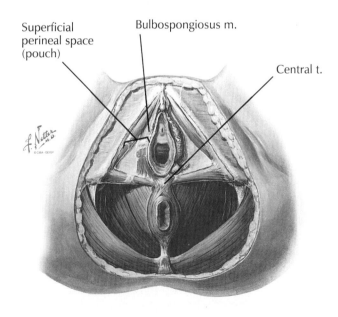

Superficial perineal space (pouch) | Bulbospongiosus m. | Central t.

PLATE 356

153

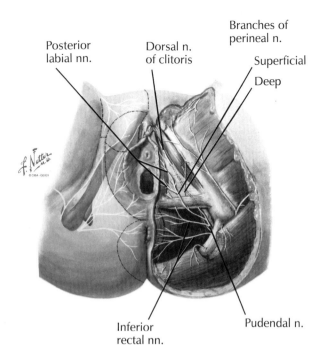

Posterior labial nn.   Dorsal n. of clitoris   Branches of perineal n.   Superficial   Deep

Inferior rectal nn.   Pudendal n.

PLATE 388

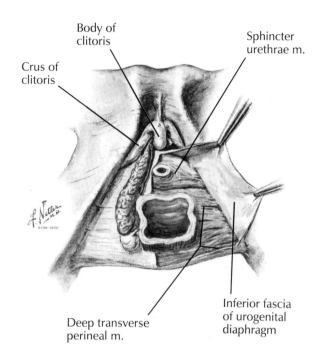

Crus of clitoris   Body of clitoris   Sphincter urethrae m.

Deep transverse perineal m.   Inferior fascia of urogenital diaphragm

PLATE 356

TRANSECT ischiocavernosus muscle and crus of clitoris at their point of emergence from ischiopubic ramus.

REFLECT ischiocavernosus muscle and crus of clitoris anteriorly to expose underlying structures.

EXAMINE cut ends of ischiocavernosus muscle and crus of clitoris to observe difference between muscle and erectile tissue.

LOOK for **deep artery** of **clitoris** and **dorsal nerve** of **clitoris** entering crus of clitoris.

CAUTION   During following steps, preserve deep artery and dorsal nerve of clitoris for use as guides.

REMOVE inferior fascia of urogenital triangle to expose **deep transverse perineal** and **sphincter urethrae muscles** around region where crus of clitoris has been reflected.

DEFINE boundaries of **deep perineal space** (**pouch**, *not labeled*), between removed inferior fascia of urogenital diaphragm and superior fascia of urogenital diaphragm.

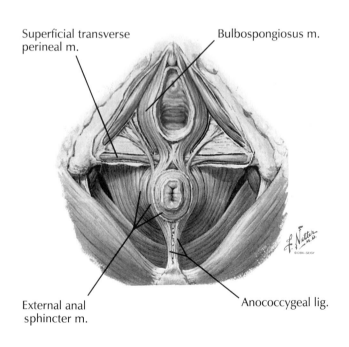

Superficial transverse perineal m.   Bulbospongiosus m.

External anal sphincter m.   Anococcygeal lig.

PLATE 371

IDENTIFY **internal pudendal artery** and its branches, **artery** to **clitoris**, and **artery** to **vestibular bulb** in deep perineal space.

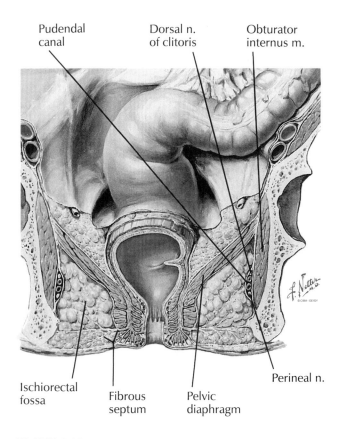

Pudendal canal

Dorsal n. of clitoris

Obturator internus m.

Ischiorectal fossa

Fibrous septum

Pelvic diaphragm

Perineal n.

PLATE 368

TRACE dorsal nerve of **clitoris** retrograde to pudendal nerve.

REIDENTIFY central tendon of perineum. Note that **external anal sphincter muscle** and superficial transverse perineal and bulbospongiosus muscles attach to it.

CAUTION During following steps, preserve inferior rectal nerves and arteries to external anal sphincter muscle.

REMOVE skin from external anal sphincter muscle, and locate **anococcygeal ligament**, which extends posteriorly to tip of coccyx.

REMOVE fat from **ischiorectal fossa**, preserving **inferior rectal nerves** and **arteries** as they cross fossa, and internal pudendal artery and **pudendal nerve** along lateral wall of fossa. Note numerous **fibrous septa** found in ischiorectal fossa.

NOTE that medial walls of ischiorectal fossa are formed by **pelvic diaphragm** and lateral walls are formed by **obturator internus muscle**. Ischiorectal fossa has an **anterior recess** that extends superior to urogenital diaphragm.

PALPATE pudendal canal in obturator fascia extending from **greater sciatic foramen** to posterior margin of urogenital triangle.

PALPATE spine of **ischium** by placing finger in rectum or vagina. Note relationship of pudendal canal to spine of ischium.

FOLLOW superficial and deep perineal nerves (found earlier in urogenital triangle) posteriorly to identify **perineal nerve**. Note that perineal nerve is located inferior to internal pudendal artery in pudendal canal.

IDENTIFY dorsal nerve of clitoris located superior to internal pudendal artery in pudendal canal.

DISSECTION 7.2
MALE PERINEUM

Complete DISSECTIONS **4.6** Posterior Abdominal Wall, **6.1** Gluteal Region, and **6.7** Joints of Lower Limb.

Read DISCUSSIONS **6.2** Bones (Pelvic Girdle), **7.1** Pelvic Diaphragm, **7.2** Urogenital Diaphragm, **7.3** Ischiorectal Fossa, **7.5** Male External Genitalia, and **7.9** Arteries.

NOTE that following directions assume that <u>both</u> hip joints have been disarticulated.

PLACE cadaver with perineum facing up.

REMEMBER that directions are given as though cadaver were in anatomical position.

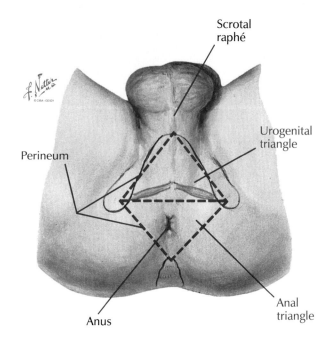

PLATE 358

PLATE 335

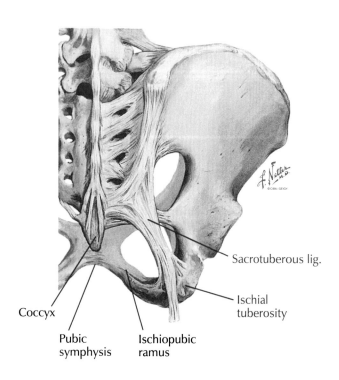

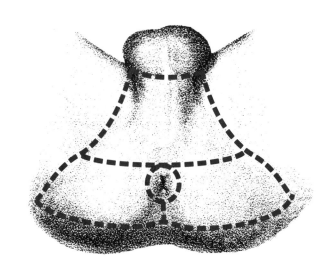

Figure 32

NOTE that bony pelvis with intact ligaments should be placed beside and in same position as cadaver.

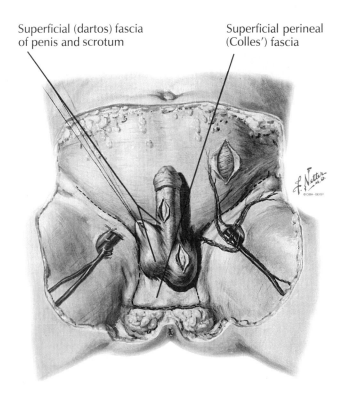

Superficial (dartos) fascia of penis and scrotum

Superficial perineal (Colles') fascia

PLATE 358

PALPATE following bony landmarks: inferior border of **pubic symphysis, coccyx, ischial tuberosity, ischiopubic ramus** (*not labeled*), and **sacrotuberous ligament**. Note that sacrotuberous ligament may have been cut on 1 side during gluteal dissection.

DEFINE boundaries of **perineum** as diamond-shaped space divided into **urogenital triangle** and **anal triangle**.

IDENTIFY **prepuce** of **penis** in uncircumcised cadaver.

IDENTIFY **glans, corona,** and **frenulum** of **penis**.

IDENTIFY **scrotal raphé**.

IDENTIFY **anus**.

CAUTION   During following steps, preserve posterior scrotal arteries and nerves and superficial dorsal vein of penis.

INCISE skin (**Figure 32**). Note that circular area of skin around anus will be dissected later.

SKIN remaining posterior wall of scrotal sac.

CAUTION   During next step, remove only skin of penis, not any fascial layers.

BLUNT DISSECT deep to skin of penis, and remove skin.

REMOVE skin from perineum with scalpel. Note that to understand varying descriptions of fascial layers, time should be afforded to careful dissection.

EXAMINE superficial fatty subcutaneous tissue covering both urogenital and anal triangles.

REMOVE as much superficial fatty subcutaneous tissue as possible with forceps and paper towels. Make an effort <u>not</u> to cut this tissue away to preserve deep membranous subcutaneous tissue, called **superficial perineal (Colles') fascia**.

PLATE 360

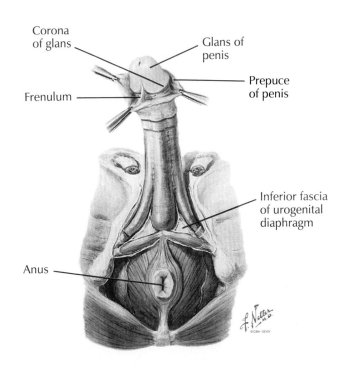

Corona of glans

Glans of penis

Prepuce of penis

Frenulum

Inferior fascia of urogenital diaphragm

Anus

157

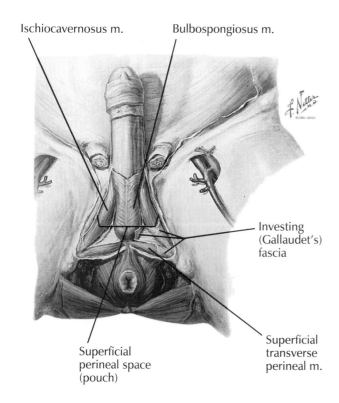

Ischiocavernosus m.   Bulbospongiosus m.

Investing
(Gallaudet's)
fascia

Superficial
perineal space
(pouch)

Superficial
transverse
perineal m.

PLATE 359

IDENTIFY **superficial dorsal vein** of **penis** within superficial fascia of penis.

TRACE **superficial (dartos) fascia** of **penis** and **scrotum** posterior to urogenital triangle.

IDENTIFY Colles' fascia, which is continuous with dartos tunic and also attaches to posterior border of urogenital triangle and laterally to ischiopubic rami.

BLUNT DISSECT deep to Colles' fascia to expose contents of **superficial perineal space (pouch)**.

CAUTION   Preserve posterior scrotal arteries and nerves to trace later.

REMOVE Colles' fascia with forceps.

DEFINE boundaries of superficial perineal space between removed Colles' fascia and exposed **inferior fascia** of **urogenital diaphragm**, to which following muscles are attached.

IDENTIFY **ischiocavernosus, bulbospongiosus,** and **superficial transverse perineal muscles** and their **investing (Gallaudet's) fascia.**

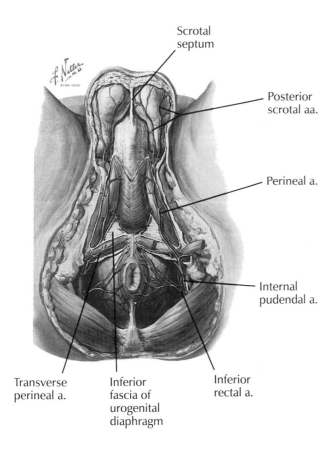

Scrotal
septum

Posterior
scrotal aa.

Perineal a.

Internal
pudendal a.

Transverse
perineal a.

Inferior
fascia of
urogenital
diaphragm

Inferior
rectal a.

PLATE 380

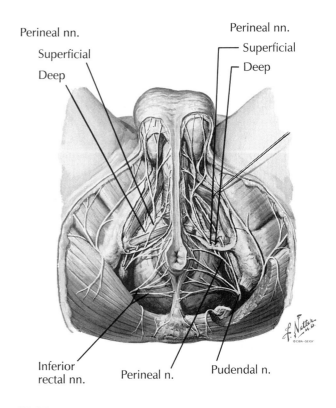

Perineal nn.

Superficial

Deep

Perineal nn.

Superficial

Deep

Inferior
rectal nn.

Perineal n.

Pudendal n.

PLATE 386

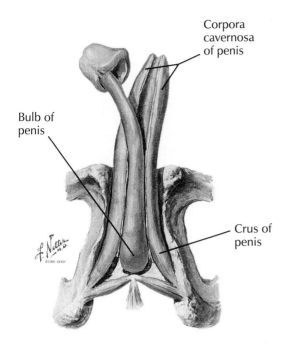

Corpora
cavernosa
of penis

Bulb of
penis

Crus of
penis

PLATE 360

IDENTIFY central tendon of **perineum**.
Note that superficial transverse perineal and
bulbospongiosus muscles attach to it.

IDENTIFY posterior scrotal arteries and **nerves**
on <u>left</u> side where testis was not dissected during
DISSECTION **2.4**.

IDENTIFY transverse perineal artery located
superficial (inferior) to superficial transverse
perineal muscle.

IDENTIFY perineal artery located superficial
(inferior) to ischiocavernosus muscle.

TRACE posterior scrotal arteries to their origin
from perineal artery.

TRACE posterior scrotal nerves to their origin from
superficial branch of **perineal nerve**.

TRACE transverse perineal artery and superficial
branch of perineal nerve to where they are found
superficial (inferior) to superficial transverse
perineal muscle at posterior margin of urogenital
triangle.

IDENTIFY branches of **deep branch** of **perineal
nerve** to bulbospongiosus muscle.

TRACE deep branch of perineal nerve and
accompanying perineal artery as they pass deep
(superior) to superficial transverse perineal muscle
to supply muscles in superficial perineal space.

TRANSECT superficial transverse perineal muscle,
and reflect cut ends medially and laterally.

BLUNT DISSECT deep to ischiocavernosus muscle
to determine extent of **crus** of **penis**.

INCISE bulbospongiosus muscle vertically along
its raphé.

IDENTIFY bulb of **penis** beneath muscle layer.

BLUNT DISSECT deep to bulbospongiosus
muscle, and reflect muscles laterally.

CAUTION   During next step, preserve corpora
cavernosa and spongiosum.

REMOVE ischiocavernosus, bulbospongiosus, and
superficial transverse perineal muscles from <u>left</u>
side with undissected testis.

FOLLOW deep investing fascia deep to
bulbospongiosus and ischiocavernosus muscles to
identify **deep (Buck's) fascia** of **penis**. Note that
fascia is substantial.

IDENTIFY suspensory ligament of **penis**
extending from pubic symphysis to surround root
of penis attaching to Buck's fascia.

EXCISE Buck's fascia carefully over components of
root of **penis** (*not labeled*).

EXAMINE bulb of penis formed of **corpus
spongiosum**, and crura of penis formed of
corpora cavernosa.

LOOK for **artery** of **bulb** of **penis** and **deep artery**
of **penis**, which enters crus. Note that both
arteries branch from internal pudendal artery as
it passes through **deep perineal space**, (**pouch**,
not labeled).

LOCATE deep dorsal vein of **penis** in midline on
dorsal surface of shaft of penis deep to Buck's
fascia. Note large size of vein.

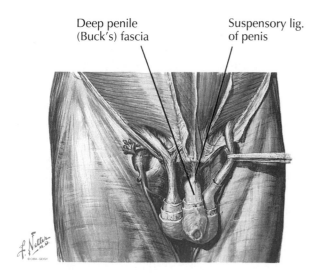

Deep penile
(Buck's) fascia

Suspensory lig.
of penis

PLATE 233

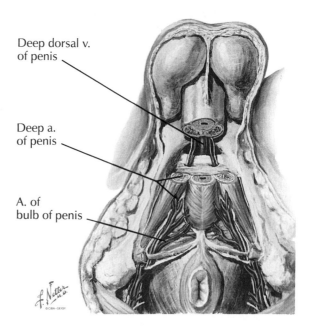

Deep dorsal v.
of penis

Deep a.
of penis

A. of
bulb of penis

PLATE 380

TRACE deep dorsal vein of penis through its passage between **arcuate pubic ligament** on inferior margin of pubic symphysis and **transverse perineal ligament**, which is anterior margin of fascia covering urogenital diaphragm. Note that penis must be detached from pubic bone to observe these structures.

LOCATE dorsal arteries of **penis** passing on either side of deep dorsal vein deep to Buck's fascia, and **dorsal nerves** of **penis** passing lateral to each dorsal artery.

BLUNT DISSECT deep to bulb of penis and <u>right</u> crus, and remove them.

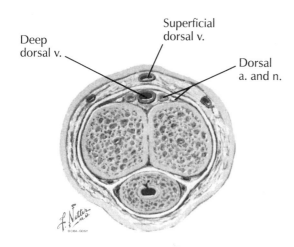

Deep
dorsal v.

Superficial
dorsal v.

Dorsal
a. and n.

PLATE 359

REMOVE inferior fascia of urogenital triangle to expose **deep transverse perineal** and **sphincter urethrae muscles**.

DEFINE boundaries of deep perineal space between removed inferior fascia of urogenital diaphragm and superior fascia of urogenital diaphragm.

LOCATE bulbourethral (Cowper's) gland.

REIDENTIFY internal pudendal artery, dorsal artery of **penis, artery** of **bulb of penis**, and **dorsal nerve** of **penis**.

REIDENTIFY central tendon of perineum. Note that **external anal sphincter muscle** and superficial transverse perineal and bulbospongiosus muscles attach to it.

CAUTION During following steps, preserve inferior rectal nerves and arteries to external anal sphincter muscle.

REMOVE skin from external anal sphincter muscle, and locate **anococcygeal ligament**, which extends posteriorly to tip of coccyx.

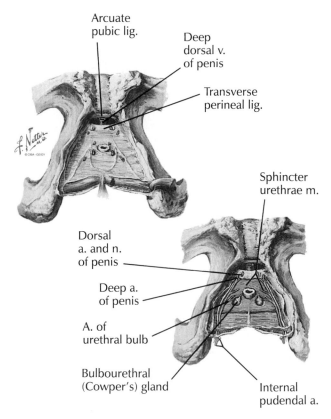

Arcuate pubic lig.

Deep dorsal v. of penis

Transverse perineal lig.

Sphincter urethrae m.

Dorsal a. and n. of penis

Deep a. of penis

A. of urethral bulb

Bulbourethral (Cowper's) gland

Internal pudendal a.

PLATE 361

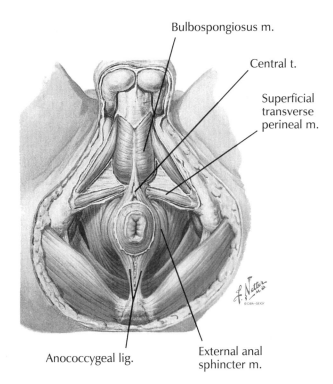

Bulbospongiosus m.

Central t.

Superficial transverse perineal m.

Anococcygeal lig.

External anal sphincter m.

PLATE 371

REMOVE fat from **ischiorectal fossa**, preserving **inferior rectal nerves** and **arteries** as they cross fossa.

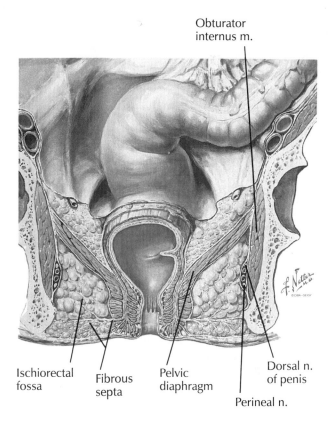

Obturator internus m.

Ischiorectal fossa

Fibrous septa

Pelvic diaphragm

Dorsal n. of penis

Perineal n.

PLATE 368

PRESERVE internal pudendal artery and **pudendal nerve** along lateral wall of fossa. Note numerous **fibrous septa** found in ischiorectal fossa.

NOTE that medial walls of ischiorectal fossa are formed by **pelvic diaphragm** and lateral walls are formed by **obturator internus muscle**. Ischiorectal fossa has an **anterior recess** that extends superior to urogenital diaphragm.

PALPATE **pudendal canal** in obturator fascia extending from **greater sciatic foramen** to posterior margin of urogenital triangle.

PALPATE **spine** of **ischium** by placing finger in rectum. Note relationship of pudendal canal to spine of ischium.

FOLLOW superficial and deep perineal nerves (found earlier in urogenital triangle) posteriorly to identify **perineal nerve**. Note that perineal nerve is located inferior to internal pudendal artery in pudendal canal.

IDENTIFY dorsal nerve of penis located superior to internal pudendal artery in pudendal canal.

DISSECTION 7.3
FEMALE PELVIC ORGANS

Complete DISSECTION **7.1** Female Perineum.

Read DISCUSSIONS **7.1** Pelvic Diaphragm, **7.2** Urogenital Diaphragm, **7.6** Pelvic Organs, **7.7** Female Pelvic Organs, and **7.9** Arteries.

NOTE that bony pelvis with intact ligaments should be placed beside and in same position as cadaver.

REMEMBER that directions are given as though cadaver were in anatomical position.

PLACE cadaver with perineum facing down. Try to dissect pelvis in anatomical position.

DEFINE boundaries of **true pelvis** (*not labeled*) below **linea terminalis**, which is formed by **sacral promontory**, and **iliopectineal line**, which is formed by **arcuate line** and **pecten pubis**.

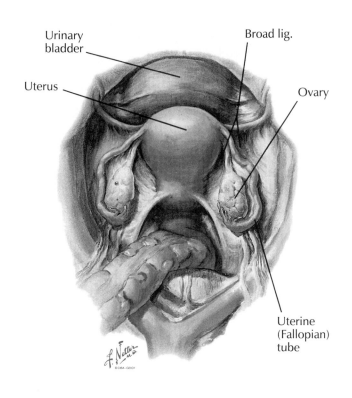

PLATE 348

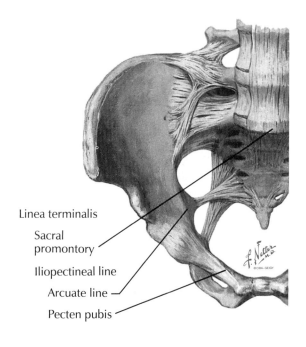

Linea terminalis
Sacral promontory
Iliopectineal line
Arcuate line
Pecten pubis

PLATE 335

INSPECT bladder, uterus, uterine (Fallopian) tubes, and **ovaries** with peritoneum intact.

IDENTIFY superior surface of bladder with peritoneum covering it and apex of bladder with **median umbilical fold** passing superiorly from it.

IDENTIFY external surface of **fundus** and **body** of **uterus, fimbria, infundibulum, ampulla**, and **isthmus** of **uterine tubes**.

IDENTIFY rectum.

EXAMINE folds and fossae in peritoneum over pelvic structures.

IDENTIFY ureteric fold, which contains ureter.

IDENTIFY uterosacral fold between posterior surface of uterus and sacrum.

EXAMINE paravesical fossa anterior to fold covering round ligament of uterus.

EXAMINE vesicouterine fossa posterior to bladder and anterior to uterus.

EXAMINE broad ligament and its component parts: **mesometrium, mesosalpinx,** and **mesovarium** (*not labeled*).

EXAMINE pararectal fossa between uterosacral fold and rectum.

EXAMINE rectouterine space (**pouch**) anterior to rectum and posterior to uterus.

PALPATE passage of **round ligament** of **uterus** across paravesical fossa to its descent posterior to bladder at uterosacral fold.

PALPATE suspensory ligament of **ovary**, which contains ovarian artery and vein.

PALPATE cardinal ligament, which contains uterine artery and vein.

CAUTION During next step, preserve neurovascular structures around pelvic organs.

REMOVE peritoneum from structures in pelvis with forceps.

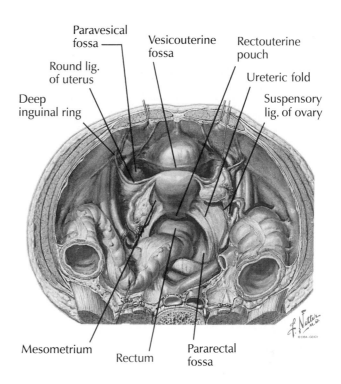

Paravesical fossa
Round lig. of uterus
Deep inguinal ring
Vesicouterine fossa
Rectouterine pouch
Ureteric fold
Suspensory lig. of ovary
Mesometrium
Rectum
Pararectal fossa

PLATE 343

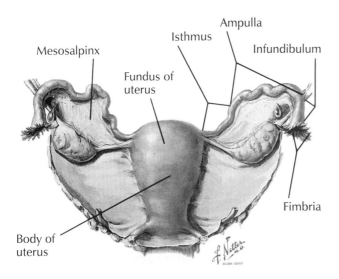

Ampulla
Isthmus
Infundibulum
Mesosalpinx
Fundus of uterus
Fimbria
Body of uterus

PLATE 350

REVIEW passage of following structures from abdominal cavity into pelvis: ovarian artery and vein, common iliac artery and vein, superior rectal artery and vein, and middle sacral artery and vein.

IDENTIFY internal iliac artery.

TRACE round ligament of uterus from deep inguinal ring as it passes superior to superior vesical artery and vein, obturator nerve and vessels, and ureter.

TRACE uterine artery from cervical end of uterus to its origin from internal iliac artery. Note spiral nature of uterine artery near uterus and that ureter passes inferior to uterine vessels.

TRACE passage of **ureter** from anterior to internal iliac artery deep to uterine vessels to posterior lateral surface of bladder.

TRACE obturator nerve from medial to psoas major muscle to **obturator canal.**

IDENTIFY obturator artery at obturator canal inferior to obturator nerve.

163

TRACE umbilical artery from **medial umbilical ligament** to its origin from internal iliac artery.

IDENTIFY superior vesical arteries branching from umbilical artery to bladder.

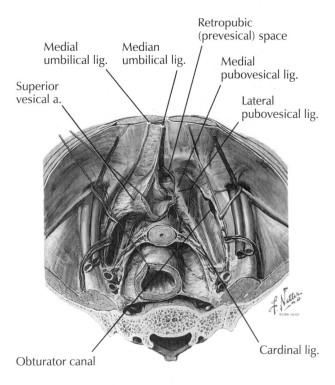

Medial umbilical lig.
Median umbilical lig.
Retropubic (prevesical) space
Medial pubovesical lig.
Superior vesical a.
Lateral pubovesical lig.
Obturator canal
Cardinal lig.

PLATE 337

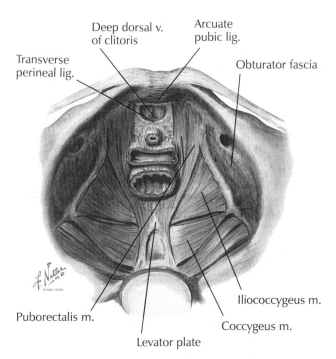

Deep dorsal v. of clitoris
Arcuate pubic lig.
Transverse perineal lig.
Obturator fascia
Puborectalis m.
Levator plate
Coccygeus m.
Iliococcygeus m.

PLATE 345

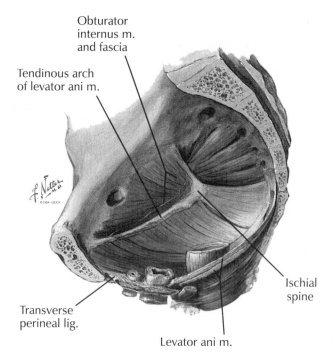

Obturator internus m. and fascia
Tendinous arch of levator ani m.
Transverse perineal lig.
Ischial spine
Levator ani m.

PLATE 337

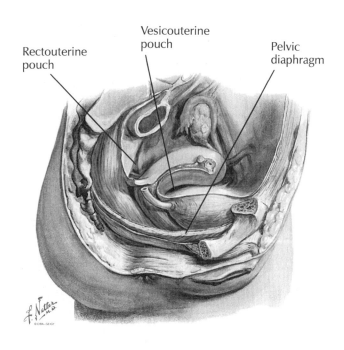

Rectouterine pouch
Vesicouterine pouch
Pelvic diaphragm

PLATE 341

REFLECT median umbilical ligament to one side.

EXAMINE retropubic (prevesical) space posterior to pubic bone and anterior to inferior lateral surface of bladder.

BLUNT DISSECT anterior to bladder, and remove areolar adipose tissue.

IDENTIFY inferior lateral and posterior surfaces (*not labeled*) of bladder.

IDENTIFY neck of **bladder** (*not labeled*) attached to **pelvic diaphragm**.

IDENTIFY medial and **lateral pubovesical ligaments** as condensation of visceral fascia between neck of bladder and pubic symphysis.

IDENTIFY deep dorsal vein of **clitoris** entering retropubic space between **arcuate pubic ligament** and **transverse perineal ligament**.

REFLECT viscera medially to expose obturator fascia and muscles forming pelvic diaphragm.

EXAMINE origin of iliacus muscle from iliac fossa in false (greater) pelvis.

REMOVE obturator fascia from internal surface of obturator internus muscle.

IDENTIFY tendinous arch of **levator ani muscle** formed from fascial attachment of pelvic diaphragm to deep fascia investing obturator internus muscle between spine of ischium and pubic bone.

IDENTIFY levator ani and **coccygeus muscles** forming pelvic diaphragm.

PLACE one hand in **ischiorectal fossa** (*not labeled*) and other hand on superior surface of levator ani muscle to establish plane of pelvic diaphragm that separates pelvic cavity from perineum.

IDENTIFY pudendal canal on inferior surface of pelvic diaphragm in relation to tendinous arch of levator ani muscle.

Bisected Pelvis

INSERT probe into urethra to establish median plane of pelvis.

SAW vertically through pubic symphysis.

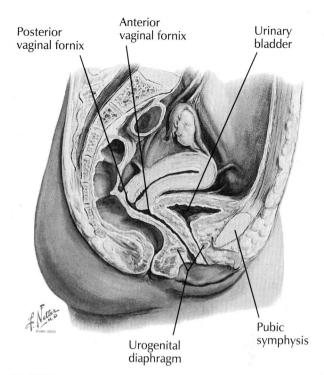

Posterior vaginal fornix · Anterior vaginal fornix · Urinary bladder · Urogenital diaphragm · Pubic symphysis

PLATE 341

SAW sacrum in median vertical plane.

EXTEND incision with scissors through pelvic diaphragm, bladder, uterus, rectum, and remaining soft tissue.

CLEAN interior of rectum by holding bisected pelvis under running water.

EXAMINE internal structures of rectum.

IDENTIFY transverse rectal folds. Note that these may be called **rectal valves**.

IDENTIFY anorectal line at pelvic diaphragm.

IDENTIFY anal columns (of **Morgagni**), **anal valves**, and **anal sinuses**.

REMOVE endopelvic fascia from structures in pelvis with forceps. Note that veins may be removed to facilitate following dissection.

TRACE superior rectal artery along posterior surface of rectum. Recall that this vessel was cut from its origin from inferior mesenteric artery during DISSECTION **4.3**.

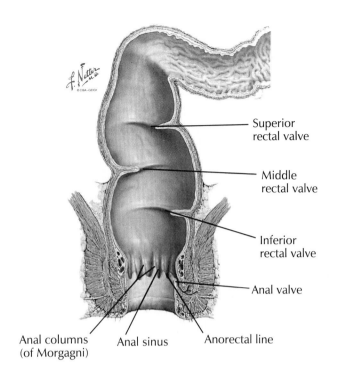

Superior
rectal valve

Middle
rectal valve

Inferior
rectal valve

Anal valve

Anal columns
(of Morgagni)   Anal sinus   Anorectal line

PLATE 369

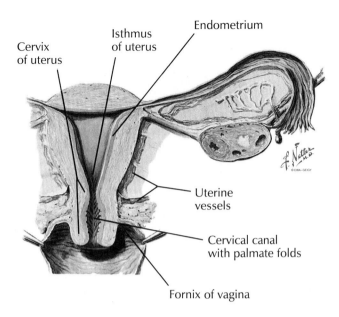

Cervix
of uterus

Isthmus
of uterus

Endometrium

Uterine
vessels

Cervical canal
with palmate folds

Fornix of vagina

PLATE 350

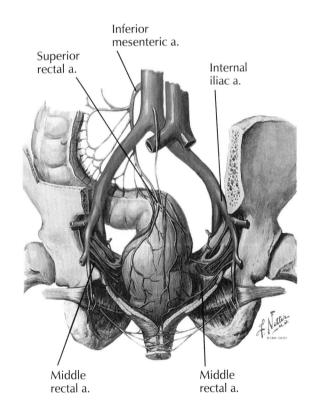

Inferior
mesenteric a.

Superior
rectal a.

Internal
iliac a.

Middle
rectal a.

Middle
rectal a.

PLATE 373

CLEAN branches of internal iliac artery to facilitate following dissection.

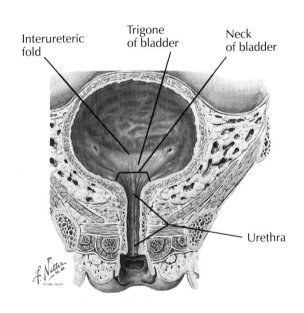

Interureteric
fold

Trigone
of bladder

Neck
of bladder

Urethra

PLATE 347

IDENTIFY middle rectal artery as it passes along superior surface of pelvic diaphragm.

TRACE middle rectal artery retrograde to its origin from internal iliac artery.

IDENTIFY scanty **rectovaginal fascia** (*not labeled*) between vagina and rectum.

EXAMINE uterus and associated structures.

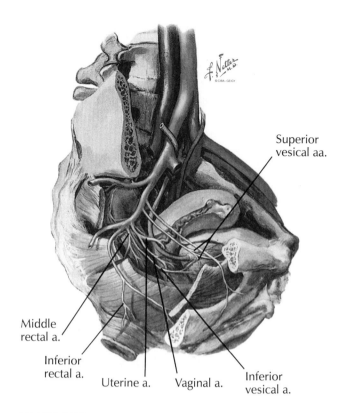

Superior
vesical aa.

Middle
rectal a.

Inferior
rectal a.

Uterine a.   Vaginal a.   Inferior
vesical a.

PLATE 377

INSPECT interior of uterus. Note that **endometrium** of fundus and body is smooth but **cervical canal** has **palmate folds**.

RETRACT bladder anteriorly and rectum posteriorly.

IDENTIFY cervix of **uterus** and **anterior** and **posterior fornices** of **vagina**. Note folds in vaginal wall.

TRACE uterine artery retrograde to its origin from internal iliac artery.

IDENTIFY vaginal artery (*not labeled*) as it originates from uterine artery to supply vagina and inferior part of cervix.

EXAMINE bladder and associated structures.

IDENTIFY trigone of **bladder** and opening of ureter into bladder. Note also bisected **interureteric fold** between entrances of right and left ureters.

DEFINE fundus, body, and **neck** of **bladder**. Note folds in mucosa of these areas.

INSPECT urethra. Note that it lies in anterior wall of vagina.

IDENTIFY inferior vesical artery on lateral inferior surface of bladder.

TRACE inferior vesical artery either to its origin from internal iliac artery or to trunk in common with middle rectal artery.

REVIEW following visceral branches of internal iliac artery: uterine, vaginal, superior and inferior vesical, and middle and inferior rectal.

FOLLOW parietal branches of internal iliac artery from their origins as listed below.

IDENTIFY superior gluteal artery as it exits pelvic cavity through greater sciatic foramen superior to piriformis muscle.

IDENTIFY inferior gluteal and **internal pudendal arteries** as they exit pelvic cavity through greater sciatic foramen inferior to piriformis muscle.

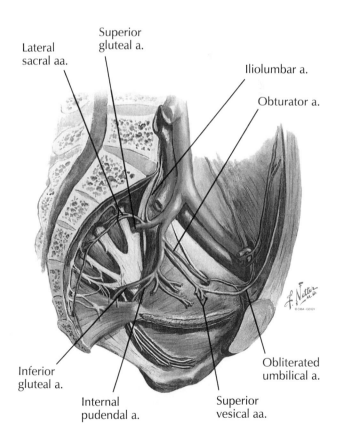

Lateral
sacral aa.

Superior
gluteal a.

Iliolumbar a.

Obturator a.

Inferior
gluteal a.

Internal
pudendal a.

Superior
vesical aa.

Obliterated
umbilical a.

PLATE 377

PLATE 387

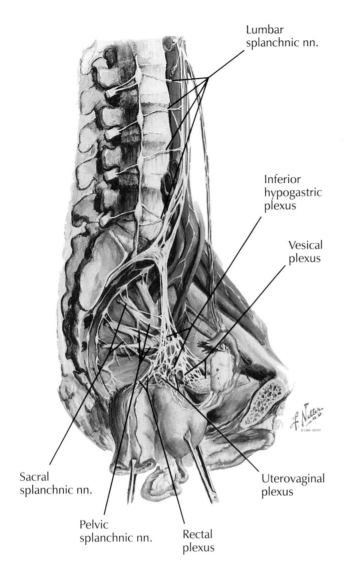

Lumbar
splanchnic nn.

Inferior
hypogastric
plexus

Vesical
plexus

Sacral
splanchnic nn.

Uterovaginal
plexus

Pelvic
splanchnic nn.

Rectal
plexus

IDENTIFY lateral sacral artery as it passes anterior to sacrum.

IDENTIFY iliolumbar artery as it passes superiorly over pelvic brim deep to common iliac artery. Its **iliac branch** (*not shown*) passes deep to psoas major muscle to supply iliacus muscle. Its **lumbar branch** (*not shown*) also passes deep to psoas major muscle to supply psoas major and quadratus lumborum muscles.

NOTE that obturator artery has already been identified.

EXAMINE nerve plexuses to pelvic structures.

REFLECT rectum, uterus, and bladder medially to expose **inferior hypogastric (pelvic) plexus**.

UNDERSTAND that different parts of pelvic plexus have regional names that correspond with organs being served.

LOOK for **pelvic splanchnic (parasympathetic) nerves** from ventral rami of spinal nerves S2–4.

LOOK for **lumbar splanchnic (sympathetic) nerves** from sympathetic trunk of vertebral levels L3, 4 and **sacral splanchnic (sympathetic) nerves** from sympathetic trunk of vertebral levels S2–4.

REIDENTIFY levator ani and coccygeus muscles and their superior and inferior fascial layers.

DISSECTION 7.4
MALE PELVIC ORGANS

Complete DISSECTION **7.2** Male Perineum.

Read DISCUSSIONS **7.1** Pelvic Diaphragm,
7.2 Urogenital Diaphragm, **7.6** Pelvic Organs,
7.8 Male Pelvic Organs, and **7.9** Arteries.

NOTE that bony pelvis with intact ligaments
should be placed beside and in same position as
cadaver.

REMEMBER that directions are given as though
cadaver were in anatomical position.

PLACE cadaver with perineum facing down. Try
to dissect pelvis in anatomical position.

DEFINE boundaries of **true pelvis** (*not labeled*)
below linea terminalis, which is formed by sacral
promontory, and iliopectineal line, which is
formed by arcuate line and pecten pubis.

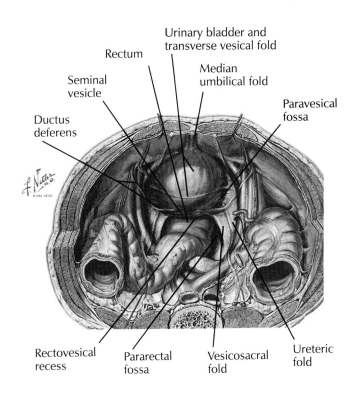

PLATE 344

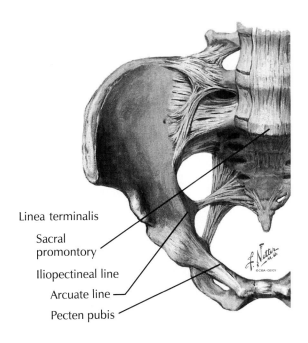

PLATE 335

INSPECT bladder and **rectum** with peritoneum
intact.

IDENTIFY superior surface of bladder with
peritoneum covering it and apex of bladder (*not
labeled*) with **median umbilical ligament** passing
superiorly from it.

EXAMINE folds and fossae in peritoneum over
pelvic structures.

IDENTIFY ureteric fold, which contains ureter.

IDENTIFY vesicosacral fold between posterior
surface of bladder and sacrum.

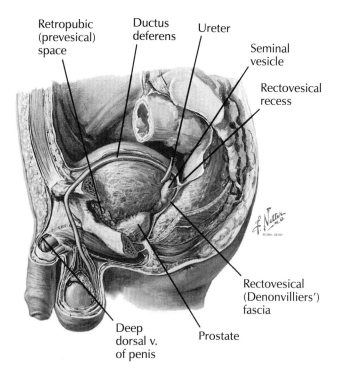

Retropubic (prevesical) space — Ductus deferens — Ureter — Seminal vesicle — Rectovesical recess — Rectovesical (Denonvilliers') fascia — Prostate — Deep dorsal v. of penis

PLATE 342

EXAMINE paravesical fossa anterior to fold covering ductus deferens.

EXAMINE pararectal fossa between vesicosacral fold and rectum.

EXAMINE rectovesical recess (space) anterior to rectum and posterior to bladder. Note that rectovesical fossa communicates with pararectal fossae on both sides.

PALPATE passage of ductus deferens across paravesical fossa to its descent posterior to bladder at rectovesical fold.

PALPATE seminal vesicles within rectovesical folds.

REMOVE peritoneum and endopelvic fascia from structures in pelvis with forceps.

NOTE that veins may be removed to facilitate dissection.

REVIEW passage of following structures from abdominal cavity into pelvis: testicular artery and vein, common iliac artery and vein, superior rectal artery and vein, and middle sacral artery and vein.

IDENTIFY internal iliac artery.

TRACE ductus deferens from deep inguinal ring as it passes superior to superior vesical artery and vein, obturator nerve and vessels, and ureter.

TRACE passage of **ureter** from anterior to internal iliac artery to posterior lateral surface of bladder.

TRACE obturator nerve (*not shown*) from medial to psoas major muscle to **obturator canal**.

IDENTIFY obturator artery at obturator canal inferior to obturator nerve.

TRACE umbilical artery from **medial umbilical ligament** to its origin from internal iliac artery.

IDENTIFY superior vesical arteries branching from umbilical artery to bladder.

REFLECT median umbilical ligament to one side.

PLATE 378

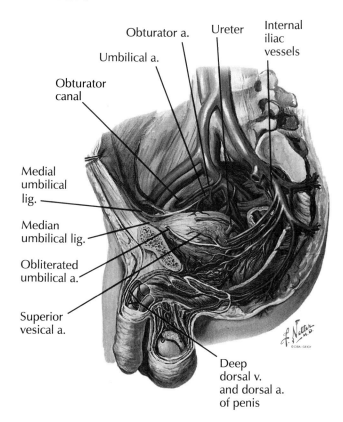

Obturator a. — Ureter — Internal iliac vessels — Umbilical a. — Obturator canal — Medial umbilical lig. — Median umbilical lig. — Obliterated umbilical a. — Superior vesical a. — Deep dorsal v. and dorsal a. of penis

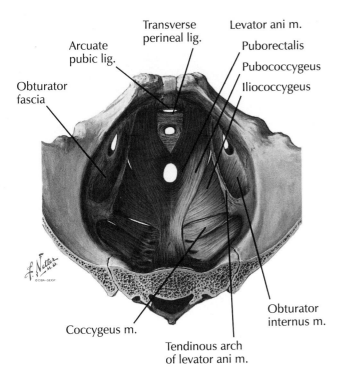

Obturator fascia

Arcuate pubic lig.

Transverse perineal lig.

Levator ani m.

Puborectalis

Pubococcygeus

Iliococcygeus

Coccygeus m.

Tendinous arch of levator ani m.

Obturator internus m.

PLATE 339

EXAMINE retropubic (prevesical) space posterior to pubic bone and anterior to inferior lateral surface of bladder.

BLUNT DISSECT anterior to bladder and remove areolar adipose tissue.

IDENTIFY inferior lateral and posterior surfaces of bladder (*not labeled*).

IDENTIFY prostate inferior to **neck** of **bladder** (*not labeled*).

IDENTIFY medial and **lateral puboprostatic ligaments** (*not shown*) as condensation of visceral fascia between neck of bladder and pubic symphysis.

IDENTIFY deep dorsal vein of **penis** entering retropubic space between **arcuate pubic ligament** and **transverse perineal ligament**.

BLUNT DISSECT posterior to bladder and prostate to locate **rectovesical (Denonvilliers') fascia** as vertical condensation of fascia anterior to rectum.

IDENTIFY seminal vesicles and terminal part of **ductus deferens** on posterior surface of bladder.

REFLECT viscera medially to expose obturator fascia and muscles forming pelvic diaphragm.

EXAMINE origin of **iliacus muscle** (*not shown*) from iliac fossa in false (greater) pelvis.

REMOVE obturator fascia from internal surface of obturator internus muscle.

IDENTIFY tendinous arch of **levator ani muscle** formed from fascial attachment of pelvic diaphragm to deep fascia investing obturator internus muscle between spine of ischium and pubic bone.

IDENTIFY levator ani and **coccygeus muscles** forming pelvic diaphragm.

PLACE one hand in **ischiorectal fossa** (*not labeled*) and other hand on superior surface of levator ani muscle to establish plane of pelvic diaphragm that separates pelvic cavity from perineum.

IDENTIFY pudendal canal on inferior surface of pelvic diaphragm in relation to tendinous arch of levator ani muscle.

Bisected Pelvis

INSERT probe into urethra to establish median plane of pelvis.

BISECT shaft and bulb of penis through **corpus spongiosum** from both dorsal and ventral surfaces of penis with scalpel.

SAW vertically through pubic symphysis.

SAW sacrum in median vertical plane.

EXTEND incision with scissors through pelvic diaphragm, bladder, rectum, and remaining soft tissue.

CLEAN interior of rectum by holding bisected pelvis under running water.

EXAMINE internal structures of rectum.

IDENTIFY transverse rectal folds. Note that these may be called **rectal valves**.

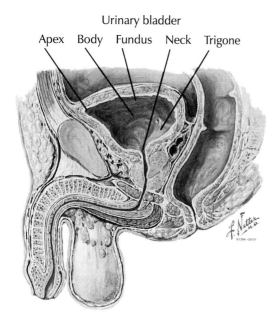

Urinary bladder

Apex Body Fundus Neck Trigone

PLATE 342

IDENTIFY **anorectal line** at pelvic diaphragm.

IDENTIFY **anal columns** (of **Morgagni**), **anal valves**, and **anal sinuses**.

TRACE **superior rectal artery** along posterior surface of rectum. Recall that this vessel was cut from its origin from inferior mesenteric artery.

IDENTIFY **middle rectal artery** as it passes along superior surface of pelvic diaphragm.

TRACE middle rectal artery to its origin from internal iliac artery.

REIDENTIFY **rectovesical (Denonvilliers') fascia** between rectum and posterior surfaces of prostate and bladder.

EXAMINE bladder and associated structures.

IDENTIFY **trigone** of **bladder** and opening of ureter into bladder. Note also **interureteric fold** between entrances of right and left ureters.

DEFINE **fundus, body,** and **neck** of **bladder** (*not labeled*). Note folds in mucosa of these areas.

IDENTIFY **inferior vesical artery** on lateral inferior surface of bladder.

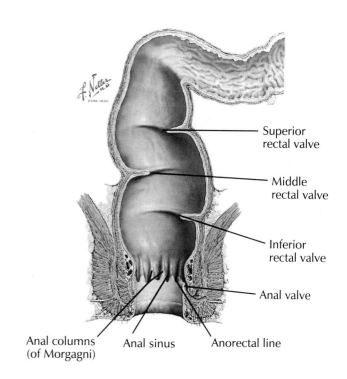

Superior rectal valve

Middle rectal valve

Inferior rectal valve

Anal valve

Anal columns (of Morgagni)   Anal sinus   Anorectal line

PLATE 369

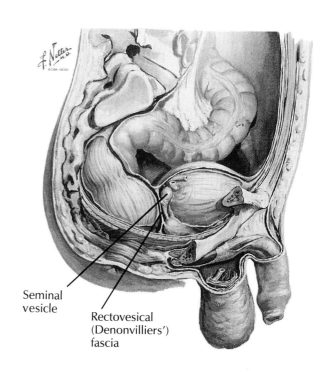

Seminal vesicle

Rectovesical (Denonvilliers') fascia

PLATE 367

TRACE inferior vesical artery to its origin from internal iliac artery or to trunk in common with middle rectal artery.

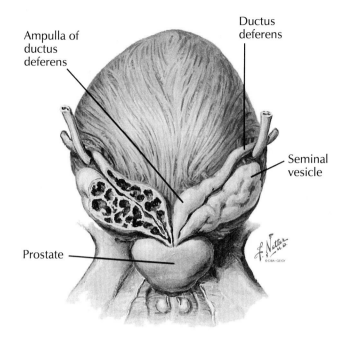

Ampulla of ductus deferens

Ductus deferens

Seminal vesicle

Prostate

PLATE 362

CONFIRM that inferior surface of prostate is supported by **urogenital diaphragm**.

EXAMINE lobulated interior of **seminal vesicle**.

TRACE excretory duct of **seminal vesicle** to its union with **ampulla** of **ductus deferens** to form **ejaculatory duct**.

TRACE ejaculatory duct through substance of prostate to its union with urethra.

EXAMINE posterior wall of **prostatic urethra** passing through prostate.

IDENTIFY medial **urethral crest**, **seminal colliculus**, and **prostatic utricle**.

IDENTIFY openings of **ejaculatory ducts** lateral to prostatic utricle.

IDENTIFY openings of **prostatic ducts** lateral to urethral crest in **prostatic sinus**.

EXAMINE membranous urethra passing through urogenital diaphragm.

EXAMINE spongy urethra passing through corpus spongiosum.

REVIEW following visceral branches of internal iliac artery: superior and inferior vesical, middle and inferior rectal, deferential, and prostatic.

FOLLOW parietal branches of internal iliac artery from their origin as listed below.

IDENTIFY superior gluteal artery as it exits pelvic cavity through greater sciatic foramen superior to piriformis muscle.

IDENTIFY inferior gluteal and **internal pudendal arteries** as they exit pelvic cavity through greater sciatic foramen inferior to piriformis muscle.

IDENTIFY lateral sacral artery as it passes anterior to sacrum.

IDENTIFY iliolumbar artery as it passes superiorly over pelvic brim deep to common iliac artery. Its **iliac branch** (*not shown*) passes deep to psoas major muscle to supply iliacus muscle. Its **lumbar branch** (*not shown*) also passes deep to psoas major muscle to supply psoas major and quadratus lumborum muscles.

PLATE 362

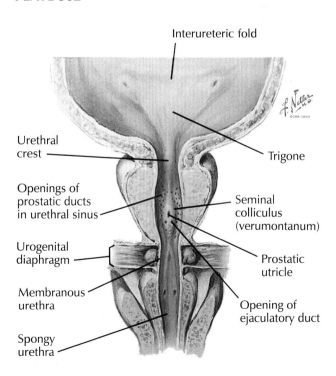

Interureteric fold

Urethral crest

Openings of prostatic ducts in urethral sinus

Urogenital diaphragm

Membranous urethra

Spongy urethra

Trigone

Seminal colliculus (verumontanum)

Prostatic utricle

Opening of ejaculatory duct

173

NOTE that obturator artery has already been identified.

EXAMINE nerve plexuses to pelvic structures.

RETRACT rectum, uterus, and bladder medially to expose **inferior hypogastric (pelvic) plexus.**

UNDERSTAND that different parts of pelvic plexus have regional names that correspond with organs being served.

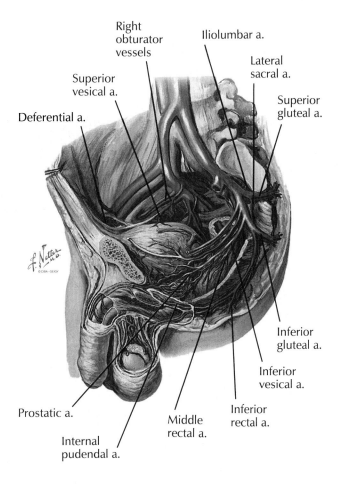

Right obturator vessels
Iliolumbar a.
Lateral sacral a.
Superior vesical a.
Superior gluteal a.
Deferential a.
Inferior gluteal a.
Inferior vesical a.
Prostatic a.
Internal pudendal a.
Middle rectal a.
Inferior rectal a.

PLATE 378

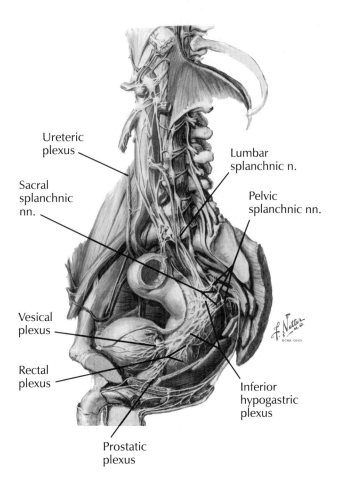

Ureteric plexus
Lumbar splanchnic n.
Sacral splanchnic nn.
Pelvic splanchnic nn.
Vesical plexus
Rectal plexus
Inferior hypogastric plexus
Prostatic plexus

PLATE 385

LOOK for **pelvic splanchnic (parasympathetic) nerves** from ventral rami of spinal nerves S2–4.

LOOK for **lumbar splanchnic (sympathetic) nerves** from sympathetic trunk of vertebral levels L3, 4 and **sacral splanchnic (sympathetic) nerves** from sympathetic trunk of vertebral levels S2–4.

REIDENTIFY levator ani and coccygeus muscles and their superior and inferior fascial layers.

Section 8

HEAD AND NECK

DISSECTIONS

DISSECTION 8.1
POSTERIOR CERVICAL TRIANGLE

Read DISCUSSIONS **8.2** Skull and **8.4** Posterior Cervical Triangle.

PLACE cadaver in supine position with boards under shoulders to extend neck.

PALPATE clavicle, acromion of **scapula, jugular notch** of **sternum, mastoid process** of **temporal bone, inferior margin** of **mandible,** and **hyoid bone.**

MARK location of cutaneous nerves and superficial veins on skin of neck with felt-tip marker.

CAUTION During skinning, preserve cutaneous nerves, superficial veins, and platysma muscle.

INCISE skin of neck (**Figure 33**). Note that dissection should be bilateral.

SKIN from anterior median cut. Note thinness of skin on neck. This step may take 30–45 minutes to do carefully.

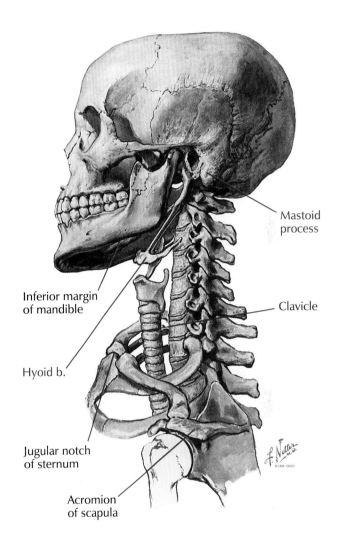

Mastoid process

Inferior margin of mandible

Clavicle

Hyoid b.

Jugular notch of sternum

Acromion of scapula

PLATE 9

REMOVE skin from both left and right sides of neck.

CAUTION As angle of mandible is approached, preserve cervical branch of facial nerve (VII).

CAUTION Preserve submandibular gland at inferior margin of mandible.

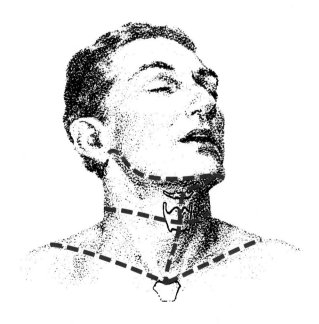

Figure 33

SEPARATE **platysma muscle** from structures deep to it, using closed scissors. Begin this separation where fibers of platysma muscle pass over clavicular origin of sternocleidomastoid muscle.

REFLECT platysma muscle superiorly.

DEFINE boundaries of **posterior cervical triangle** as posterior margin of sternocleidomastoid muscle, anterior margin of trapezius muscle, and middle 1/3 of clavicle.

NOTE that this dissection involves careful removal of substantial membranous fascia investing structures within neck. Note that this fascia is <u>deep</u> fascia investing muscles and their accompanying neurovascular components. Unfortunately, term commonly used for this fascia is "<u>superficial</u> cervical fascia."

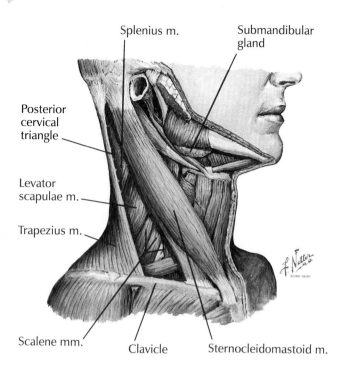

PLATE 22

PLATE 21

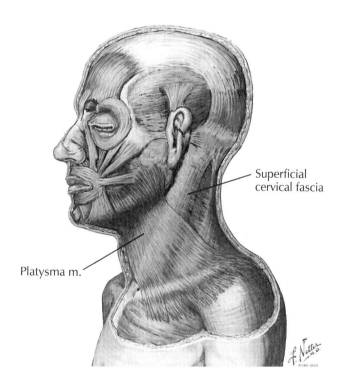

IDENTIFY **spinal accessory nerve (XI)** as it emerges from posterior margin of **sternocleido-mastoid muscle**, and trace spinal accessory nerve as it crosses posterior cervical triangle on surface of levator scapulae muscle to 2 finger-widths above clavicular attachment of anterior margin of trapezius muscle.

CAUTION   Preserve spinal accessory nerve during its cleaning.

REMOVE cervical fascia from around spinal accessory nerve in posterior cervical triangle.

IDENTIFY **lesser occipital nerve** (C2, 3) as it passes along posterior margin of sternocleido-mastoid muscle.

IDENTIFY **great auricular nerve** (C2, 3) as it accompanies external jugular vein superficial to sternocleidomastoid muscle toward parotid gland.

IDENTIFY **transverse cervical nerve** (C2, 3) as it crosses sternocleidomastoid muscle superficially toward thyroid gland to supply skin of anterior cervical triangle.

IDENTIFY medial, intermediate, and lateral branches of **supraclavicular nerves** (C3, 4). Note that medial supraclavicular nerve passes superficial to inferior part of sternocleidomastoid muscle, and intermediate supraclavicular nerve passes over clavicle and upper part of pectoralis major muscle. Lateral supraclavicular nerve passes over acromion and upper part of deltoid muscle.

IDENTIFY external jugular vein as it passes superficial to sternocleidomastoid muscle between angle of mandible and clavicle. Note that it communicates with anterior jugular vein, which will be examined in DISSECTION **8.2**.

CUT external jugular vein where it drains into **subclavian vein**, and reflect cut end of external jugular vein superiorly.

LOCATE external jugular lymph nodes (**lateral superficial cervical lymph nodes**) around vessel, and remove and discard them.

CAUTION   During following step, preserve omohyoid muscle.

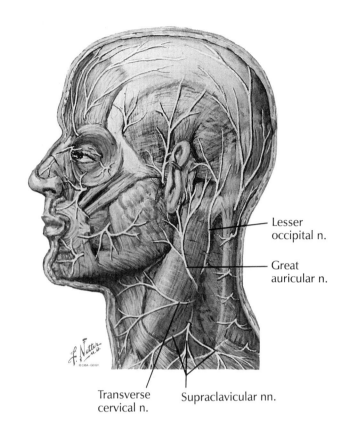

Lesser occipital n.

Great auricular n.

Transverse cervical n.

Supraclavicular nn.

PLATE 18

PLATE 27

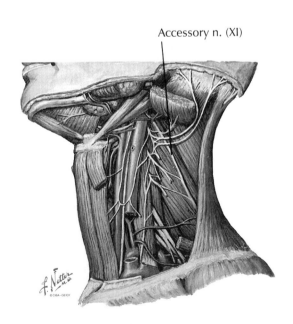

Accessory n. (XI)

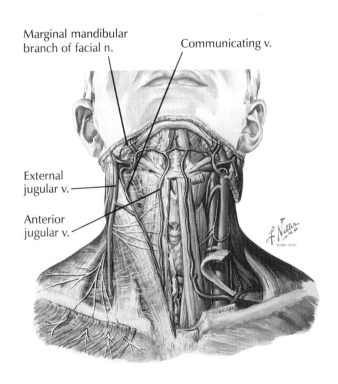

Marginal mandibular branch of facial n.

Communicating v.

External jugular v.

Anterior jugular v.

PLATE 26

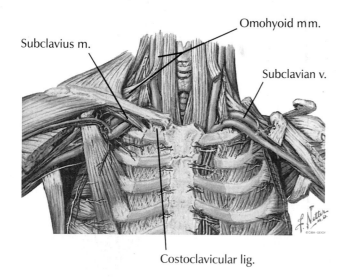

Subclavius m.

Omohyoid mm.

Subclavian v.

Costoclavicular lig.

PLATE 175 detail

BLUNT DISSECT deep to sternoclavicular origin of sternocleidomastoid muscle if DISSECTION **3.2** has <u>not</u> been completed.

DETACH clavicular and sternal heads of sternocleidomastoid muscle.

REMOVE subclavius muscle to facilitate dissection if DISSECTION **3.2** has <u>not</u> been completed.

IDENTIFY inferior belly of **omohyoid muscle**.

LOCATE intermediate tendon of omohyoid between its superior and inferior bellies and clavicle.

IDENTIFY costoclavicular ligament between cartilage of rib 1 and inferior surface of costal tubercle of clavicle if DISSECTION **5.7** has <u>not</u> been completed.

CUT clavicle at 2 points. Make lateral cut just medial to clavicular attachment of trapezius muscle, and make medial cut just lateral to clavicular attachment of sternoclavicular muscle. Note that clavicle was cut initially in DISSECTION **3.2**. Completing these 2 cuts facilitates dissection.

REMOVE middle section of clavicle.

CAUTION Preserve nerves as cleaning proceeds.

IDENTIFY splenius capitis muscle and levator scapulae muscle if DISSECTIONS **1.1** and **1.2** have <u>not</u> been completed.

IDENTIFY posterior scalene muscle (*not shown*). Note that it inserts to rib 2.

IDENTIFY anterior and **middle scalene muscles**. Note that both insert to rib 1.

SEVER intermediate tendon of **omohyoid** (*not shown*) to expose arteries and veins deep to it.

IDENTIFY subclavian vein, which passes anterior to anterior scalene muscle.

REMOVE subclavian vein to facilitate dissection.

IDENTIFY subclavian artery, which passes between anterior and middle scalene muscles.

IDENTIFY suprascapular vein, which passes posterior to clavicle, and **transverse cervical vein** (*not shown*), which passes toward back of neck.

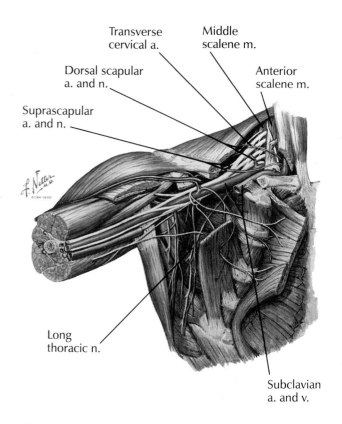

Transverse cervical a.

Middle scalene m.

Dorsal scapular a. and n.

Anterior scalene m.

Suprascapular a. and n.

Long thoracic n.

Subclavian a. and v.

PLATE 404

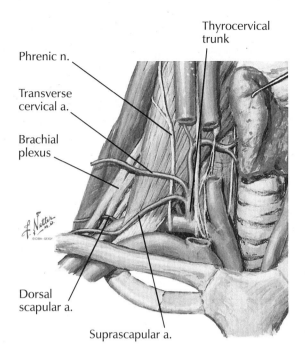

Phrenic n.

Transverse cervical a.

Brachial plexus

Thyrocervical trunk

Dorsal scapular a.

Suprascapular a.

PLATE 28

REMOVE suprascapular and transverse cervical veins to facilitate dissection.

IDENTIFY transverse cervical artery, which passes parallel to and 2 finger-widths above clavicle from **thyrocervical trunk** toward levator scapulae muscle. Note that thyrocervical trunk is branch of subclavian artery and that transverse cervical artery passes anterior to anterior scalene muscle.

TRACE superficial branch of **transverse cervical artery** (*not labeled*) deep to trapezius muscle.

TRACE deep branch of **transverse cervical artery** between levator scapulae and middle scalene muscles. Note that if deep branch originates directly from subclavian artery, it is called **dorsal scapular artery**.

IDENTIFY suprascapular artery as it passes anterior to anterior scalene muscle in lower part of posterior cervical triangle. Note that it accompanies suprascapular nerve near superior border of scapula and that it crosses anterior scalene muscle at lower level than transverse cervical artery does.

IDENTIFY phrenic nerve as it passes anterior to anterior scalene muscle to enter thorax. Note that it may be easier to trace phrenic nerve from thorax retrograde up through neck. Phrenic nerve passes deep to both transverse cervical and suprascapular arteries.

LOCATE roots of **brachial plexus** (ventral rami of C5–T1), which pass between anterior and middle scalene muscles.

TRACE formation of **superior, middle,** and **inferior trunks** of brachial plexus as roots pass anterior to middle scalene muscle.

IDENTIFY suprascapular nerve as branch of superior trunk (C5, 6) of brachial plexus. Note that no nerves originate from middle and inferior trunks of brachial plexus.

IDENTIFY dorsal scapular nerve, which is branch of C5 root. Note that its origin cannot be seen yet. Dorsal scapular and long thoracic nerves cross posterior scalene muscle, and dorsal scapular nerve and part of long thoracic nerve pierce middle scalene muscle.

REIDENTIFY long thoracic nerve (C5–7), which was examined in DISSECTION **5.1**.

DISSECTION 8.2
ANTERIOR CERVICAL TRIANGLE

Complete DISSECTION **8.1** Posterior Cervical Triangle.

Read DISCUSSION **8.5** Anterior Cervical Triangle.

PLACE cadaver in supine position with boards under shoulders to extend neck.

PALPATE clavicle, jugular notch of **sternum, mastoid** and **styloid processes** of **temporal bone, inferior margin** of **mandible, hyoid bone,** and **thyroid** and **cricoid cartilages.**

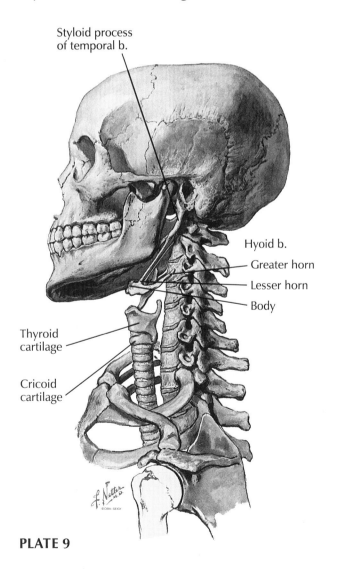

Styloid process
of temporal b.

Hyoid b.
— Greater horn
— Lesser horn
— Body

Thyroid
cartilage

Cricoid
cartilage

PLATE 9

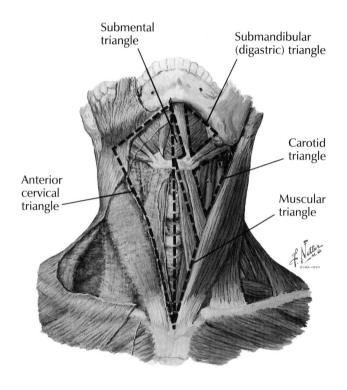

Submental
triangle

Submandibular
(digastric) triangle

Carotid
triangle

Anterior
cervical
triangle

Muscular
triangle

PLATE 23

DEFINE boundaries of **anterior cervical triangle** as anterior margin of sternocleidomastoid muscle, inferior margin of mandible, and anterior median line between jugular notch and mental symphysis of mandible.

DEFINE boundaries of following 4 triangles that are formed by omohyoid and digastric muscles within anterior cervical triangle.

DEFINE muscular triangle formed by superior belly of omohyoid muscle, anterior border of sternocleidomastoid muscle, and midline of neck.

DEFINE carotid triangle formed by superior belly of omohyoid muscle, anterior border of sternocleidomastoid muscle, and posterior belly of digastric muscle.

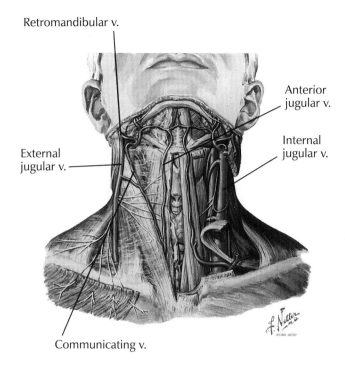

Retromandibular v.

Anterior jugular v.

Internal jugular v.

External jugular v.

Communicating v.

PLATE 26

DEFINE submandibular (digastric) triangle
formed by anterior and posterior bellies of
digastric muscle and inferior margin of mandible.
Note that there is communication between
digastric triangle and sublingual space of oral
cavity by gap between mylohyoid and hyoglossus
muscles.

DEFINE submental triangle formed by anterior
bellies of left and right digastric muscles and hyoid
bone. Note that submental triangle is shared by
both sides of neck.

IDENTIFY anterior jugular veins as they course
parallel to each other near midline of neck, and
communicating veins between anterior and
external jugular veins.

NOTE that this dissection involves careful removal
of deep investing fascia. Success requires
patience.

LOCATE connection (*not shown*) between right
and left anterior jugular veins in **suprasternal
space** (of **Burns**) superior to manubrium.

LOCATE anterior jugular lymph nodes (**anterior
superficial lymph nodes**, *not shown*), and remove
and discard them.

CUT anterior jugular veins near **mental symphysis**
of **mandible** (*not shown*).

CUT external jugular vein from **retromandibular
vein** and **posterior auricular vein** (*not shown*).

REMOVE anterior and external jugular veins to
facilitate dissection.

IDENTIFY costoclavicular ligament between
cartilage of rib 1 and inferior surface of costal
tubercle of clavicle if DISSECTION **8.1** has <u>not</u>
been completed.

CLEAN capsule of **sternoclavicular joint** if
DISSECTION **5.7** has <u>not</u> been completed.

OPEN sternoclavicular joint around entire
circumference with scalpel if DISSECTION **5.7**
has <u>not</u> been completed.

IDENTIFY articular disc between manubrium and
clavicle and rib 1 if DISSECTION **5.7** has <u>not</u> been
completed.

CAUTION During following step, free cutaneous
branches of cervical plexus.

BLUNT DISSECT deep to **sternocleidomastoid
muscle** to free fascial attachments.

REFLECT cut end of sternocleidomastoid muscle
as superiorly as possible.

NOTE that sensory nerve branches (*not shown*) to
sternocleidomastoid muscle, which pass directly
from 2 loops formed between C2, 3 and C3, 4,
must be cut to complete dissection. Branch from
occipital artery to sternocleidomastoid muscle
must also be cut. Note that artery to sternocleidomastoid muscle curves over hypoglossal
nerve (XII).

REMOVE any deep cervical lymph nodes that are
embedded in fascia deep to sternocleidomastoid
muscle.

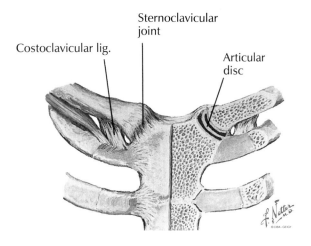

Costoclavicular lig.

Sternoclavicular joint

Articular disc

PLATE 395

CAUTION Preserve nerve loops forming ansa cervicalis, which may lie either superficial or deep to internal jugular vein.

IDENTIFY internal jugular vein deep to sternocleidomastoid muscle from posterior belly of digastric muscle to its union with subclavian vein to form brachiocephalic vein.

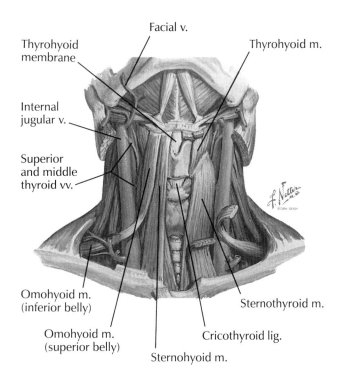

Thyrohyoid membrane

Facial v.

Thyrohyoid m.

Internal jugular v.

Superior and middle thyroid vv.

Omohyoid m. (inferior belly)

Omohyoid m. (superior belly)

Sternohyoid m.

Cricothyroid lig.

Sternothyroid m.

PLATE 24

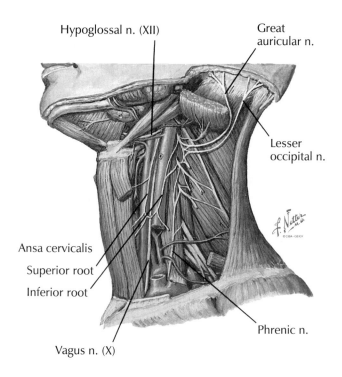

Hypoglossal n. (XII)

Great auricular n.

Lesser occipital n.

Ansa cervicalis
Superior root
Inferior root

Phrenic n.

Vagus n. (X)

PLATE 27

LOCATE internal jugular lymph nodes (deep lateral cervical lymph nodes, *not shown*), and remove and discard them.

LOCATE sites of drainage of **common facial, lingual, superior,** and **middle thyroid veins** into internal jugular vein. These tributaries, but not internal jugular vein, may be removed to expose field of dissection.

IDENTIFY body and **greater** and **lesser horns** of **hyoid bone, thyroid** and **cricohyoid cartilages, thyrohyoid membrane,** and **cricothyroid ligament** on skeleton and cadaver.

IDENTIFY infrahyoid muscles by their attachments.

RELOCATE inferior belly of **omohyoid muscle** and its origin from scapula, and review its insertion to clavicle by its intermediate tendon, which was cut in DISSECTION **8.1**.

IDENTIFY superior belly of **omohyoid muscle,** review its origin from clavicle by its intermediate tendon, and locate its insertion to body of hyoid bone.

IDENTIFY sternohyoid muscle, its origin from manubrium, and its insertion to body of hyoid bone.

RETRACT sternohyoid muscle and superior belly of omohyoid muscle laterally or medially to expose deeper infrahyoid muscles.

IDENTIFY sternothyroid muscle, its origin from manubrium, and its insertion to oblique line of thyroid cartilage.

IDENTIFY thyrohyoid muscle, its origin from oblique line of thyroid cartilage, and its insertion to body of hyoid bone.

LOCATE nerves to sternohyoid and sternothyroid muscles and superior belly of omohyoid muscle. Note that these nerves approach muscles posteriorly.

TRACE these nerves retrograde to their origins from **ansa cervicalis**.

LOCATE nerve to thyrohyoid muscle, and trace its origin retrograde to **hypoglossal nerve (XII)**. Note that nerve to thyrohyoid muscle originates from spinal nerve C1 and accompanies hypoglossal nerve. Note that hypoglossal nerve passes inferior to posterior belly of digastric muscle, external to internal carotid artery, and between mylohyoid and hyoglossus muscles.

ELEVATE superior part of internal jugular vein to facilitate following step.

TRACE superior root of **ansa cervicalis** to loop between C1, 2 and **inferior root** to loop between C2, 3. Note that superior root passes deep to posterior belly of digastric muscle and joins hypoglossal nerve, which will be inspected further within oral cavity in DISSECTION **8.10**.

LOCATE loop between spinal nerves C2, 3, and trace origin of **lesser occipital**, **great auricular**, and **transverse cervical nerves** distal from it. Note that these cutaneous branches of cervical plexus were inspected in DISSECTION **8.1**.

LOCATE loop between spinal nerves C3, 4, and trace origin of trunk of medial, lateral, and intermediate supraclavicular nerves from it.

IDENTIFY origins of **phrenic nerve** from C3–5.

NOTE that you may be able to locate branches to scalene, longus colli, and rectus capitis muscles directly from ventral rami of cervical plexus levels C2–4.

SEVER sternohyoid and sternothyroid muscles from manubrium.

REFLECT sternohyoid muscle and superior belly of omohyoid muscle superiorly.

SEVER thyrohyoid muscle from hyoid bone.

REFLECT thyrohyoid muscle inferiorly toward thyroid cartilage.

CAUTION   As fascia of carotid sheath is dissected free from its contents, preserve vagus nerve (X) within carotid sheath and sympathetic trunk deep to carotid sheath.

CLEAN common carotid artery to its division into **external** and **internal carotid arteries**.

IDENTIFY carotid sinus (*not shown*) and **carotid sinus branch** of **glossopharyngeal nerve (IX)**.

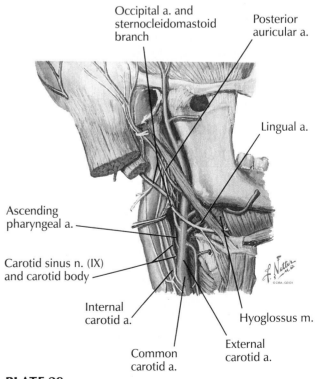

Occipital a. and sternocleidomastoid branch

Posterior auricular a.

Lingual a.

Ascending pharyngeal a.

Carotid sinus n. (IX) and carotid body

Internal carotid a.

Common carotid a.

External carotid a.

Hyoglossus m.

PLATE 29

185

SEVER posterior belly of digastric muscle and stylohyoid muscle from lesser horn of hyoid bone. Cut both muscles approximately 1 finger-width lateral to their attachment to hyoid bone to preserve intermediate tendon of digastric, which will be examined later.

REFLECT posterior bellies of digastric and stylohyoid muscles superiorly to expose structures deep to them.

IDENTIFY branches of external carotid artery.

LOCATE origin of **superior thyroid artery** from anterior surface of external carotid artery slightly inferior to greater horn of hyoid bone.

TRACE superior thyroid artery to thyroid gland.

TRACE superior laryngeal branch of **superior thyroid artery** to where it pierces thyrohyoid membrane.

PLATE 63

LOCATE origin of **ascending pharyngeal artery** from medial surface of external carotid artery. Note that this artery is named for its ascent between internal carotid artery and pharynx.

LOCATE origin of **lingual artery** on anterior surface of external carotid artery posterior to greater horn of hyoid bone.

TRACE lingual artery to where it passes deep to **hyoglossus muscle**.

NOTE that hyoglossus muscle will be studied in DISSECTION **8.10**. Its origin from greater horn of hyoid bone is visible in anterior cervical triangle.

LOCATE origin of **facial artery** from anterior surface of external carotid artery, slightly superior to origin of lingual artery, or from common trunk with lingual artery.

TRACE facial artery to its passage deep to reflected posterior belly of digastric muscle. Note that facial artery passes deep to **submandibular gland**, which is supplied by its branches.

RECALL that **facial vein** passes posterior to facial artery as they cross inferior margin of mandible. Facial vein is superficial to submandibular gland.

CAUTION Preserve submental branch of facial artery, which lies close to submandibular gland.

PLATE 30

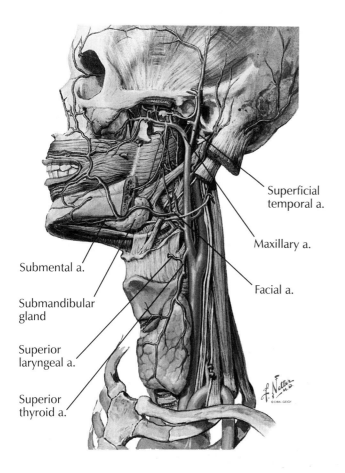

Superficial temporal a.

Maxillary a.

Submental a.

Facial a.

Submandibular gland

Superior laryngeal a.

Superior thyroid a.

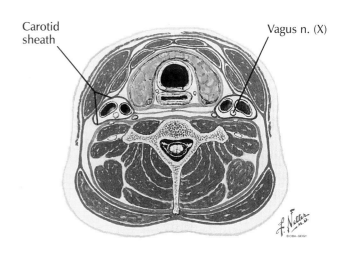

Carotid sheath

Vagus n. (X)

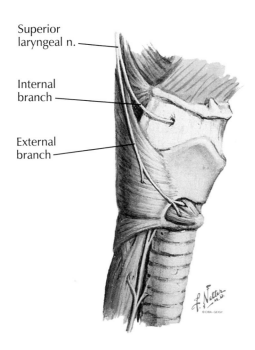

Superior
laryngeal n.

Internal
branch

External
branch

PLATE 74

LOCATE submental branch of **facial artery** anteriorly. Note that submental artery accompanies nerve to mylohyoid (V_3).

LOCATE origin of occipital artery on posterior surface of external carotid artery close to posterior belly of digastric muscle.

TRACE occipital artery to where it passes deep to posterior belly of digastric muscle.

NOTE that branch of occipital artery that hooks over hypoglossal nerve to supply sternocleido-mastoid muscle was cut during reflection of muscle.

NOTE that origin of posterior auricular artery from posterior surface of external carotid artery just superior to posterior belly of digastric muscle will be examined in DISSECTION **8.5**.

NOTE that maxillary and superficial temporal arteries (2 terminal branches of external carotid) will be studied in DISSECTIONS **8.4** and **8.5**.

SEPARATE internal jugular vein and internal carotid artery by retracting internal jugular vein laterally and internal carotid artery medially.

BLUNT DISSECT vagus nerve (X) free from **fascia** of **carotid sheath**.

TRACE internal laryngeal nerve retrograde from where it passes through thyrohyoid membrane just inferior to greater horn of hyoid bone to its origin from **superior laryngeal nerve**, which is branch of vagus nerve. Note that internal laryngeal nerve passes superficial to middle pharyngeal constrictor muscle and deep to thyrohyoid muscle.

CAUTION During next step, preserve cervical sympathetic trunk.

TRACE superior laryngeal nerve retrograde to its origin from vagus nerve. Note that superior laryngeal nerve passes deep to external and internal carotid arteries.

IDENTIFY cut end of **common facial vein**, which passes superficial to posterior belly of digastric and stylohyoid muscles.

TRACE formation of common facial vein retrograde to facial vein.

PLATE 55

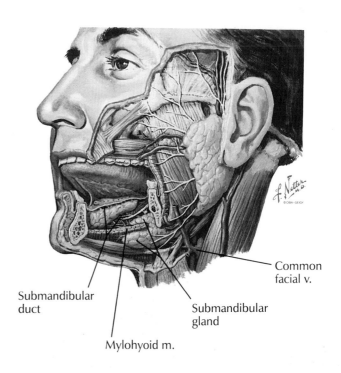

Common facial v.

Submandibular duct

Submandibular gland

Mylohyoid m.

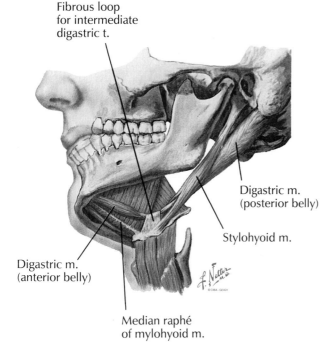

Fibrous loop
for intermediate
digastric t.

Digastric m.
(posterior belly)

Stylohyoid m.

Digastric m.
(anterior belly)

Median raphé
of mylohyoid m.

f. Netter
©CIBA-GEIGY

PLATE 47

CUT all branches of facial artery to and tributaries of facial vein from submandibular gland.

IDENTIFY superficial part of **submandibular gland**.

RETRACT submandibular gland by gently pulling it inferiorly from submandibular triangle to expose **submandibular duct**, which passes deep to mylohyoid muscle. Note that deep part of submandibular gland accompanies its duct and will be inspected in DISSECTION **8.10**.

TRANSECT superficial part of submandibular gland external to **mylohyoid muscle**.

REMOVE superficial part of submandibular gland.

REPLACE posterior bellies of digastric and stylohyoid muscles to perform following steps.

IDENTIFY anterior and posterior bellies of **digastric muscle**. Note that origin of anterior belly is digastric fossa of mandible and origin of posterior belly is mastoid notch of temporal bone.

LOCATE insertion of **intermediate tendon** of **digastric**, which passes through tendon of stylohyoid and attaches near junction of greater horn and body of hyoid bone.

IDENTIFY stylohyoid muscle. Note that its origin is styloid process of temporal bone and that its tendon of insertion is pierced by intermediate tendon of digastric.

LOOK for branches of **facial nerve** (VII, *not shown*) to posterior bellies of digastric and stylohyoid muscles by separating muscles and gently pulling both inferiorly to expose their nerves.

LOOK for branch of **nerve** to **mylohoid** (V₃) to anterior belly of digastric muscle by gently pulling muscle inferiorly to expose nerve.

IDENTIFY left and right **mylohyoid muscles** and their **median raphé**. Note attachments of mylohyoid muscle to **mylohyoid line** of **mandible** and hyoid bone.

LOCATE nerve to mylohyoid superficial to mylohyoid muscle along margin of body of mandible.

DISSECTION 8.3
ROOT OF NECK

Complete DISSECTIONS **8.1** Posterior Cervical Triangle and **8.2** Anterior Cervical Triangle.

Read DISCUSSION **8.6** Root of Neck.

PLACE cadaver in supine position with boards under shoulders to extend neck.

NOTE that dissection is to be completed bilaterally.

PALPATE thyroid cartilage.

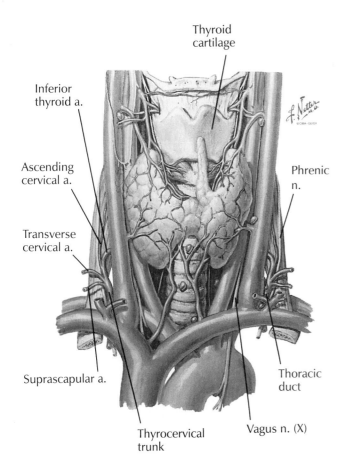

Thyroid cartilage

Inferior thyroid a.

Ascending cervical a.

Transverse cervical a.

Phrenic n.

Suprascapular a.

Thoracic duct

Thyrocervical trunk

Vagus n. (X)

PLATE 68

BLUNT DISSECT deep to manubrium to free attached fascia if DISSECTION **3.1** has <u>not</u> been completed.

REMOVE cut medial end of clavicle and manubrium from field of dissection.

IDENTIFY cut ends of **subclavian veins** draining into **brachiocephalic veins**.

IDENTIFY vertebral veins (*not shown*), which descend anterior to **vertebral** and **subclavian arteries** to join subclavian vein.

IDENTIFY thoracic duct as it empties into beginning of left brachiocephalic vein at union of **internal jugular vein** and subclavian vein. Note that thoracic duct passes between vertebral vessels and carotid arteries before descending anterior to <u>left</u> **phrenic nerve**.

RELOCATE thoracic duct in thorax, and trace it toward its termination to confirm its identification.

CUT vertebral vein as high as possible in neck.

REMOVE internal jugular, vertebral, and subclavian veins to facilitate dissection.

IDENTIFY origin of vertebral artery from 1st part of subclavian artery.

LOCATE passage of vertebral artery into transverse foramen of C6. Note that further course of vertebral artery will be examined in DISSECTION **8.8**.

RELOCATE transverse cervical and **suprascapular arteries**.

TRACE transverse cervical and suprascapular arteries retrograde to their origins from **thyrocervical trunk**. Note that thyrocervical trunk originates from 1st part of subclavian artery.

TRACE inferior thyroid artery from its origin from thyrocervical trunk to its passage posterior to common carotid artery to supply thyroid gland.

TRACE origin of **ascending cervical artery** from inferior thyroid artery. Note that ascending cervical artery is named for its ascent on anterior surface of **anterior scalene muscle**.

IDENTIFY origin of cut end of **internal thoracic artery** from inferior surface of 1st part of subclavian artery.

OBSERVE that phrenic nerve, **vagus nerve (X)**, and vertebral vein pass anterior to 1st part of subclavian artery.

CAUTION During next step, preserve structures deep to anterior scalene muscle.

RETRACT phrenic nerve medially.

SEVER insertion of anterior scalene muscle to rib 1.

REFLECT anterior scalene muscle superiorly.

PLATE 28

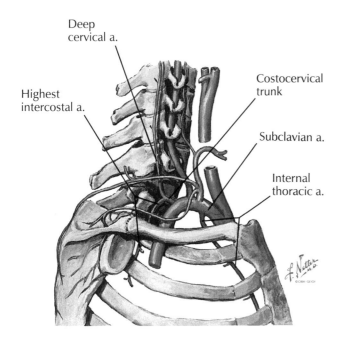

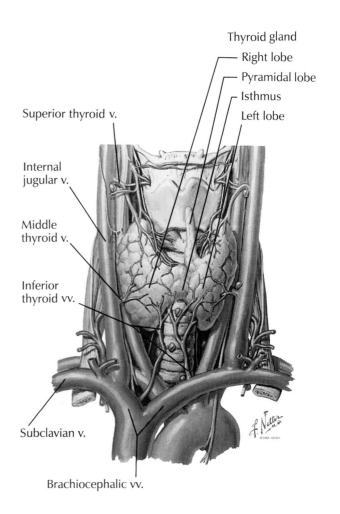

Thyroid gland
— Right lobe
— Pyramidal lobe
— Isthmus
— Left lobe

Superior thyroid v.

Internal jugular v.

Middle thyroid v.

Inferior thyroid vv.

Subclavian v.

Brachiocephalic vv.

PLATE 68

CAUTION During following steps, preserve sympathetic trunk running deep to structures to be examined.

IDENTIFY costocervical trunk deep to insertion of anterior scalene muscle. Note that costocervical trunk is branch of 2nd part of subclavian artery.

TRACE origin of **deep cervical artery** from costocervical trunk, and note that it goes deep to **middle scalene muscle**.

TRACE origin of **highest intercostal artery** from costocervical trunk to its descent to intercostal spaces 1–2, where it forms first 2 posterior intercostal arteries. Note that it may have been cut in thorax during earlier dissections.

NOTE that 1st and 2nd parts of subclavian artery pass anterior to cervical parietal pleura (cupula) over apex of lung.

OBSERVE that usually no branches originate from 3rd part of subclavian artery. Occasionally **dorsal scapular artery** or suprascapular artery may arise from it.

EXAMINE **thyroid gland** and associated structures.

IDENTIFY **lateral lobes** and **median isthmus** of **thyroid gland**. Note that isthmus passes anterior to tracheal rings 3, 4.

LOOK for inconstant **pyramidal lobe** of **thyroid gland**, which ascends from isthmus toward hyoid bone.

RETRACE **superior thyroid artery** retrograde from thyroid gland to confirm origin from **external carotid artery**.

RETRACE **inferior thyroid artery** retrograde from thyroid gland to confirm origin from thyrocervical trunk.

TRACE **inferior thyroid veins** to their union and drainage into left brachiocephalic vein.

TRANSECT isthmus of thyroid gland.

BLUNT DISSECT deep to lateral lobes of thyroid gland.

REFLECT medial cut ends of lateral lobes of thyroid gland laterally to expose trachea.

LOOK for pale-colored **parathyroid glands** embedded in posterior surface of lateral lobes of thyroid gland. Note 2 superior and 2 inferior parathyroid glands; these may be very difficult to see in cadaver.

INSPECT C-shaped semirings of cartilage that form skeleton of **trachea**.

CAUTION During next step, preserve recurrent laryngeal nerves.

ELEVATE trachea from anterior surface of **esophagus** to expose fibroelastic and muscular connections.

NOTE muscle fibers joining free ends of cartilage rings posteriorly in trachea.

CLEAN anterior surface of esophagus to observe its outer longitudinal layer of muscle.

IDENTIFY **recurrent laryngeal nerve**, which passes between trachea and esophagus.

TRACE <u>right</u> recurrent laryngeal nerve retrograde to its origin from vagus nerve as vagus crosses 1st part of <u>right</u> subclavian artery.

TRACE <u>left</u> recurrent laryngeal nerve retrograde to its origin from vagus nerve as vagus crosses arch of aorta.

BLUNT DISSECT deep to esophagus to establish **retropharyngeal space** (*not shown*). Continue this dissection posterior to esophagus down into thorax to free esophagus until its cut end is mobile. Note that retropharyngeal space extends to mediastinum.

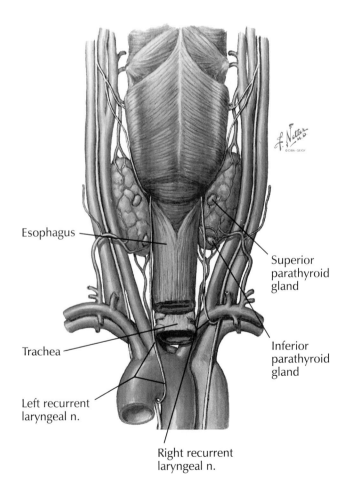

Esophagus

Superior parathyroid gland

Trachea

Inferior parathyroid gland

Left recurrent laryngeal n.

Right recurrent laryngeal n.

PLATE 69

EXAMINE sympathetic trunk in neck.

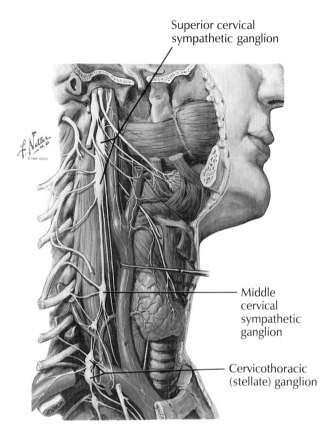

Superior cervical
sympathetic ganglion

Middle
cervical
sympathetic
ganglion

Cervicothoracic
(stellate) ganglion

PLATE 124

IDENTIFY inferior cervical sympathetic ganglion, and determine whether it is fused with 1st thoracic paravertebral sympathetic ganglion to form **cervicothoracic (stellate) sympathetic ganglion**.

LOOK for inconstant **middle cervical sympathetic ganglion** at level of cricoid cartilage.

IDENTIFY superior cervical sympathetic ganglion at vertebral level C1, 2.

SEVER connection between sympathetic ganglia and vagus nerve on right side.

BLUNT DISSECT anterior to right sympathetic trunk to preserve its relationship with prevertebral muscles.

BLUNT DISSECT posterior to left sympathetic trunk to preserve its connections with vagus nerve and its relationship with viscera.

CUT left sympathetic trunk just distal to stellate ganglion to mobilize left cervical sympathetic trunk with great vessels and nerves on left side of neck.

NOTE that separation of visceral and somatic neck will be completed in DISSECTION **8.8**.

DISSECTION 8.4

SUPERFICIAL FACE AND SCALP

Read DISCUSSIONS **8.1** Surface Anatomy, **8.2** Skull, and **8.7** Superficial Face and Scalp.

NOTE that dried skull should be kept at dissection table for reference.

IDENTIFY individual bones and labeled bony landmarks (**Plates 1, 2,** and **4**).

IDENTIFY sutures in skull of adult and fontanelles in neonate (**Plate 8**).

MARK location of cutaneous nerves on skin with felt-tip marker (**Plate 18**).

PLACE cadaver in supine position to skin face.

TURN cadaver to prone position to complete skinning scalp posterior to bregma.

NOTE that skinning time is extremely long because it must be done carefully.

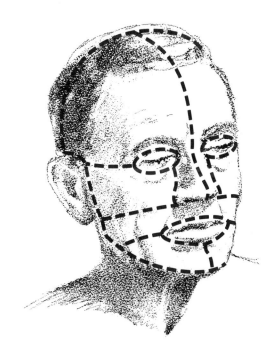

Figure 34

INCISE skin of face and scalp (**Figure 34**). Do not remove skin of eyelids, lips, and auricles yet.

CAUTION During skinning, preserve cutaneous branches of trigeminal nerve (V) and branches of facial nerve (VII) to muscles of facial expression.

BEGIN vertical median incision at bregma to establish layers of scalp and to determine plane between skin and subcutaneous tissue.

ESTABLISH plane between skin and **platysma muscle** at inferior margin of body of mandible.

REFLECT skin laterally from initial vertical incision over face, using scalpel to separate skin carefully from insertion of muscles to skin. Continue skinning laterally to coronal incision between auricle and bregma and inferiorly to plane between skin and platysma muscle. Note that area around bregma has very little subcutaneous tissue.

REMOVE skin of face and discard it.

ESTABLISH plane between subcutaneous tissue and **galea aponeurotica** with its attaching **frontalis** and **occipitalis muscles**.

CAUTION During following steps, preserve superficial temporal artery and vein over temporal region and greater and lesser occipital nerves and occipital artery over posterior skull.

REFLECT skin and subcutaneous tissue of scalp posterior to bregma.

REMOVE skin of scalp and discard it.

IDENTIFY individual **muscles** of **facial expression**. Note that emphasis of preservation of muscles is to be on <u>right</u> side of face.

NOTE that small veins should be removed from muscles to facilitate observation.

NOTE that emphasis of preservation of nerves and arteries is to be on <u>left</u> side of face.

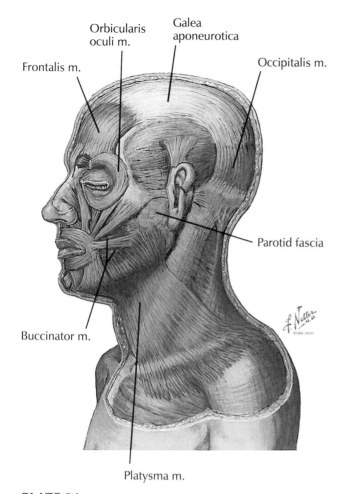

Frontalis m.

Orbicularis oculi m.

Galea aponeurotica

Occipitalis m.

Parotid fascia

Buccinator m.

Platysma m.

PLATE 21

CAUTION   During next step, preserve facial artery and vein and branches of facial nerve.

BLUNT DISSECT deep to insertion of platysma muscle over lower border of mandible.

REMOVE platysma muscle and discard it.

IDENTIFY parotid fascia investing **parotid gland**, and identify **masseter muscle**.

CAUTION   During next step, preserve zygomatic and buccal branches of facial nerve (VII).

LOCATE parotid duct, which emerges from anterior surface of parotid gland and passes 2 finger-widths inferior to and parallel with zygomatic arch.

TRACE parotid duct deep toward cheek by removing **buccal fat pad** (*not shown*). Note that parotid duct pierces **buccinator muscle**.

EXAMINE following branches of facial nerve.

LOCATE temporal and **zygomatic branches** of **facial nerve** (**VII**) as they emerge from superior margin of parotid gland.

LOCATE buccal and **mandibular branches** of **facial nerve** (**VII**) as they emerge from anterior margin of parotid gland.

TRACE cervical branch of **facial nerve** (**VII**) from margin of mandible to where it emerges from inferior margin of parotid gland. Recall that cervical branch supplies platysma muscle.

TRACE temporal branch as it passes superiorly toward temporal region to supply **superior** and **anterior auricular muscles**.

TRACE zygomatic branch as it passes over **zygomatic bone** to supply **orbicularis oculi muscle**.

TRACE buccal branches as they pass over cheek to supply buccinator muscle and muscles of upper lip and nostril. Note that buccal branches pass lateral to masseter muscle.

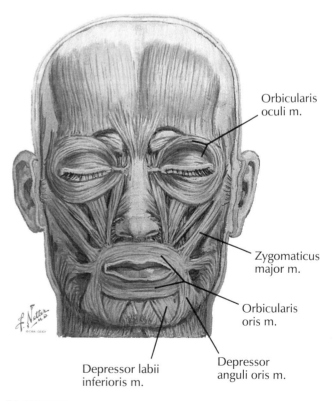

Orbicularis oculi m.

Zygomaticus major m.

Orbicularis oris m.

Depressor labii inferioris m.

Depressor anguli oris m.

PLATE 20

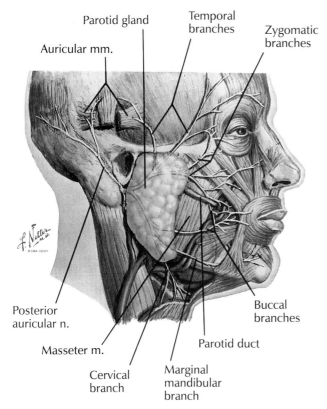

Parotid gland
Temporal branches
Zygomatic branches
Auricular mm.
Posterior auricular n.
Masseter m.
Cervical branch
Marginal mandibular branch
Parotid duct
Buccal branches

PLATE 19

TRACE mandibular branch as it passes along margin of mandible to supply **depressor anguli oris** and **depressor labii inferioris muscles.**

NOTE that facial nerve will be traced retrograde through substance of parotid gland to establish passage of its trunks in DISSECTION **8.5.** Posterior auricular branch will be considered then.

TRACE facial vein from angle of eye to where it crosses inferior margin of mandible.

NOTE that facial vein is joined by anterior branch of **retromandibular vein** to form internal jugular vein. Posterior branch of retromandibular vein joins **posterior auricular vein** to form external jugular vein. Origin of retromandibular vein will be examined in DISSECTION **8.5.**

TRACE facial artery from anterior border of masseter muscle to angle of eye where it is called **angular artery.**

LOCATE origins of **superior** and **inferior labial** and **lateral nasal arteries** as they branch from facial artery.

LOCATE superficial temporal artery and **vein** as they pass anterior to ear.

IDENTIFY frontal and **parietal branches** of **superficial temporal artery.**

LOOK for origin of **middle temporal artery** as it branches from superficial temporal artery and pierces fascia over temporal muscle. Note that middle temporal artery comes off immediately after superficial temporal artery emerges from parotid gland.

NOTE that origin of superficial temporal artery from external carotid artery and drainage of superficial temporal vein into retromandibular vein will be examined in DISSECTION **8.5.**

LOCATE transverse facial artery as it passes superior and parallel to parotid duct. Note that transverse facial artery branches from superficial temporal artery.

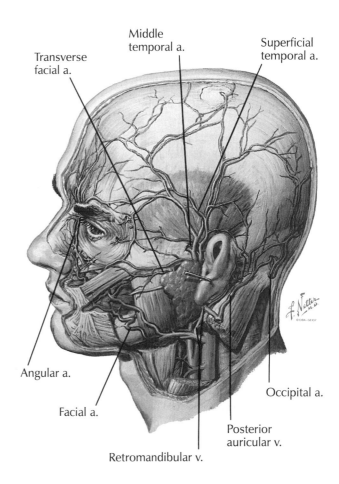

Transverse facial a.
Middle temporal a.
Superficial temporal a.
Angular a.
Facial a.
Retromandibular v.
Posterior auricular v.
Occipital a.

PLATE 17

195

EXAMINE following cutaneous branches of **trigeminal nerve (V)**.

IDENTIFY auriculotemporal nerve (V₃), which accompanies superficial temporal artery.

IDENTIFY supraorbital nerve (V₁) as it exits supraorbital foramen or notch.

IDENTIFY supratrochlear nerve (V₁) as it passes superior to medial angle of orbit.

IDENTIFY infratrochlear nerve (V₁) as it passes medial to angle of orbit just inferior to supratrochlear nerve.

IDENTIFY external nasal nerve (V₁) as it emerges between nasal bone and nasal cartilages.

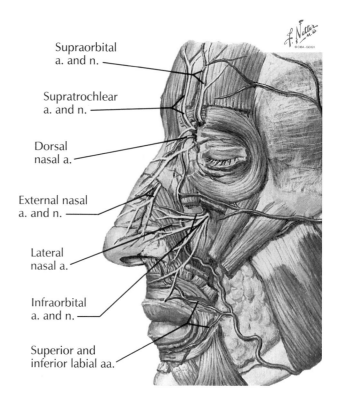

Supraorbital a. and n.

Supratrochlear a. and n.

Dorsal nasal a.

External nasal a. and n.

Lateral nasal a.

Infraorbital a. and n.

Superior and inferior labial aa.

PLATE 31

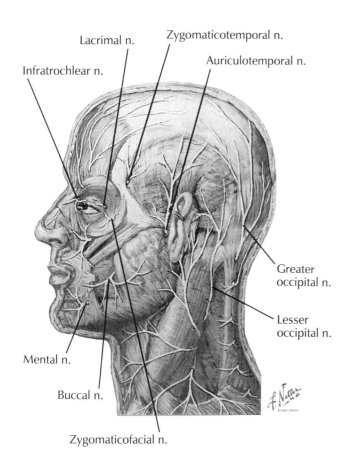

Lacrimal n.

Zygomaticotemporal n.

Infratrochlear n.

Auriculotemporal n.

Greater occipital n.

Lesser occipital n.

Mental n.

Buccal n.

Zygomaticofacial n.

PLATE 18

IDENTIFY lacrimal nerve (V₁) as it passes superior to lateral angle of orbit.

IDENTIFY infraorbital nerve (V₂) as it exits infraorbital foramen.

IDENTIFY zygomaticofacial nerve (V₂) as it passes out of its named foramen from zygomatic arch.

IDENTIFY zygomaticotemporal nerve (V₂) in anterior part of temporal region.

IDENTIFY mental nerve (V₃) as it exits mental foramen.

IDENTIFY buccal nerve (V₃) as it passes lateral to buccinator muscle. It is located deep to anterior border of masseter muscle. Distinguish between this buccal nerve and **buccal branch** of **facial nerve (VII)** examined earlier.

DISSECTION 8.5
INFRATEMPORAL FOSSA

Complete DISSECTION **8.4** Superficial Face and Scalp.

Read DISCUSSION **8.8** Infratemporal Fossa.

PALPATE mastoid process, styloid process, inferior margin of **external auditory meatus** of **temporal bone**, and **angle** of **mandible**.

INSPECT superficial extent of **parotid gland**.

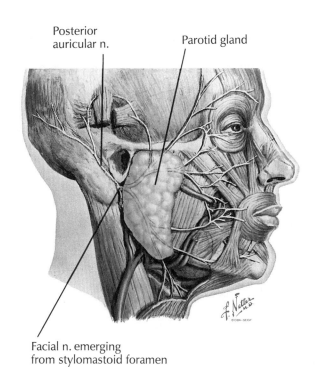

Posterior auricular n.

Parotid gland

Facial n. emerging from stylomastoid foramen

PLATE 19

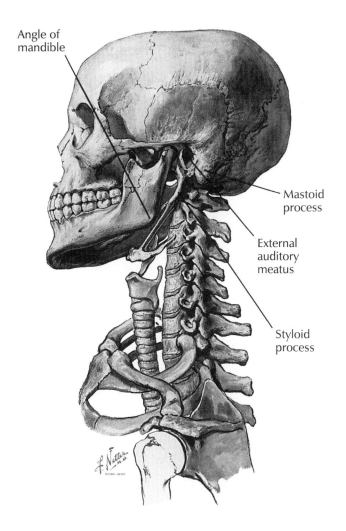

Angle of mandible

Mastoid process

External auditory meatus

Styloid process

PLATE 9

CAUTION During next steps, preserve trunks of facial nerve (VII).

ELEVATE parotid gland slightly by blunt dissection and with hemostat to inspect structures deep to it.

IDENTIFY stylomandibular ligament between **styloid process** and **angle** of **mandible**. Note that stylomandibular ligament separates parotid and submandibular glands.

TRACE either **temporal, zygomatic,** and **buccal branches** or buccal, mandibular, and cervical branches of **facial nerve** (**VII**) retrograde into substance of parotid gland, blunt dissecting glandular tissue away from nerve.

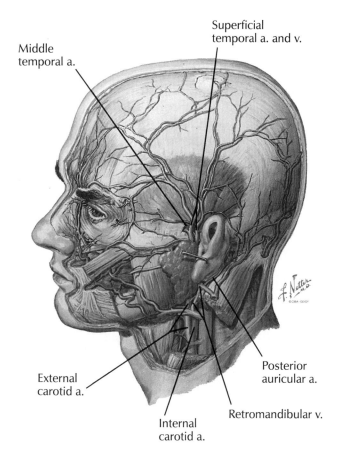

Middle temporal a.

Superficial temporal a. and v.

External carotid a.

Internal carotid a.

Posterior auricular a.

Retromandibular v.

PLATE 17

NOTE that temporal, zygomatic, and buccal branches form upper trunk of facial nerve and **buccal**, **mandibular**, and **cervical branches** form a lower trunk.

NOTE that common trunk of facial nerve passes superficial to **external carotid artery** and **retromandibular vein** within substance of parotid gland.

CAUTION Preserve origin of posterior auricular branch (VII) from trunk of facial nerve just distal to stylomastoid foramen. Note that posterior auricular nerve accompanies posterior auricular artery to supply occipitalis and posterior auricular muscles.

CAUTION During next step, preserve superficial temporal artery.

TRACE facial nerve to its exit from base of skull through **stylomastoid foramen** by removing parotid tissue around nerve.

NOTE that retromandibular vein is formed by union of **superficial temporal vein** and **maxillary vein**.

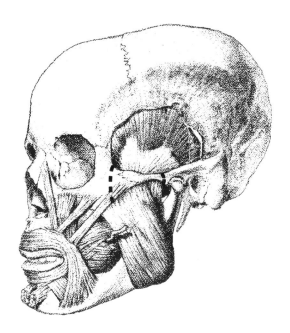

Figure 35

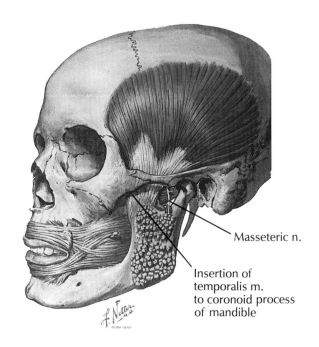

Masseteric n.

Insertion of temporalis m. to coronoid process of mandible

PLATE 48

198

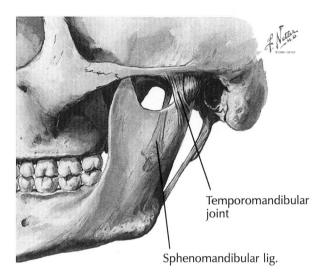

Temporomandibular joint

Sphenomandibular lig.

PLATE 11

REMOVE retromandibular vein and its immediate tributaries to facilitate dissection.

IDENTIFY origin of **superficial temporal artery** and **maxillary artery** (*not shown*) from external carotid artery.

IDENTIFY origin of **posterior auricular artery** from external carotid artery just superior to posterior belly of digastric muscle.

NOTE that styloid process separates external carotid artery from **internal carotid artery** in parotid region.

IDENTIFY superficial and deep heads of **masseter muscle**. Note that superficial fibers insert to coronoid process and angle of mandible while deep fibers are oriented vertically and insert to ramus.

CLEAN area deep to zygomatic arch from its superior margin.

CUT zygomatic arch (**Figure 35**).

BLUNT DISSECT between origin of masseter muscle and insertion of temporalis muscle.

REFLECT masseter muscle and attached part of zygomatic arch inferiorly.

IDENTIFY masseteric nerve passing through mandibular notch.

CLEAN posterior and lateral parts of capsule of **temporomandibular joint (TMJ)** with scalpel. Note **lateral ligament** of **temporomandibular joint**.

OPEN temporomandibular joint posteriorly with scalpel to demonstrate fibrous **articular disc**.

CUT condylar process of mandible distal to capsular attachment with mallet and chisel, rongeur forceps, or Stryker saw (**Figure 35**). Note that this cut is to be made to leave temporomandibular joint *in situ*.

IDENTIFY buccal nerve (V_3) and **auriculotemporal nerve** (V_3). Buccal nerve is located deep to superior part of ramus, passing through medial and lateral heads of lateral pterygoid muscles. Auriculotemporal nerve passes posterior to condylar process of mandible.

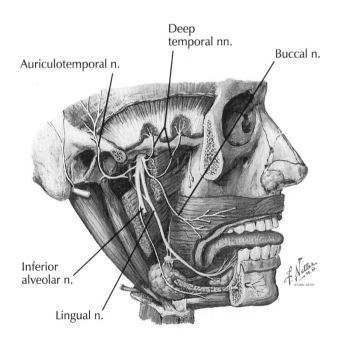

Auriculotemporal n.

Deep temporal nn.

Buccal n.

Inferior alveolar n.

Lingual n.

PLATE 41

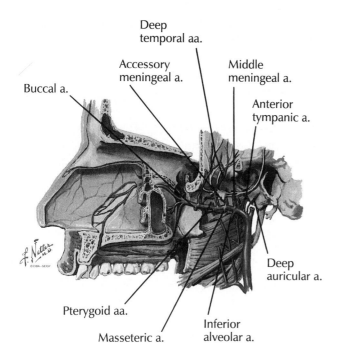

Deep
temporal aa.

Accessory
meningeal a.

Middle
meningeal a.

Buccal a.

Anterior
tympanic a.

Deep
auricular a.

Pterygoid aa.

Inferior
alveolar a.

Masseteric a.

PLATE 35

REMOVE temporalis fascia from its muscle.

CUT coronoid process of **mandible** inferior to insertion of **temporalis muscle.**

REFLECT temporalis muscle with attached coronoid process of mandible superiorly.

LOOK for **middle** and **deep temporal arteries** and **deep temporal nerves** (V₃) to temporalis muscle, deep to muscle fibers.

NOTE that middle temporal artery is branch of superficial temporal artery and deep temporal artery is branch of maxillary artery.

DETACH (scrape) temporalis muscle from **temporal fossa** enough to reflect temporalis muscle superiorly.

REMOVE ramus of mandible piece by piece with chisel and hammer.

IDENTIFY origins of following branches of 1st and 2nd parts of maxillary artery: **deep auricular, anterior tympanic, middle meningeal, accessory meningeal, inferior alveolar, deep temporal, pterygoid, masseteric,** and **buccal.**

LOCATE deep branches of mandibular nerve (V₃) as parts of mandible are removed.

IDENTIFY lingual nerve (V₃) and **inferior alveolar nerve** (V₃) as they pass between inferior part of ramus and medial pterygoid muscle.

IDENTIFY sphenomandibular ligament between the spine of sphenoid bone and lingula of mandible as it passes between medial and lateral pterygoid muscles. Note that sphenomandibular ligament passes between lingual and inferior alveolar nerves.

REMOVE pterygoid venous plexus and its connections to facilitate dissection.

EXAMINE 2 heads of **lateral pterygoid muscle.** Confirm that they attach to mandible capsule and articular disc of temporomandibular joint.

CAUTION During following steps, preserve arteries and nerves around temporomandibular joint.

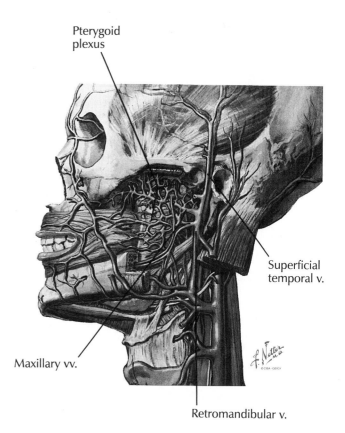

Pterygoid
plexus

Superficial
temporal v.

Maxillary vv.

Retromandibular v.

PLATE 64 detail

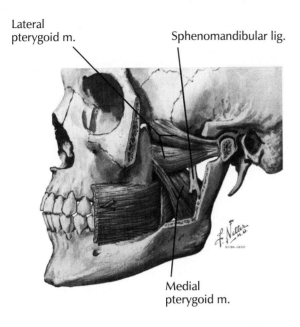

Lateral
pterygoid m.

Sphenomandibular lig.

Medial
pterygoid m.

PLATE 49

SEVER tendon of lateral pterygoid from its insertion to capsule of temporomandibular joint.

REFLECT capsular attachment of lateral pterygoid muscle anteriorly toward maxilla.

NOTE that anterior and posterior divisions of mandibular nerve (V_3) can be identified only after lateral pterygoid muscle is reflected.

IDENTIFY medial pterygoid muscle and arteries and nerves to it.

DISSECTION 8.6
CRANIAL CONTENTS

Complete DISSECTION **8.4** Superficial Face and Scalp.

Read DISCUSSIONS **8.2** Skull, **8.3** Cranial Nerves, and **8.9** Cranial Contents.

NOTE that dried skull should be kept at dissection table for reference.

PLACE cadaver so that head is upright in anatomical position.

INCISE galea aponeurotica and posterior scalp to bone (**Figure 36**), extending from nasion to inion along sagittal suture and from bregma laterally to right and left auricles along coronal suture if DISSECTION **8.4** has <u>not</u> been completed.

REFLECT 4 triangular flaps of scalp inferiorly, pulling anterior half of scalp and **frontalis muscle** down over upper face.

SCRAPE temporalis fascia and **temporalis muscle** free from temporal lines to expose bone for dissection if DISSECTION **8.5** has <u>not</u> been completed.

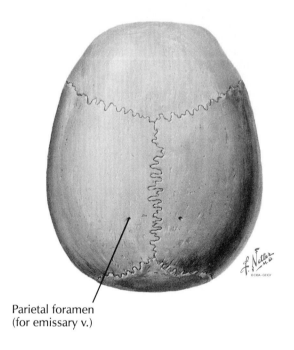

Parietal foramen
(for emissary v.)

PLATE 4

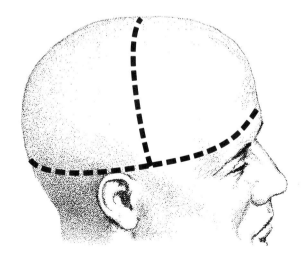

Figure 36

SEPARATE halves of posterior scalp in nuchal region by pulling halves to left and right.

REVIEW 5 layers of scalp in DISCUSSION **8.7**.

IDENTIFY sutures on exposed calvaria.

LOCATE parietal foramen for emissary veins.

REVIEW drainage of emissary and diploic veins.

MARK entire circumference of calvaria, (**Figure 37**).

NOTE that line is to pass 1 finger-width superior to superior margin of orbit and to inion (*not labeled*).

202

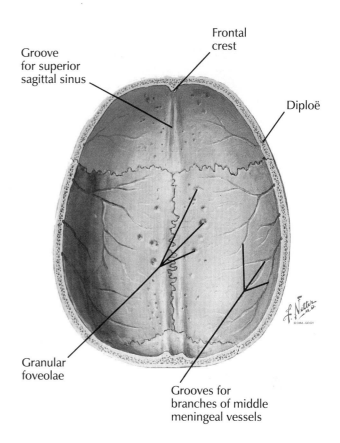

Groove
for superior
sagittal sinus

Frontal
crest

Diploë

Granular
foveolae

Grooves for
branches of middle
meningeal vessels

PLATE 4

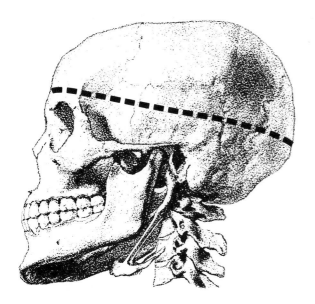

Figure 37

PLACE cadaver in either supine or prone position as needed for following steps to remove calvaria and occipital bone.

SAW through calvaria along marked line, permitting saw to break only outer lamina of calvaria during initial pass with saw. Note that entrance into **diploë** is apparent when congealed blood is seen on saw blade.

CAUTION   During following steps, protect meninges and brain deep to calvaria.

BREAK through inner lamina of calvaria, using mallet and chisel or Stryker saw.

PULL calvaria free from skull using fingers to separate calvaria and **dura mater**. Take time by circling entire head and applying pressure at many different locations. This is not exercise in force. It may take strength, but it demands patience and gentle persuasion.

EXAMINE interior of calvaria.

IDENTIFY **frontal crest** and **groove** for **superior sagittal sinus**, **grooves** for **branches** of **middle meningeal vessels**, and **granular foveolae**.

PLACE cadaver in prone position.

IDENTIFY following foramina on interior of dried skull: **foramen magnum**, **hypoglossal canal**, and **jugular foramen**.

IDENTIFY **occipital condyles** and **stylomastoid** and **jugular foramina** on external base of dried skull.

REMOVE (scrape) muscle fibers and fascia from external surface of occipital bone with scalpel.

REFLECT muscles inferiorly to expose posterior view of base of skull and atlas.

MARK incision line on occipital bone (**Figure 38**). Note that incision is to go as far laterally as possible without damaging external ear and should connect with lateral part of foramen magnum.

CAUTION   During following step, protect meninges and brain deep to cut.

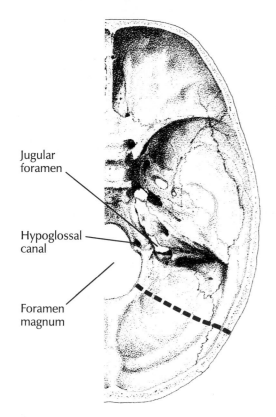

Jugular
foramen

Hypoglossal
canal

Foramen
magnum

Figure 38

SAW through outer lamina of occipital wedge line with Stryker saw.

BREAK through inner lamina of occipital wedge using mallet and chisel or Stryker saw.

CAUTION During next step, preserve spinal cord deep to atlantooccipital membrane.

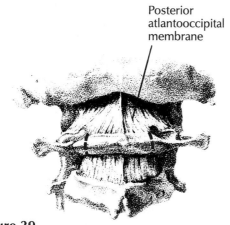

Posterior
atlantooccipital
membrane

Figure 39

SEVER posterior atlantooccipital membrane horizontally (**Figure 39**).

CAUTION Preserve transverse, sigmoid, and occipital sinuses within dura mater.

PULL occipital wedge free from anterior part of skull, using fingers to separate bone from dura mater.

EXAMINE dura mater *in situ*.

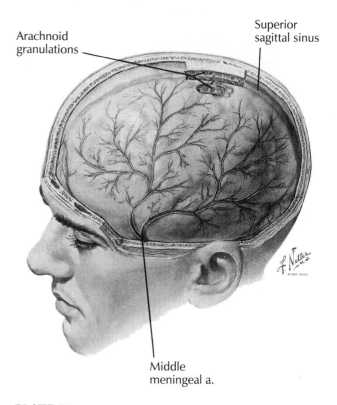

Arachnoid
granulations

Superior
sagittal sinus

Middle
meningeal a.

PLATE 95

IDENTIFY middle meningeal artery and its anterior and posterior branches.

LOCATE passage of **superior sagittal sinus** within dura mater.

CUT 4-inch sagittal incision in superior sagittal sinus near site of bregma.

REFLECT cut edges of superior sagittal sinus.

IDENTIFY arachnoid granulations (**villi**) within opened superior sagittal sinus.

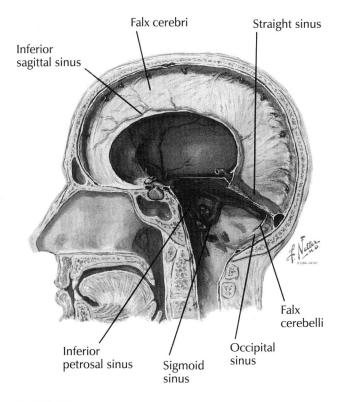

Inferior sagittal sinus

Falx cerebri

Straight sinus

Inferior petrosal sinus

Sigmoid sinus

Occipital sinus

Falx cerebelli

PLATE 97

IDENTIFY following bony landmarks in interior of dried skull: **crista galli**; **internal occipital protuberance**; and **grooves** for **occipital, transverse, sigmoid,** and **superior petrosal sinuses**.

CUT right side of dura mater along right circumference of cut edge of skull extending from anterior edge to posterior edge of superior sagittal sinus.

CUT left side of dura mater along left circumference of cut edge of skull extending from anterior edge to posterior edge of superior sagittal sinus to meet cut on right side. Note that these 2 cuts permit superior part of dura mater to be removed and inferior part of dura mater to remain *in situ* with cranial base.

ELEVATE frontal lobes of **cerebrum** gently (**Figure 40**) to expose attachment of dura mater to crista galli and frontal crest.

SEVER anterior attachment of **falx cerebri** from crista galli and frontal crest with scalpel or scissors.

PULL anterior cut end of falx cerebri posteriorly by grasping dura mater from top of brain.

RETRACT right **cerebral hemisphere** to right to expose attachment of falx cerebri to **tentorium cerebelli.**

SEVER attachment of falx cerebri to tentorium cerebelli by cutting along **straight sinus** with scalpel or scissors.

REMOVE freed dura mater and falx cerebri from brain.

NOTE that falx cerebri separates cerebral hemispheres and that **inferior sagittal sinus** is enclosed in free margin of falx cerebri.

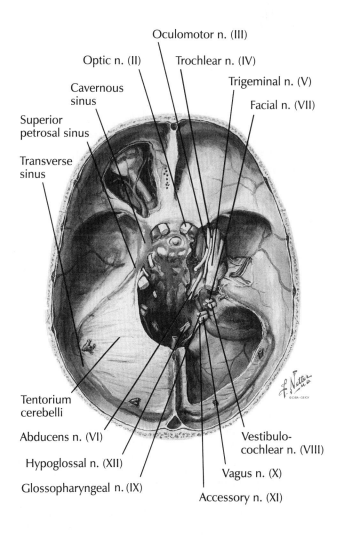

Optic n. (II)

Cavernous sinus

Oculomotor n. (III)

Trochlear n. (IV)

Trigeminal n. (V)

Facial n. (VII)

Superior petrosal sinus

Transverse sinus

Tentorium cerebelli

Abducens n. (VI)

Hypoglossal n. (XII)

Glossopharyngeal n. (IX)

Vestibulo-cochlear n. (VIII)

Vagus n. (X)

Accessory n. (XI)

PLATE 98

205

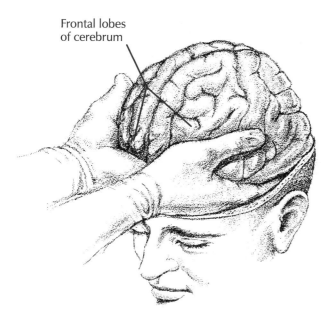

Frontal lobes
of cerebrum

Figure 40

ELEVATE occipital lobes of **cerebrum** gently to expose attachment of tentorium cerebelli to groove for transverse sinus.

NOTE that tentorium cerebelli separates occipital lobes of cerebrum from **cerebellum** and that its anterior and medial borders form **tentorial notch** (*not labeled*), which surrounds midbrain.

CUT both right and left sides of tentorium cerebelli obliquely from part of transverse sinus next to cut end of occipital bone to tentorial notch.

CUT cerebellar dura mater on both right and left sides from transverse sinus to foramen magnum along cut edge of occipital wedge.

REMOVE cerebellar dura mater with attached part of tentorium cerebelli and falx cerebelli.

NOTE that **falx cerebelli** separates hemispheres of cerebellum.

POSITION cadaver to see beneath brain as it is gently elevated by another student.

ELEVATE frontal lobes of cerebrum again (**Figure 40**).

REEXAMINE following structures after brain has been removed.

CUT olfactory nerve (I) as it passes through **cribriform plate** to **olfactory bulbs**.

CUT optic nerve (II) as it exits **optic canal**.

CUT internal carotid artery as it enters cranial cavity.

CUT infundibulum of **hypophysis (pituitary gland)** above **diaphragma sellae**.

CONTINUE to gently and carefully elevate and support frontal lobes of brain, including temporal lobes, to expose attachment of tentorium cerebelli to petrous part of temporal bone along groove for superior petrosal sinus.

CUT along superior petrosal sinus to pull free edge of tentorium cerebelli posteriorly from between cerebrum and cerebellum.

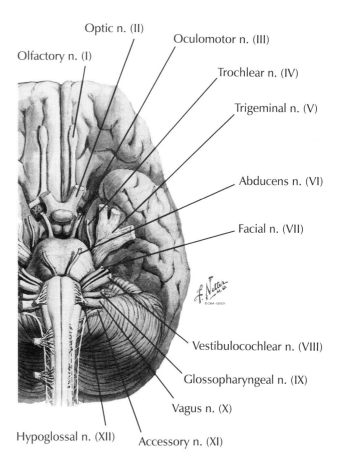

Optic n. (II)

Olfactory n. (I)

Oculomotor n. (III)

Trochlear n. (IV)

Trigeminal n. (V)

Abducens n. (VI)

Facial n. (VII)

Vestibulocochlear n. (VIII)

Glossopharyngeal n. (IX)

Vagus n. (X)

Hypoglossal n. (XII)

Accessory n. (XI)

PLATE 112

NOTE that **trochlear nerve (IV)** may have been cut during above step.

CUT oculomotor nerve (III) from ventral surface of pons. Leave short stub of nerve for later identification.

CUT trigeminal nerve (V) as it enters its **trigeminal cavity (Meckel's cave)**.

CUT abducens nerve (VI) as it enters dura mater covering **clivus**.

CUT facial (VII) and **vestibulocochlear (VIII) nerves** as they enter **internal auditory meatus**.

CUT roots of **glossopharyngeal (IX)**, **vagus (X)**, and **spinal accessory (XI) nerves** as they enter jugular foramen.

CUT hypoglossal nerve (XII) as it enters **hypoglossal canal**.

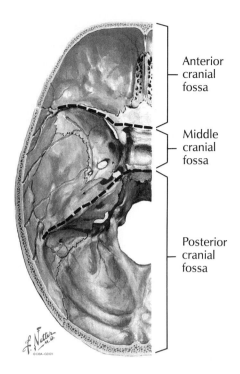

Anterior cranial fossa

Middle cranial fossa

Posterior cranial fossa

PLATE 6

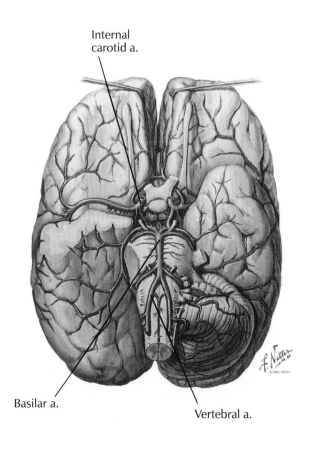

Internal carotid a.

Basilar a.

Vertebral a.

PLATE 132

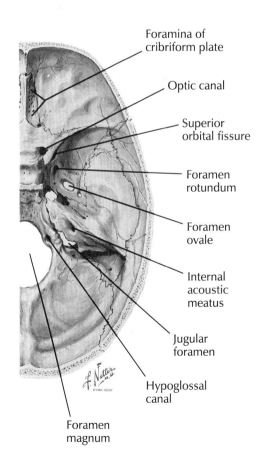

Foramina of cribriform plate

Optic canal

Superior orbital fissure

Foramen rotundum

Foramen ovale

Internal acoustic meatus

Jugular foramen

Hypoglossal canal

Foramen magnum

PLATE 7

CUT **right** and **left vertebral arteries** proximal to where they join to form **basilar artery**.

LOWER brain back into cranial vault.

CUT posterior arch of atlas with Stryker saw or chisel and mallet (**Figure 39**). Note that cut is to be same width as foramen magnum.

REMOVE posterior arch of atlas, removing fascial attachments adherent to it.

INCISE dura mater vertically from cranium to previous vertical cut in spinal cord dura mater made in DISSECTION **1.4**.

REFLECT brain to <u>right</u> to ensure that tentorium cerebelli has been severed. Repeat inspection of <u>left</u> tentorium cerebelli.

REMOVE brain with attached segment of spinal cord. Note that nerves, vessels, and meningeal reflections are to be severed as brain is lifted.

EXAMINE interior of cranial base.

DEFINE boundaries of **anterior**, **middle**, and **posterior cranial fossae**.

IDENTIFY cut ends of cranial nerves as they enter dura mater.

REVIEW foramina for exit of cranial nerves from cranial base.

IDENTIFY superior and inferior petrosal, occipital, and cavernous sinuses.

STORE brain in separate container for later inspection.

DISSECTION 8.7
ORBITAL CONTENTS

Complete DISSECTION **8.6** Cranial Contents.

Read DISCUSSION **8.10** Orbital Contents.

NOTE that dried skull should be kept at dissection table for reference.

IDENTIFY orbital surface of following bones on dried skull: **frontal, greater** and **lesser wings** of **sphenoid, zygomatic, ethmoid, lacrimal, palatine,** and **maxilla**.

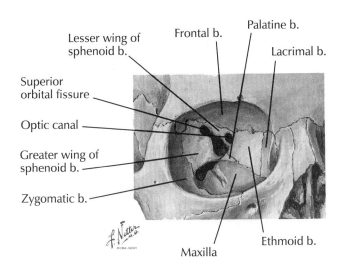

Lesser wing of sphenoid b.

Frontal b.

Palatine b.

Lacrimal b.

Superior orbital fissure

Optic canal

Greater wing of sphenoid b.

Zygomatic b.

Maxilla

Ethmoid b.

PLATE 1

PLACE cadaver so that head is upright in anatomical position.

PEEL away dura mater from floor of anterior cranial fossa to expose cranial surface of orbital plate of frontal bone.

CAUTION During next step, do not damage orbital contents, since orbital plate of frontal bone is thin and does not require much force to break.

BREAK through center of roof of orbital cavity by tapping with chisel and mallet. Continue breaking orbital plate carefully into small bone chips.

REMOVE roof of orbit piece by piece.

REFER to dried skull for orientation, and refer to anterior aspect of orbit for dissection.

CAUTION During next step, preserve supraorbital nerve (V_1) and artery while reflecting muscle.

PULL down superior part of **orbicularis oculi muscle** over eyelids.

LOCATE superior orbital notch or **foramen**.

Figure 41

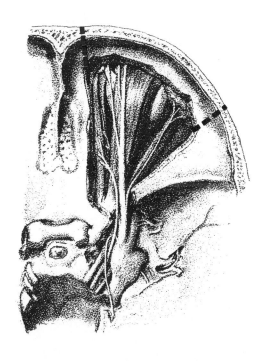

INSERT probe between anterior margin of roof of orbit and **supraorbital nerve**.

SAW through cut edge of squamous part of frontal bone at lateral and medial limits of orbit (**Figure 41**).

REMOVE superior margin of roof of orbit to expose anterior superior part of **periorbita** lining orbit. Note that if cadaver has superior orbital <u>notch</u>, free **supraorbital artery** and nerve by dissection. However, if cadaver has <u>foramen,</u> pull artery and nerve through it before removing bone.

LOCATE **frontal paranasal sinus** within section of squamous part of frontal bone.

INSERT probe from middle cranial fossa through **superior orbital fissure** between superior margin of fossa and contents of fissure.

CAUTION   During next step, do not damage orbital contents, since lesser wing of sphenoid bone is thin and does not require much force to break.

CUT through superior margin of superior orbital fissure with chisel and mallet.

INSERT probe from middle cranial fossa through **optic canal** between superior margin of canal and optic nerve (**II**).

CUT through superior margin of optic canal with chisel and mallet.

REMOVE lesser wing of sphenoid bone, piece by piece.

INCISE periorbita of orbit sagittally from anterior to posterior and coronally from lateral to medial. Note that periorbita is direct continuation of dura mater.

REMOVE flaps of periorbita to expose contents of orbit embedded in fat.

NOTE that most of dissection time is required for careful removal of **orbital fat**, lobule by lobule.

IDENTIFY **frontal nerve** (**V₁**) and its division into **supraorbital** and **supratrochlear nerves**.

IDENTIFY **supraorbital artery**, which travels with supraorbital nerve.

IDENTIFY **trochlear nerve** (**IV**) as it passes medially in orbit to supply superior oblique muscle.

IDENTIFY **superior oblique muscle** and its trochlea attached to medial angle of orbital margin.

IDENTIFY **lacrimal nerve** (**V₁**) as it enters orbit lateral to frontal nerve.

IDENTIFY **lacrimal gland**.

TRACE branch of lacrimal nerve to lacrimal gland and branch onto face (*not shown*).

IDENTIFY **levator palpebrae superioris muscle**.

CUT levator palpebrae superioris muscle from its insertion to superior tarsal plate of **upper eyelid**.

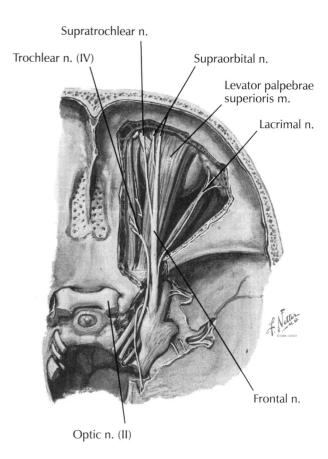

Supratrochlear n.

Trochlear n. (IV)

Supraorbital n.

Levator palpebrae superioris m.

Lacrimal n.

Frontal n.

Optic n. (II)

PLATE 81

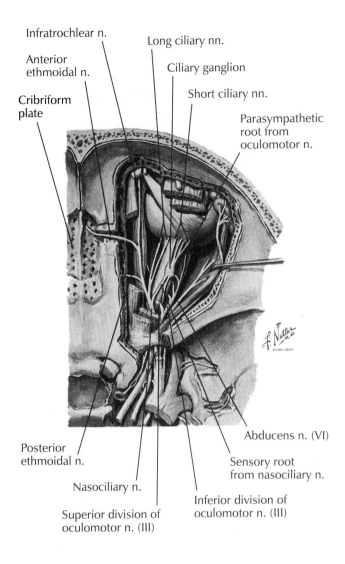

Infratrochlear n.
Anterior ethmoidal n.
Cribriform plate
Long ciliary nn.
Ciliary ganglion
Short ciliary nn.
Parasympathetic root from oculomotor n.

Posterior ethmoidal n.
Nasociliary n.
Superior division of oculomotor n. (III)
Inferior division of oculomotor n. (III)
Sensory root from nasociliary n.
Abducens n. (VI)

PLATE 81

REFLECT cut end of levator palpebrae superioris muscle posteriorly to expose **superior rectus muscle**.

IDENTIFY branches of **oculomotor nerve (III)** on deep surface of levator palpebrae superioris muscle.

CUT superior rectus muscle from its insertion to eyeball.

REFLECT cut end of superior rectus muscle posteriorly.

IDENTIFY branches of oculomotor nerve on deep surfaces of superior rectus muscle.

NOTE that branches to superior rectus and levator palpebrae superioris muscles originate from **superior division** of **oculomotor nerve (III)**.

IDENTIFY superior ophthalmic vein in superior part of orbit.

IDENTIFY optic nerve (II).

IDENTIFY lateral rectus muscle and its **abducens nerve (VI)**.

LOCATE 2 heads of lateral rectus muscle originating from **common annular tendon** over superior orbital fissure.

IDENTIFY nasociliary nerve (V_1) passing between 2 heads of lateral rectus muscle.

TRACE nasociliary nerve from its entrance into orbit lateral to optic nerve, to its passage to medial side of orbit above optic nerve, and to its passage between superior oblique and medial rectus muscles.

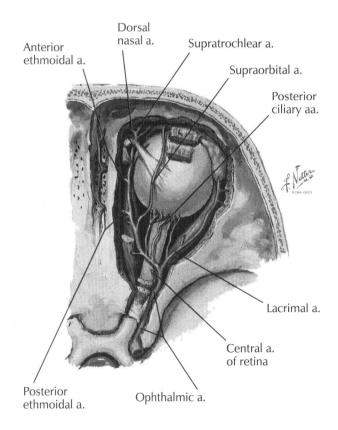

Anterior ethmoidal a.
Dorsal nasal a.
Supratrochlear a.
Supraorbital a.
Posterior ciliary aa.
Lacrimal a.
Central a. of retina
Posterior ethmoidal a.
Ophthalmic a.

PLATE 80

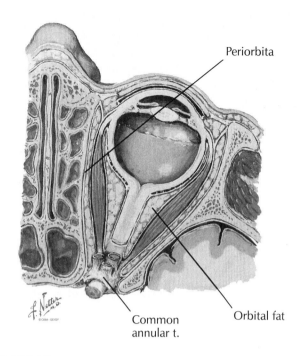

Periorbita

Common annular t.

Orbital fat

PLATE 78

IDENTIFY origins of **posterior** and **anterior ethmoidal nerves (V₁)** branching from nasociliary nerve.

TRACE posterior and anterior ethmoidal nerves to their exit from orbit through foramina of same name.

CAUTION During next step, do not damage ethmoidal air cells, since ethmoid bone is thin and does not require much force to break.

BREAK lateral and superior parts of **cribriform plate** of ethmoid bone into small chips by tapping with chisel and mallet.

REMOVE lateral and superior parts of cribriform plate of ethmoid bone, piece by piece.

INSPECT ethmoidal air cells (*not shown*) located in medial wall of orbit.

IDENTIFY continuation of anterior and posterior ethmoidal nerves into ethmoidal air cells.

TRACE infratrochlear nerve (V₁) onto face from point anterior to origin of anterior ethmoidal nerve from nasociliary nerve.

IDENTIFY ciliary ganglion positioned posteriorly in orbit between optic nerve and lateral rectus muscle.

LOOK for **sensory root** to **ciliary ganglion**, which is branch of nasociliary nerve.

LOOK for **long ciliary nerves** branching from nasociliary nerve to posterior eyeball.

LOOK for **parasympathetic root** to **ciliary ganglion**, which is branch of **inferior division** of **oculomotor nerve (III)**.

LOOK for **short ciliary nerves** from ciliary ganglion to posterior eyeball.

IDENTIFY ophthalmic artery as it passes in company with nasociliary nerve. Note that entrance of ophthalmic artery into orbit is inferior to optic nerve but that ophthalmic artery passes optic nerve superiorly from lateral to medial.

IDENTIFY following branches of ophthalmic artery: **central artery** of **retina, lacrimal, posterior ciliary, supraorbital, anterior** and **posterior ethmoidal, supratrochlear,** and **dorsal nasal**. Note that most of these arteries accompany nerves of same names.

PLATE 79

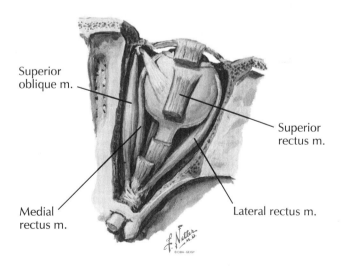

Superior oblique m.

Superior rectus m.

Medial rectus m.

Lateral rectus m.

REMOVE branches of superior ophthalmic vein to clean field of dissection. Note connections between superior ophthalmic vein and veins on face and cavernous sinus. **Inferior ophthalmic veins** (which cannot be inspected successfully from superior approach) have connections with **pterygoid venous plexus** and **cavernous sinus.**

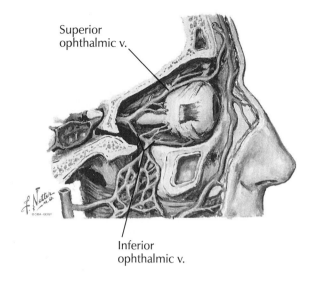

Superior ophthalmic v.

Inferior ophthalmic v.

PLATE 80

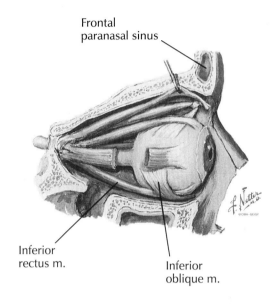

Frontal paranasal sinus

Inferior rectus m.

Inferior oblique m.

PLATE 79

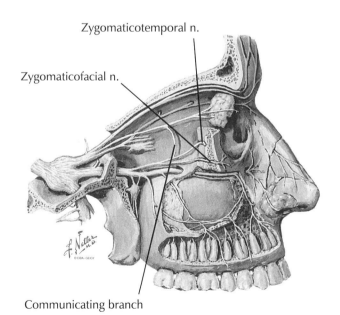

Zygomaticotemporal n.

Zygomaticofacial n.

Communicating branch

PLATE 40

RETRACT optic nerve (II) laterally to expose **inferior rectus** and **inferior oblique muscles.** Note that severing optic nerve and elevating cut end of optic nerve and eyeball will expose structures inferior to optic nerve.

LOCATE branches of oculomotor nerve to medial rectus, inferior rectus, and inferior oblique muscles. Note that these branches originate from **inferior division** of **oculomotor nerve (III).**

BLUNT DISSECT periorbita free from lateral wall of orbit.

RETRACT contents of orbit medially by reflecting lateral periorbita with hemostat.

NOTE that following structures may not be visible in some cadavers because of normal variations in their locations. They may be traveling within bone.

IDENTIFY zygomatic nerve (V_2), which passes along lateral wall of orbit.

LOOK for division of zygomatic nerve into **zygomaticotemporal** and **zygomaticofacial nerves.**

LOOK for **communicating branch** between zygomaticotemporal (V_2) and **lacrimal** (V_1)**nerves.**

NOTE that following dissections require careful removal of dura mater because nerves and arteries are traced retrograde to their entrances into orbit.

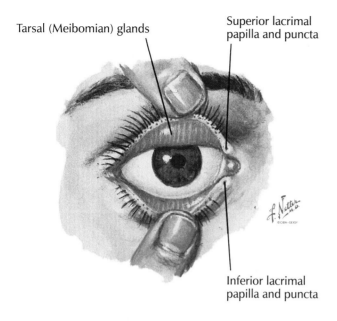

Tarsal (Meibomian) glands

Superior lacrimal papilla and puncta

Inferior lacrimal papilla and puncta

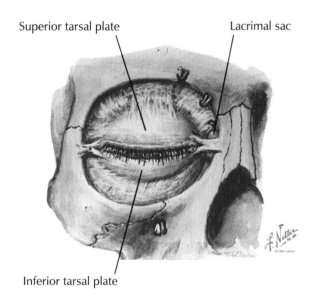

Superior tarsal plate

Lacrimal sac

Inferior tarsal plate

PLATE 76

TRACE frontal nerve retrograde to where nasociliary and lacrimal nerves branch from ophthalmic nerve (V₁). Continue tracing ophthalmic nerve through cavernous sinus to trigeminal ganglion in **trigeminal cavity (Meckel's cave**, *not labeled*; **Plate 98**).

TRACE oculomotor nerve (III) retrograde through cavernous sinus to its passage between anterior and posterior clinoid processes.

TRACE trochlear nerve (IV) retrograde through cavernous sinus to its passage in anterior part of free margin of tentorium cerebelli.

TRACE abducens nerve (VI) retrograde through cavernous sinus to its passage deep to dura mater covering clivus.

TRACE ophthalmic artery retrograde to **internal carotid artery** within cavernous sinus.

NOTE that eyelid dissection, which follows, should be done only if time permits.

EXAMINE facial aspect of orbit.

REPOSITION superior part of orbicularis oculi muscle to expose eyelids.

INSPECT eyelids from frontal view. Note **superior** and **inferior lacrimal puncta**.

INCISE skin along entire length of **superior tarsal fold** (*not labeled*).

BLUNT DISSECT between skin of superior eyelid and **superior tarsal plate** to expose attachment of superior tarsal plate.

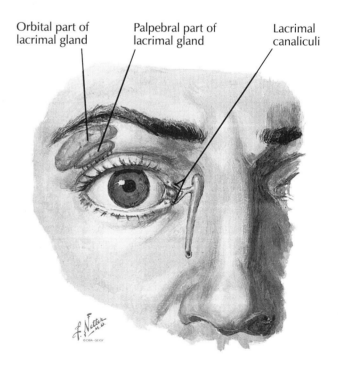

Orbital part of lacrimal gland

Palpebral part of lacrimal gland

Lacrimal canaliculi

PLATE 77

LOOK for medial and lateral fat pads between superior tarsal plate and conjunctival lining of superior eyelid.

ELEVATE upper eyelid with hemostat.

INSPECT lacrimal ducts piercing **conjunctiva**.

INCISE through superior palpebral conjunctiva, fat pads, and attachment of superior tarsal plate to **orbital septum**. Begin incision within conjunctival sac, and continue for length of tarsal fold.

REMOVE upper eyelid.

EXAMINE inner aspect of eyelid both on cadaver and on self or fellow student.

IDENTIFY tarsal (Meibomian) glands located in lower part of eyelid.

EXAMINE lacrimal gland *in situ*.

IDENTIFY orbital and **palpebral parts** of **lacrimal gland**.

RETRACT eyeball laterally with hemostat.

IDENTIFY trochlea of superior oblique muscle from frontal view.

INCISE skin along entire length of ciliary margin of lower eyelid.

BLUNT DISSECT between skin of inferior eyelid and **inferior tarsal plate**.

PULL skin of lower eyelid inferiorly to expose inferior tarsal plate.

LOOK for medial, middle, and lateral fat pads between inferior tarsal plate and conjunctival lining of inferior eyelid.

INCISE through inferior palpebral conjunctiva, fat pads, and attachment of inferior tarsal plate to orbital septum.

REMOVE lower eyelid.

RETRACT eyeball superiorly with hemostat.

IDENTIFY origin of **inferior oblique muscle** from maxilla in anterior medial wall of orbit.

LOCATE insertion of extrinsic muscles of eyeball to sclera. Note that inferior oblique muscle passes inferior to inferior rectus muscle.

LOCATE branches of inferior ophthalmic vein.

DISSECTION 8.8
PHARYNX AND PALATE

Complete DISSECTION **8.6** Cranial Contents.

Read DISCUSSION **8.11** Pharynx and Palate.

NOTE that dried skull should be kept at dissection table for reference.

DIRECT attention during following steps to separation of prevertebral and pharyngeal regions.

PLACE head of cadaver in prone position.

INCISE dura mater transversely over anterior margin of foramen magnum.

BLUNT DISSECT deep to dura mater.

PEEL away dura mater over foramen magnum to expose **tectorial membrane**.

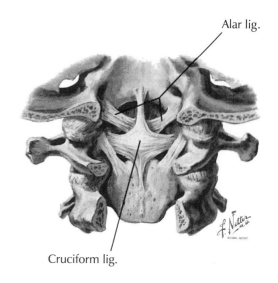

Alar lig.

Cruciform lig.

PLATE 15

PLATE 15

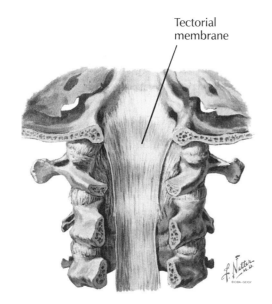

Tectorial membrane

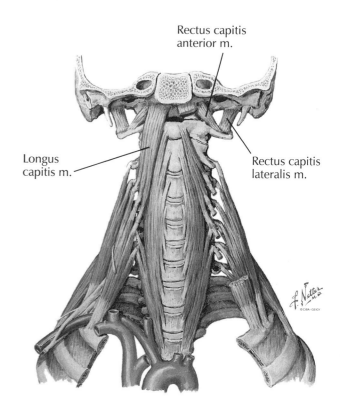

Rectus capitis anterior m.

Longus capitis m.

Rectus capitis lateralis m.

PLATE 25

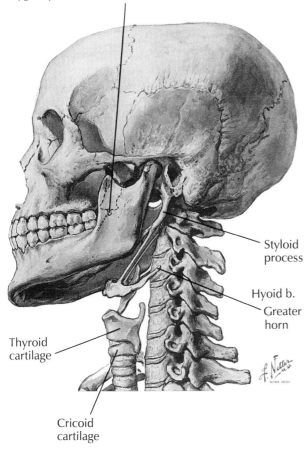

Hamulus of medial
pterygoid plate (*broken line*)

Styloid
process

Hyoid b.
Greater
horn

Thyroid
cartilage

Cricoid
cartilage

PLATE 9 detail

INCISE tectorial membrane transversely over anterior margin of foramen magnum.

BLUNT DISSECT deep to tectorial membrane.

PEEL away tectorial membrane to expose components of **cruciform** and **alar ligaments**. Note that rotating and tilting head assists observation of ligaments.

SEVER superior and inferior longitudinal fibers of cruciform ligament and right and left limbs of transverse ligament of atlas.

SEVER right and left alar ligaments.

TURN head of cadaver to supine position.

FLEX head on neck to relax tension on viscera and prevertebral muscles. Note that this maneuver requires strenuous manipulation.

SEPARATE visceral neck from somatic neck by extending fingers as deep to esophagus as possible.

BLUNT DISSECT if necessary to complete separation. Note that separation has occurred within **retropharyngeal space** (*not labeled*).

INSERT scalpel between anterior arch of atlas and cranium to make following incisions. Note that structures to be cut cannot be seen but may be palpated. Again, strenuous manipulation is required.

SEVER longus capitis muscle to free its occipital attachment.

SEVER rectus capitis anterior and **lateralis muscles**.

INCISE anterior atlantooccipital membrane (*not shown*) horizontally from posterior approach.

PLATE 130

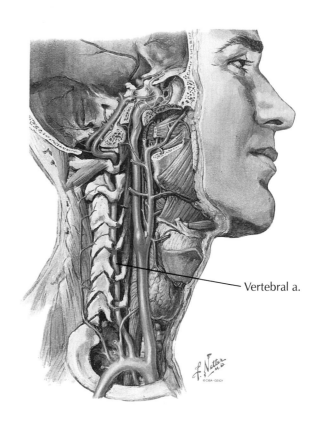

Vertebral a.

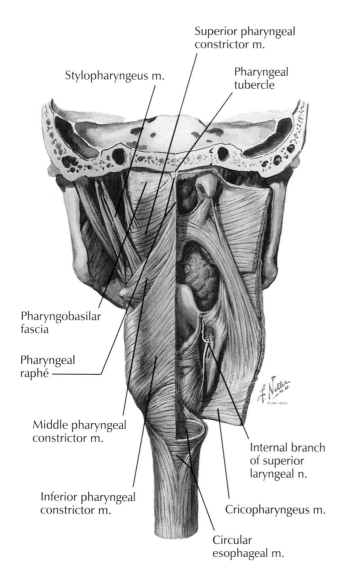

Stylopharyngeus m.

Superior pharyngeal constrictor m.

Pharyngeal tubercle

Pharyngobasilar fascia

Pharyngeal raphé

Middle pharyngeal constrictor m.

Inferior pharyngeal constrictor m.

Internal branch of superior laryngeal n.

Cricopharyngeus m.

Circular esophageal m.

PLATE 61

SEPARATE cervical vertebral column from visceral neck and attached anterior part of cranial base and skull.

INSPECT passage of **vertebral artery** through transverse foramina of cervical vertebrae.

PALPATE greater horn of **hyoid bone** and **thyroid** and **cricoid cartilages** on cadaver from posterior approach.

DIRECT attention to **pharynx.**

PLACE anterior part of head in prone position so that posterior pharynx is exposed.

IDENTIFY following structures on dried skull: **pharyngeal tubercle, styloid process,** and **hamulus** of **medial pterygoid plate.**

REMOVE buccopharyngeal fascia (*not shown*) from posterior pharynx. Note that **pharyngeal plexus** (*not shown*) of nerves and veins passes in buccopharyngeal fascia.

IDENTIFY circular muscle fibers of **esophagus** continuing inferior to **inferior pharyngeal constrictor muscle.**

NOTE that **cricopharyngeus muscle** acts as sphincter to restrict swallowing of air.

DEFINE superior boundary of **inferior pharyngeal constrictor muscle,** which originates from thyroid and cricoid cartilages. Note that inferior pharyngeal constrictor muscle overlaps caudal fibers of middle pharyngeal constrictor muscle.

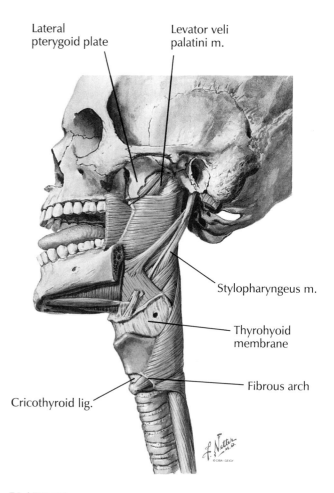

Lateral pterygoid plate

Levator veli palatini m.

Stylopharyngeus m.

Thyrohyoid membrane

Fibrous arch

Cricothyroid lig.

PLATE 62

DEFINE boundaries of **middle pharyngeal constrictor muscle**, which originates from greater horn of hyoid bone. Note that middle pharyngeal constrictor muscle overlaps caudal fibers of superior pharyngeal constrictor muscle.

DEFINE anterior boundary of **superior pharyngeal constrictor muscle**, which originates from pterygomandibular raphé. Note that this may be inspected more easily after bisection of head, which will be done later in this dissection.

NOTE that superior attachment of **median pharyngeal raphé** is to pharyngeal tubercle of occipital bone.

Glossopharyngeal n. (IX)

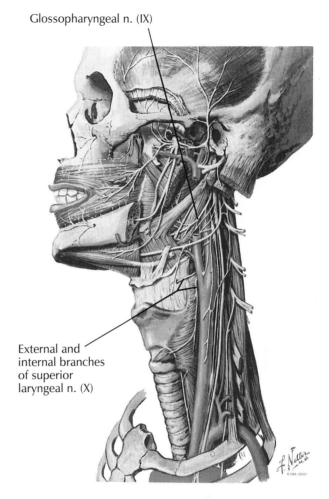

External and internal branches of superior laryngeal n. (X)

PLATE 65

Glossopharyngeal n. (IX)

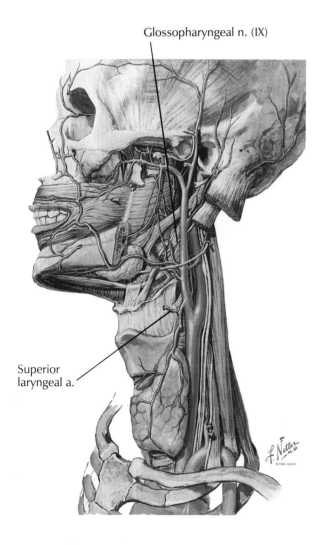

Superior laryngeal a.

PLATE 63

LOCATE, with fingers, lateral spaces devoid of muscle fibers between adjacent pharyngeal constrictor muscles. These gaps are covered with **pharyngobasilar fascia**.

IDENTIFY internal laryngeal nerve and **superior laryngeal artery** and **vein** (*not labeled*) as they enter **thyrohyoid membrane** below inferior border of middle pharyngeal constrictor muscle.

IDENTIFY stylopharyngeus muscle and **glossopharyngeal nerve** (**IX**) as they enter pharyngeal wall below inferior border of superior pharyngeal constrictor muscle.

NOTE that stylohyoid ligament also passes between inferior border of superior pharyngeal constrictor muscle and superior border of middle pharyngeal constrictor muscle.

219

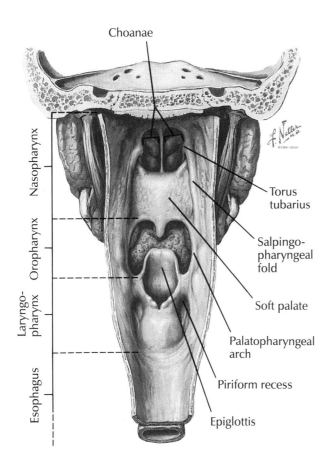

Choanae

Nasopharynx

Oropharynx

Laryngo-pharynx

Esophagus

Torus tubarius

Salpingo-pharyngeal fold

Soft palate

Palatopharyngeal arch

Piriform recess

Epiglottis

PLATE 60

DIRECT attention to lateral view of pharynx.

REMOVE medial and lateral pterygoid muscles, branches of mandibular division of trigeminal nerve, and branches of maxillary artery on exposed side of infratemporal fossa.

IDENTIFY **levator veli palatini muscle** and **cartilage** of **auditory tube** (*not shown*) passing above superior border of superior pharyngeal constrictor muscle.

IDENTIFY **tensor veli palatini muscle** lateral to superior pharyngeal constrictor muscle.

TRACE tendon of tensor veli palatini inferior to superior pharyngeal constrictor muscle and around hamulus of medial pterygoid plate.

REDIRECT attention to posterior view of pharynx.

INCISE posterior wall of esophagus and pharynx with scissors, using median vertical incision.

RETRACT cut edges of pharynx to expose its interior surface.

DEFINE inferior boundary of nasopharynx as **soft palate**.

DEFINE open anterior wall of nasopharynx as **choanae** of nasal cavity.

IDENTIFY **torus tubarius** in **nasopharynx**.

TRACE **salpingopharyngeal fold** inferiorly to where it joins palatopharyngeal arch.

DEFINE boundaries of **oropharynx** between soft palate and epiglottis.

DEFINE open anterior wall of oropharynx as passage between **fauces** of oral cavity.

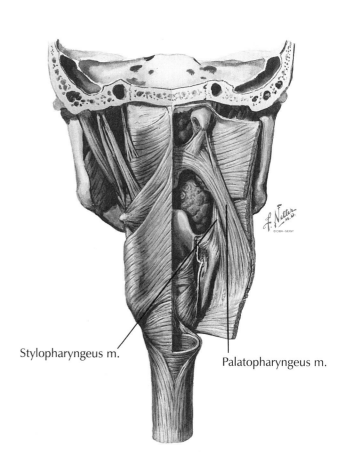

Stylopharyngeus m.

Palatopharyngeus m.

PLATE 61

IDENTIFY palatopharyngeal arch between soft palate and thyroid cartilage.

DEFINE boundaries of **laryngopharynx** between epiglottis and cricoid cartilage.

DEFINE closed anterior wall of laryngopharynx as posterior wall of larynx.

IDENTIFY piriform recess in laryngopharynx.

BLUNT DISSECT deep to mucosa of internal surface of pharynx and deep to superior surface of soft palate.

IDENTIFY palatopharyngeus muscle extending from soft palate vertically and attaching to thyroid cartilage.

IDENTIFY stylopharyngeus muscle passing between superior and middle pharyngeal constrictor muscles and joining palatopharyngeus muscle.

DIRECT attention to inferior lateral aspect of inferior pharyngeal constrictor muscle.

LOCATE fibrous arch of inferior pharyngeal constrictor muscle overlapping **cricothyroid muscle**.

DIRECT attention to bisection of head.

EXAMINE nasal septum and lateral nasal wall in bisected dried skull.

PLACE head of cadaver so that it can be held steady during bisection.

CAUTION Do <u>not</u> extend bisection through tongue, mandible, epiglottis, and larynx.

EXAMINE nasal septum in cadaver to determine whether septum deviates to right or left.

PLACE probe through nostril of nasal cavity opposite from nostril to which septum deviates. Use probe as guide toward which to direct cut.

BISECT head in midsagittal plane slightly to opposite side of head from side to which septum deviates. Use saw on bony elements and scalpel on soft tissue.

BEGIN saw cut at cribriform plate of ethmoid bone.

EXTEND cut through nasal bones and cartilages and through palate.

SEPARATE head into right and left halves, leaving tongue, epiglottis, and larynx intact.

REMOVE mucosa from remainder of nasopharynx and oropharynx to identify following structures.

LOCATE region in nasopharynx where **pharyngeal tonsil** (**adenoid**) is found in child.

IDENTIFY palatoglossal arch and palatopharyngeal arch in anterior part of oropharynx.

LOCATE region in fauces where **palatine tonsil** is found in child.

EXAMINE root of **tongue** (*not labeled*), and locate **lingual tonsil**.

IDENTIFY levator veli palatini muscle extending from medial side of cartilage of auditory tube to superior surface of soft palate.

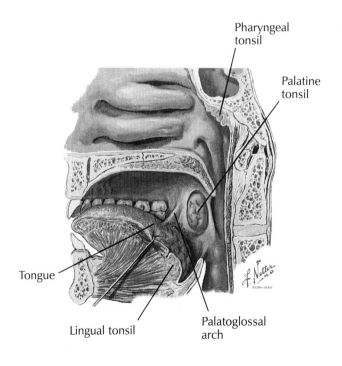

Pharyngeal tonsil

Palatine tonsil

Tongue

Lingual tonsil

Palatoglossal arch

PLATE 58

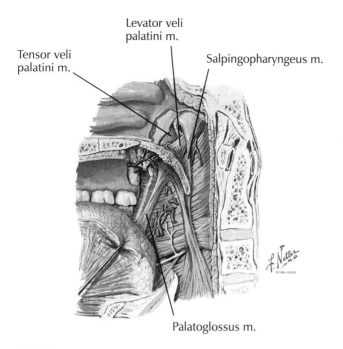

Tensor veli palatini m.

Levator veli palatini m.

Salpingopharyngeus m.

Palatoglossus m.

PLATE 58

IDENTIFY salpingopharyngeus muscle extending from medial side of cartilage of auditory tube to join palatopharyngeus muscle.

BLUNT DISSECT deep to levator veli palatini muscle to identify **aponeurosis** of tensor veli palatini muscle forming fibrous base for soft palate.

TRACE tendon of tensor veli palatini from soft palate to hamulus of lateral pterygoid plate.

REMOVE mucosa covering **palatoglossus muscle**, and trace its muscle fibers forward toward sides of tongue as far as possible.

NASAL REGION

Complete DISSECTION **8.8** Pharynx and Palate.

Read DISCUSSION **8.12** Nasal Cavity and Paranasal Sinuses.

NOTE that bisected dried skull should be kept at dissection table for reference.

EXAMINE nasal septum in dried skull.

EXAMINE nasal septum in cadaver, identifying cartilaginous portion absent in dried skull.

CAUTION   Preserve nerves and arteries during removal of mucosa from nasal region.

BLUNT DISSECT mucosa free from exposed side of nasal septum. Note that mucosa has spongy texture.

IDENTIFY perpendicular plate of **ethmoid bone**, **palatine process** of **maxilla**, **horizontal plate** of **palatine bone**, and **vomer** in both dried skull and cadaver.

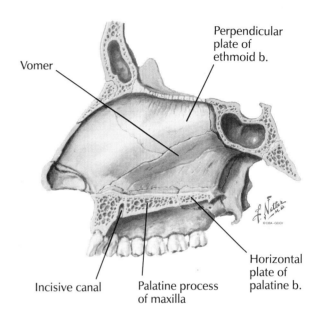

PLATE 34

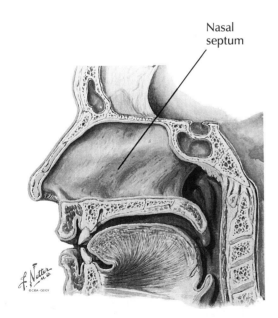

PLATE 34

LOOK for **medial internal nasal branch** of **anterior ethmoidal nerve (V₁)**, which supplies anterior 1/3 of nasal septum. Note that it is accompanied by **anterior septal branch** of **anterior ethmoidal artery**.

LOCATE nasopalatine nerve (V₂), which supplies posterior 2/3 of nasal septum. Note that it is accompanied by **sphenopalatine artery**.

IDENTIFY incisive canal in dried skull and in side of cadaver that has intact nasal septum.

TRACE both nasopalatine nerve and sphenopalatine artery to incisive canal.

IDENTIFY branches of **superior labial artery** from facial artery at entrance to nasal cavity.

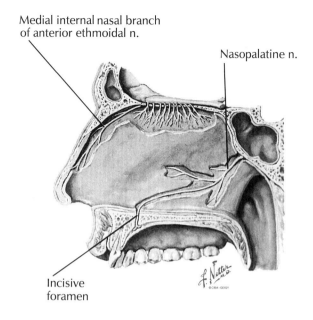

Medial internal nasal branch
of anterior ethmoidal n.

Nasopalatine n.

Incisive
foramen

PLATE 38

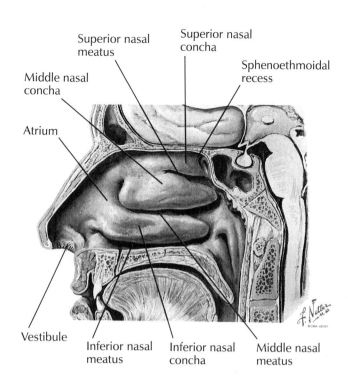

Superior nasal
meatus

Superior nasal
concha

Sphenoethmoidal
recess

Middle nasal
concha

Atrium

Vestibule

Inferior nasal
meatus

Inferior nasal
concha

Middle nasal
meatus

PLATE 32

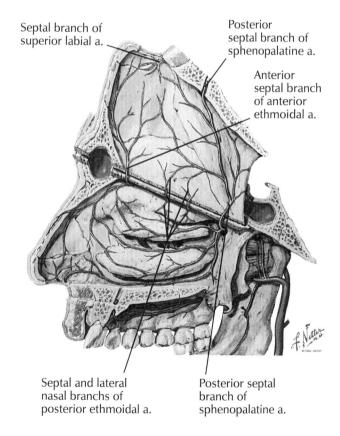

Septal branch of
superior labial a.

Posterior
septal branch of
sphenopalatine a.

Anterior
septal branch
of anterior
ethmoidal a.

Septal and lateral
nasal branchs of
posterior ethmoidal a.

Posterior septal
branch of
sphenopalatine a.

PLATE 36

IDENTIFY branches of **posterior ethmoidal artery** on superior part of nasal septum midway in cavity.

EXAMINE lateral wall of nasal cavity.

IDENTIFY nasal vestibule by presence of hairs.

IDENTIFY atrium as area between vestibule and conchae lying anterior to **middle nasal concha**.

IDENTIFY superior, **middle**, and **inferior nasal conchae** in cadaver.

IDENTIFY sphenoethmoidal recess and **superior**, **middle**, and **inferior nasal meatus**.

IDENTIFY middle and **superior nasal conchae** of **ethmoid bone, frontal process** of **maxilla, perpendicular plate** of **palatine bone,** and **inferior concha** in dried skull.

CAUTION Preserve nerves and arteries during removal of mucosa covering conchae.

BLUNT DISSECT mucosa free from conchae of lateral nasal wall.

IDENTIFY posterior nasal nerves (V₂), which supply posterior part of lateral nasal wall. Note that there are **posterior superior, posterior middle** (*not shown*), and **posterior inferior nasal nerves**.

IDENTIFY posterior lateral nasal artery, which is branch of sphenopalatine artery that accompanies posterior nasal nerves.

IDENTIFY lateral nasal branches of **anterior ethmoidal nerve (V_1)**, which supplies anterior part of lateral nasal wall.

IDENTIFY greater palatine and **sphenopalatine foramina** in both dried skull and cadaver.

CAUTION During next steps, use only gentle force to preserve structures within pterygopalatine fossa.

INSERT probe into greater palatine foramen from oral surface of hard palate. Note that its course is directly posterior to conchae in vertical orientation.

BREAK vertical opening in posterior lateral nasal wall from sphenopalatine foramen directly posterior to conchae. Use chisel and mallet to expose **greater** and **lesser palatine nerves**, which lie lateral to vertical opening in perpendicular plate of palatine bone. Begin break close to greater palatine foramen.

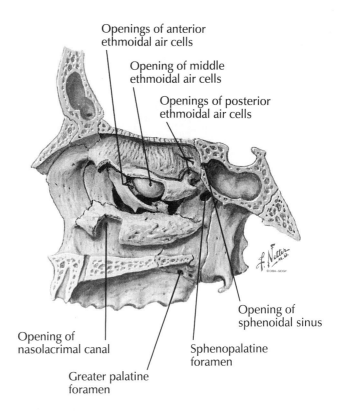

Openings of anterior ethmoidal air cells

Opening of middle ethmoidal air cells

Openings of posterior ethmoidal air cells

Opening of sphenoidal sinus

Sphenopalatine foramen

Greater palatine foramen

Opening of nasolacrimal canal

PLATE 33

TRACE posterior superior nasal nerves to their origin from **pterygopalatine ganglion**.

TRACE posterior middle (*not shown*) and inferior nasal nerves to their origin from greater palatine nerve.

BLUNT DISSECT mucosa from oral surface of hard palate to expose **greater palatine nerve** and **artery**.

CUT off nasal conchae as close to their roots as possible to expose openings into their corresponding nasal meatus.

LOCATE opening of **sphenoidal sinus** into sphenoethmoidal recess.

LOCATE opening of **posterior ethmoidal air cells** into superior nasal meatus.

LOCATE opening from **nasofrontal duct** of **frontal sinus** into middle nasal meatus. Note that opening is into space called **infundibulum**.

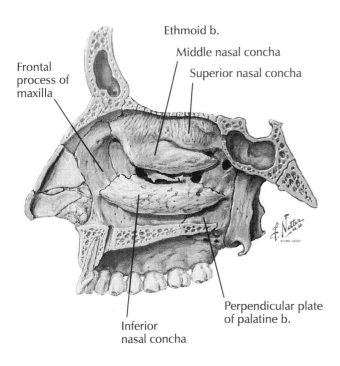

Ethmoid b.

Middle nasal concha

Superior nasal concha

Frontal process of maxilla

Perpendicular plate of palatine b.

Inferior nasal concha

PLATE 33

225

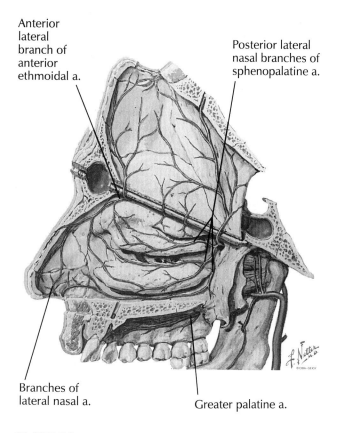

Anterior lateral branch of anterior ethmoidal a.

Posterior lateral nasal branches of sphenopalatine a.

Branches of lateral nasal a.

Greater palatine a.

PLATE 36

LOCATE opening of **maxillary sinus** and **anterior ethmoidal air cells** into **semilunar hiatus**, which is posterior to infundibulum in middle nasal meatus. Note that opening of maxillary sinus is posterior to opening for anterior ethmoidal air cells.

IDENTIFY ethmoidal bulla, which bulges superior to semilunar hiatus.

LOCATE opening of **middle ethmoidal air cells** onto **ethmoidal bulla** in **middle nasal meatus**.

LOCATE opening of **nasolacrimal duct** into inferior nasal meatus.

EXAMINE paranasal sinuses.

CAUTION During following 2 steps, use only gentle force.

BREAK through superior and middle nasal conchae on one side of head with chisel and mallet to expose ethmoidal air cells.

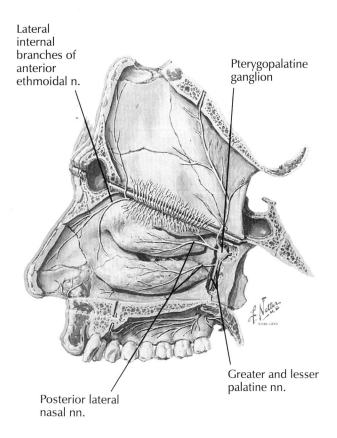

Lateral internal branches of anterior ethmoidal n.

Pterygopalatine ganglion

Posterior lateral nasal nn.

Greater and lesser palatine nn.

PLATE 37

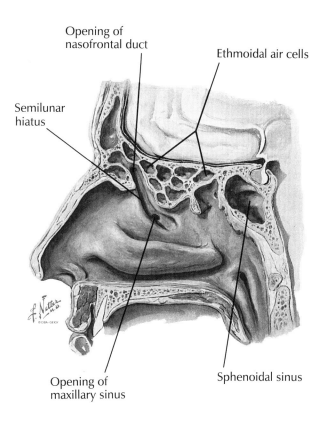

Opening of nasofrontal duct

Ethmoidal air cells

Semilunar hiatus

Opening of maxillary sinus

Sphenoidal sinus

PLATE 43

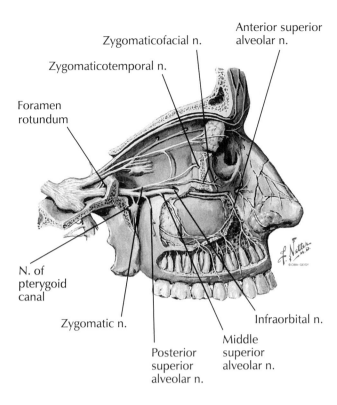

Zygomaticofacial n.
Zygomaticotemporal n.
Anterior superior alveolar n.
Foramen rotundum
N. of pterygoid canal
Zygomatic n.
Posterior superior alveolar n.
Middle superior alveolar n.
Infraorbital n.

PLATE 40

BREAK through inferior nasal concha on one side of head with chisel and mallet to expose maxillary sinus.

LOCATE sphenoidal sinus in body of bisected sphenoid bone.

REVIEW location of **frontal sinus**.

DEFINE boundaries of **pterygopalatine fossa** in dried skull.

CAUTION   During following steps, preserve maxillary nerve (V₂).

PEEL back dura mater from floor of middle cranial fossa.

PLACE probe through **foramen rotundum** from middle cranial fossa through pterygopalatine fossa into **inferior orbital fissure, groove**, and **canal** passing superior to **maxillary nerve (V₂)**.

CAUTION   During next step, use only gentle force.

BREAK through floor of orbit (roof of maxillary sinus) with chisel and mallet from orbital approach to expose **infraorbital nerve (V₂)**.

LOOK for origins of **anterior** and **middle superior alveolar nerves (V₂)** as they branch from infraorbital nerve. Note that transillumination (shining light into sinus from facial side of maxilla while looking into sinus from bisected medial side) aids observation of these nerves.

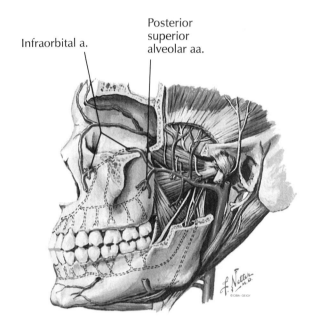

Infraorbital a.
Posterior superior alveolar aa.

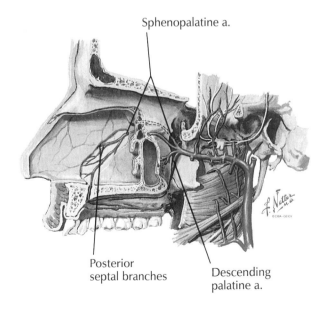

Sphenopalatine a.
Posterior septal branches
Descending palatine a.

PLATE 35

227

TRACE zygomatic (V$_2$) and **posterior superior alveolar (V$_2$) nerves** as they pass laterally out of **pterygomaxillary fissure**.

RETRACE zygomaticotemporal and **zygomaticofacial branches** of zygomatic nerve to their respective foramina in lateral wall of orbit.

EXAMINE pterygopalatine ganglion suspended from maxillary nerve through opening in lateral wall of nasal cavity.

LOOK for **nerve** of **pterygoid canal**, which joins pterygopalatine ganglion from pterygoid canal in posterior wall of pterygopalatine fossa.

LOOK for **pharyngeal branch** (V$_2$, *not shown*), which originates from pterygopalatine ganglion and passes through foramen in posterior wall of pterygopalatine fossa medial to pterygoid canal.

BREAK through floor of sphenoidal sinus to expose nerve of pterygoid canal.

EXAMINE branches of 3rd part of maxillary artery from opening in lateral wall of nasal cavity.

IDENTIFY sphenopalatine artery and descending palatine artery divided into greater and lesser palatine arteries.

EXAMINE additional branches of 3rd part of maxillary artery from lateral view through **pterygomaxillary fissure**.

IDENTIFY infraorbital and **posterior superior alveolar arteries**.

LOOK for **artery** of **pterygoid canal** and **pharyngeal artery**.

DISSECTION 8.10

ORAL REGION

Complete DISSECTION **8.9** Nasal Region.

Read DISCUSSION **8.13** Oral Region.

EXAMINE mandible, palate, and upper jaw in dried skull.

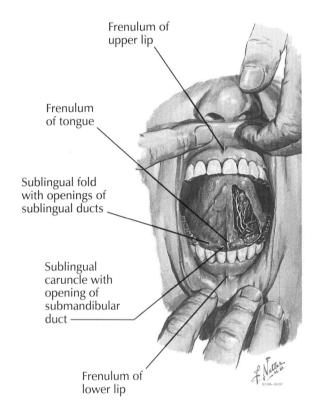

Frenulum of upper lip

Frenulum of tongue

Sublingual fold with openings of sublingual ducts

Sublingual caruncle with opening of submandibular duct

Frenulum of lower lip

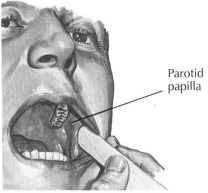

Parotid papilla

PLATE 45

USE mirror to study own oral cavity, or study oral cavity of fellow student using following steps.

DEFINE boundaries of **vestibule** (*not labeled*) and **oral cavity proper** (*not labeled*).

RETRACT lips and identify **frenula** of **upper** and **lower lips**.

IDENTIFY parotid papilla and **pterygomandibular raphé** in buccal mucosa.

IDENTIFY incisive papilla, transverse palatine folds, longitudinal palatine raphé, uvula, and **palatoglossal** and **palatopharyngeal arches** associated with palate.

EXAMINE tongue as it rests on floor of mouth.

IDENTIFY foramen cecum, sulcus terminalis, and **vallate papillae.**

LOOK for **filiform** and **fungiform papillae.**

NOTE that posterior 1/3 of tongue will be reexamined in cadaver later in this dissection.

ELEVATE tongue to expose following sublingual structures.

IDENTIFY frenulum of **tongue, sublingual fold** with openings of **sublingual ducts,** and **sublingual caruncle** with opening of **submandibular duct.**

EXAMINE teeth (**Plate 51**).

REVIEW eruption pattern of deciduous and permanent teeth (**Plate 50**).

REPEAT all preceding steps on cadaver, then continue with dissection.

DIRECT attention to bisection of tongue and floor of mouth.

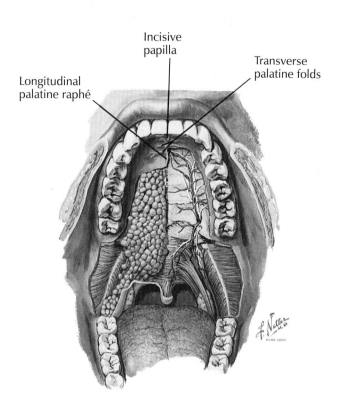

PLATE 46

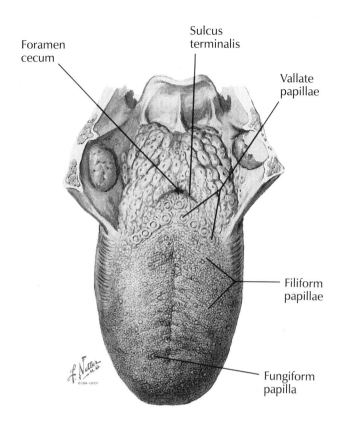

PLATE 52

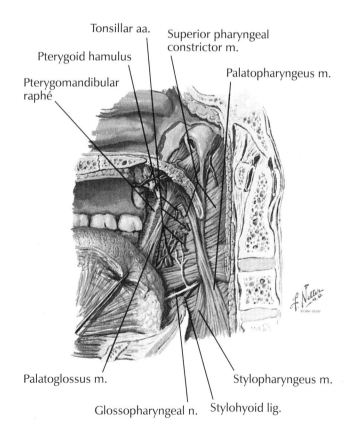

PLATE 58

PLACE head so that it can be held steady during bisection.

CAUTION Do <u>not</u> extend following bisection through epiglottis and larynx.

SAW through **jugum** (*not labeled*) of **mandible**.

BISECT tongue and soft tissue in sublingual region along midsagittal plane with scalpel, leaving epiglottis and larynx intact.

SEPARATE tongue and floor of mouth into right and left halves.

RETRACT bisected tongue medially with hemostat.

CLEAN mucosa completely from **palatopharyngeus** and **palatoglossus muscles**.

REMOVE palatine tonsil if present by blunt dissection. Note that inferior part of palatine tonsil is continuous with **lingual tonsil**.

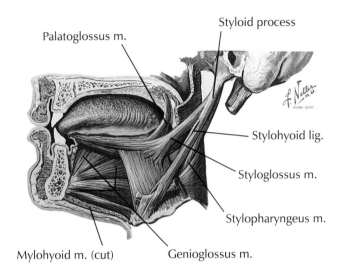

Palatoglossus m.

Styloid process

Stylohyoid lig.

Styloglossus m.

Stylopharyngeus m.

Mylohyoid m. (cut)

Genioglossus m.

PLATE 53

REMOVE pharyngobasilar fascia from bed of tonsil to expose **superior pharyngeal constrictor muscle.**

LOOK for **tonsillar branches** of **lesser palatine, ascending pharyngeal, ascending palatine, dorsal lingual,** and **facial arteries.** Note that origins of branches may be difficult to determine.

EXAMINE superior pharyngeal constrictor muscle from lateral view to determine its inferior border. Note that passage of glossopharyngeal nerve (IX), stylopharyngeus muscles, and stylohyoid ligament (*not shown*) delineates that border.

INSERT probe from lateral side of cadaver into oral region below inferior border of superior pharyngeal constrictor muscle.

EXAMINE passage of probe from medial view.

CLEAN stylopharyngeus muscle, and reconfirm its association with palatopharyngeus muscle.

IDENTIFY glossopharyngeal nerve, and trace its lingual branches to posterior 1/3 of tongue.

PALPATE styloid process and **hyoid bone** on both skeleton and cadaver.

LOCATE stylohyoid ligament stretching from styloid process to lesser horn of hyoid bone and passing between inferior margin of superior pharyngeal constrictor muscle and superior margin of middle pharyngeal constrictor muscle.

PALPATE hamulus of **medial pterygoid plate** and **mylohyoid line** (*not shown*) on both dried skull and cadaver.

LOCATE pterygomandibular raphé between hamulus of medial pterygoid plate and posterior edge of mylohyoid line.

REPOSITION probe from lateral side of cadaver into oral region below inferior border of superior pharyngeal constrictor muscle.

RETRACT inferior border of superior pharyngeal constrictor muscle superiorly to expose origin of **styloglossus muscle** from medial view.

TRACE styloglossus muscle from styloid process to lateral side of tongue.

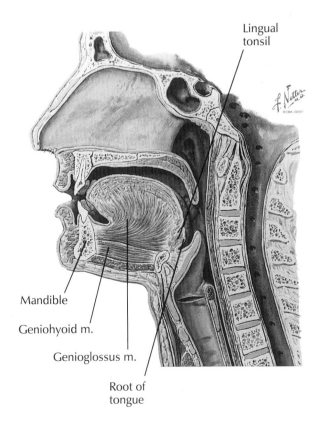

Lingual tonsil

Mandible

Geniohyoid m.

Genioglossus m.

Root of tongue

PLATE 57 detail

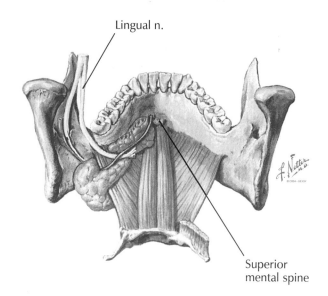

Lingual n.

Superior
mental spine

PLATE 47

BLUNT DISSECT between **mylohyoid muscle** and **geniohyoid muscle** deep (superior) to mylohyoid muscle. Note that both muscles attach between mandible and hyoid bone. Mylohyoid muscle originates from mylohyoid line (*not shown*), and geniohyoid muscle originates from **inferior mental spine** (*not labeled*).

IDENTIFY fibers of **genioglossus muscle**, which fan out in body of tongue from their origin on **superior mental spine**.

EXAMINE structures in sublingual region from inferior view of submandibular triangle.

CAUTION   During next step, preserve hypoglossal nerve (XII) deep to mylohyoid muscle.

REMOVE anterior bellies of digastric and mylohyoid muscles from one side of cadaver to expose origin of **hyoglossus muscle** from hyoid bone.

IDENTIFY lingual (V_3) and hypoglossal (XII) **nerves**, which pass lateral to hyoglossus muscle. Note that lingual nerve passes superior to hypoglossal nerve.

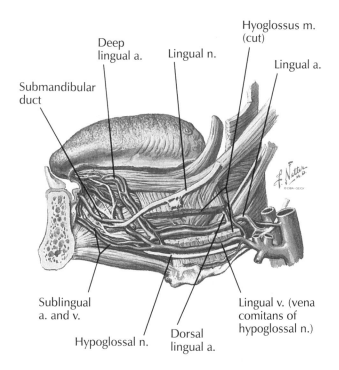

Submandibular duct

Deep lingual a.

Lingual n.

Hyoglossus m. (cut)

Lingual a.

Sublingual a. and v.

Hypoglossal n.

Dorsal lingual a.

Lingual v. (vena comitans of hypoglossal n.)

PLATE 53

TRACE fibers of palatoglossus muscle into body of tongue.

EXAMINE muscles of floor of mouth and sublingual region from medial view in bisected head.

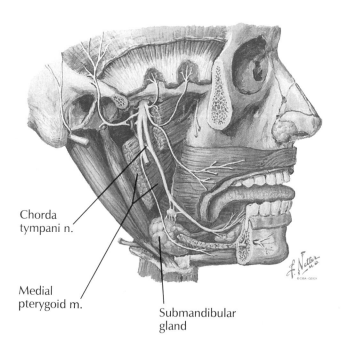

Chorda tympani n.

Medial pterygoid m.

Submandibular gland

PLATE 41

PLATE 55

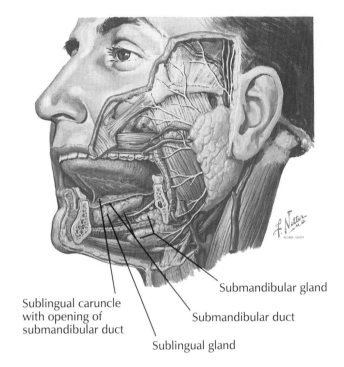

Sublingual caruncle
with opening of
submandibular duct

Submandibular gland

Submandibular duct

Sublingual gland

TRACE lingual nerve posteriorly from where it is crossed by submandibular duct to where it passes between **medial pterygoid muscle** and ramus of mandible.

TRACE lingual nerve retrograde to where it is joined by **chorda tympani nerve** in infratemporal fossa. Note that lingual nerve passes inferior to inferior border of superior pharyngeal constrictor muscle to enter oral cavity.

LOCATE submandibular ganglion suspended from lingual nerve close to **submandibular gland**.

IDENTIFY submandibular duct inferior to lingual nerve traveling toward frenulum of tongue.

PLACE probe deep to medial side of hyoglossus muscle.

EXAMINE extrinsic muscles of tongue from medial view.

REMOVE attachment of genioglossus muscle from hyoid bone on one side to expose probe and hyoglossus muscle.

LOCATE lingual artery, which passes medial to hyoglossus muscle.

IDENTIFY origin of **dorsal lingual arteries** from lingual artery.

TRACE dorsal lingual arteries as they ascend into posterior part of tongue.

IDENTIFY origin of **deep lingual artery** from lingual artery.

TRACE deep lingual artery as it passes to tip of tongue.

TRACE sublingual artery as it passes superior to genioglossus muscle to supply **sublingual gland**.

EXAMINE sublingual region on side of bisected head that has intact mylohyoid muscle. During identification of structures, it may be useful to refer to other side of mouth for structures already identified.

ELEVATE tongue with hemostat.

CAUTION During removal of mucosa, preserve sublingual caruncle.

INCISE mucosa in sublingual region between body of mandible and sublingual fold.

BLUNT DISSECT deep to sublingual mucosa, and remove it to expose sublingual gland and deep part of submandibular gland.

LOCATE series of short sublingual ducts, which open into sublingual fold.

RETRACT sublingual gland laterally and body of tongue medially.

REIDENTIFY submandibular duct as it passes medial to sublingual gland.

TRACE submandibular duct from sublingual caruncle near anterior end of sublingual gland and then posteriorly to deep part of submandibular gland.

IDENTIFY lingual nerve as it passes deep to sublingual gland.

TRACE branches of lingual nerve deep to anterior 2/3 of tongue.

LOCATE hypoglossal nerve (XII) lateral to hyoglossus muscle between submandibular gland and hyoglossus muscle. Note that hypoglossal nerve is inferior to lingual nerve.

LOCATE lingual vein, which accompanies hypoglossal nerve. Note that lingual vein passes lateral to hyoglossus muscle and lingual artery passes medial to hyoglossus muscle.

TRACE hypoglossal nerve anteriorly to its branches to genioglossus and intrinsic muscles of tongue.

LOOK for branches of cervical plexus, which appear to be branches of hypoglossal nerve to geniohyoid and thyrohyoid muscles.

DISSECTION 8.11

LARYNX

Complete DISSECTION **8.8** Pharynx and Palate.

Read DISCUSSION **8.14** Larynx.

IDENTIFY following structures on model of larynx: **thyroid**, **cricoid**, **arytenoid**, and **epiglottic cartilages**.

PALPATE same structures on cadaver.

STUDY locations of **corniculate** and **cuneiform cartilages** (*not shown*) on model.

DEFINE actions at **cricothyroid** and **crico-arytenoid joints** (*not labeled*) on model.

MANIPULATE arytenoid cartilages on model to illustrate their rotation and gliding movements.

IDENTIFY muscular and **vocal processes** of **arytenoid muscles** on model.

IDENTIFY thyrohyoid membrane and **cricothyroid ligament** on model.

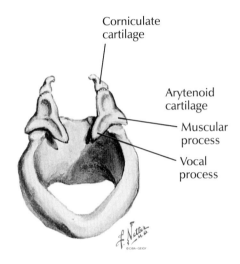

Corniculate cartilage

Arytenoid cartilage

Muscular process

Vocal process

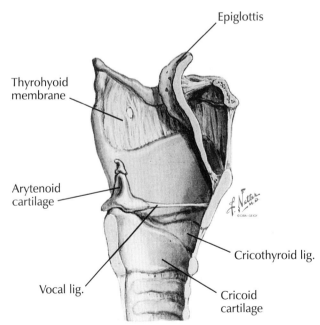

Epiglottis

Thyrohyoid membrane

Thyroid cartilage

Arytenoid cartilage

Cricoid cartilage

Epiglottis

Thyrohyoid membrane

Arytenoid cartilage

Vocal lig.

Cricothyroid lig.

Cricoid cartilage

PLATE 71

PLATE 71

DEFINE attachments of **conus elasticus** (*not shown*) on model between superior border of cricoid cartilage and vocal ligaments.

DEFINE attachments of **quadrangular membrane** (*not shown*) on model between epiglottic and arytenoid cartilages.

NOTE that inferior border of quadrangular membrane is **vestibular fold** (false vocal cord) and superior border of conus elasticus is **vocal ligament** (true vocal cord).

CAUTION As dissection proceeds, preserve laryngeal nerves.

DIRECT attention to posterior view of larynx in cadaver.

IDENTIFY piriform recess and fold covering **internal branch** of **superior laryngeal nerve**, which passes through piriform recess.

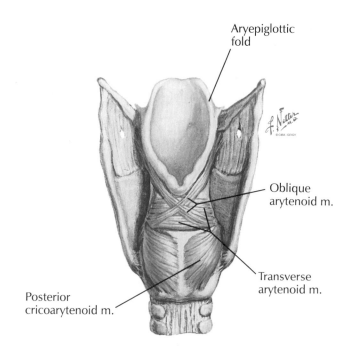

PLATE 72

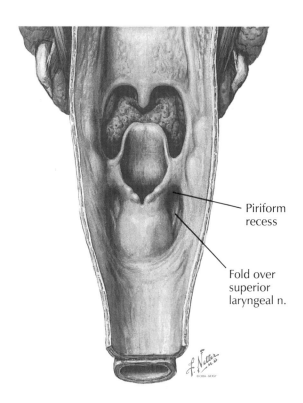

PLATE 60 detail

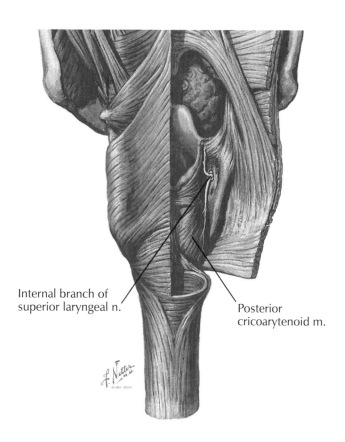

PLATE 61 detail

BLUNT DISSECT mucosa from anterior wall of laryngopharynx to expose **posterior cricoarytenoid** and **transverse** and **oblique arytenoid muscles**. Note that posterior cricoarytenoid muscle abducts vocal cords and transverse and oblique arytenoid muscles adduct them.

IDENTIFY internal branch of superior laryngeal nerve.

IDENTIFY inferior laryngeal nerve above cricoid cartilage.

TRACE anterior and posterior branches of inferior laryngeal nerve retrograde between pharynx and trachea to establish its source as **recurrent laryngeal nerve**.

IDENTIFY attachment of posterior cricoarytenoid muscle to muscular process of arytenoid cartilage. Note that it is only muscle that can abduct vocal folds.

DIRECT attention to lateral view of larynx.

IDENTIFY thyrohyoid membrane.

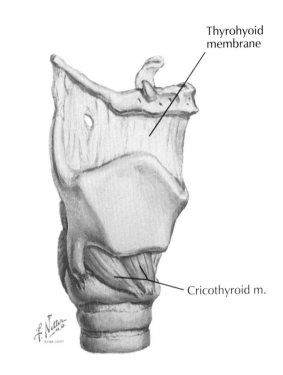

Thyrohyoid membrane

Cricothyroid m.

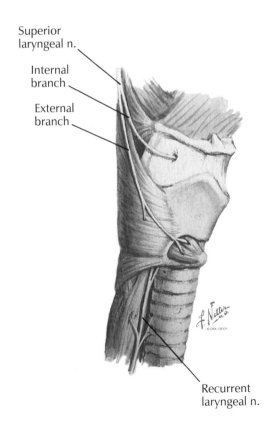

Superior laryngeal n.

Internal branch

External branch

Recurrent laryngeal n.

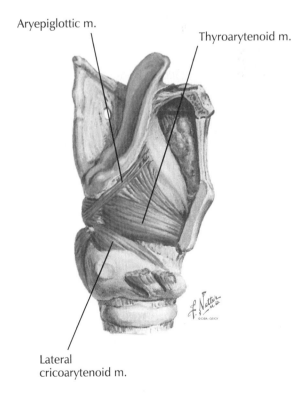

Aryepiglottic m.

Thyroarytenoid m.

Lateral cricoarytenoid m.

PLATE 74

PLATE 72

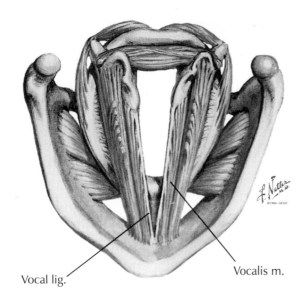

Vocal lig.   Vocalis m.

PLATE 72

TRACE internal laryngeal nerve retrograde to establish its source as **superior laryngeal nerve.**

FOLLOW external branch of **superior laryngeal nerve** distally to **cricothyroid muscle.** Note that external laryngeal nerve passes superficial to inferior pharyngeal constrictor muscle and deep to sternothyroid muscle.

CLEAN external surface of lamina of thyroid cartilage on one side by removing any fascia and all muscles.

CAUTION During next step, preserve internal branch of superior laryngeal nerve.

SEVER inferior border of thyrohyoid membrane from thyroid cartilage on cleaned side.

IDENTIFY cricothyroid muscle, its origin from anterior surface of arch of cricoid cartilage, and its insertion to internal surface of lamina of thyroid cartilage. Note that cricothyroid muscle lengthens vocal cords.

BLUNT DISSECT to separate cricothyroid and lateral cricoarytenoid muscles.

TRANSECT cricothyroid muscle and cricothyroid joint on cleaned side by cutting between thyroid and cricoid cartilages with scissors.

MAKE median vertical incision between right and left lamina of thyroid cartilage with scissors.

BLUNT DISSECT deep to cleaned lamina of thyroid cartilage.

REMOVE cleaned lamina of thyroid cartilage.

IDENTIFY attachment of **lateral cricoarytenoid muscle** to muscular process of arytenoid cartilage. Note that lateral cricoarytenoid muscle a<u>d</u>ducts vocal cords.

LOOK for fibers of **thyroarytenoid muscle.** Note that thyroarytenoid muscle shortens vocal cords.

TRACE fibers of oblique arytenoid muscle laterally as **aryepiglottic muscle.**

IDENTIFY aryepiglottic fold superior to aryepiglottic muscle. Note that superior border of quadrangular membrane forms aryepiglottic fold.

REMOVE lateral cricoarytenoid and thyroarytenoid muscles to expose conus elasticus.

IDENTIFY vocal ligament in medial border of **vocalis muscle.** Note that vocalis muscle is medial part of thyroarytenoid muscle.

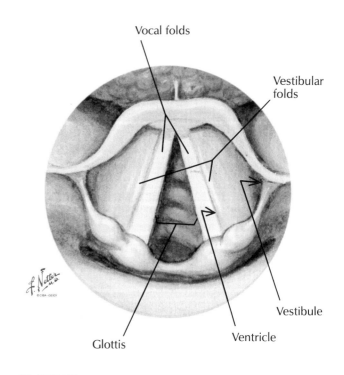

Vocal folds

Vestibular folds

Vestibule

Ventricle

Glottis

PLATE 75

MAKE median vertical incision in posterior wall of trachea and larynx.

RETRACT cut ends of larynx laterally to expose interior.

DIRECT attention to interior of larynx.

IDENTIFY 3 compartments of cavity of larynx that are formed by vestibular and vocal folds.

DEFINE boundaries of **vestibule** between epiglottis and vestibular folds.

DEFINE boundaries of **ventricle** between vestibular and vocal folds. Note presence of saccules in anterior part of ventricle.

DEFINE boundaries of **infraglottic cavity** (*not labeled*) between vocal folds and trachea.

IDENTIFY glottis as opening between vocal folds.

BLUNT DISSECT mucosa free from 1/2 of interior of larynx.

IDENTIFY conus elasticus and vocal ligament from interior of larynx.

BLUNT DISSECT mucosa free from 1/2 of epiglottic cartilage.

REIDENTIFY quadrangular membrane.

REVIEW actions of intrinsic muscles of larynx (**Plate 73**).

DISSECTION 8.12

EAR

Complete all Head and Neck DISSECTIONS **8.1** through **8.11**.

Read DISCUSSION **8.15** Ear.

NOTE that dissection should be restricted to just one side to preserve other side for review.

NOTE that dried skull should be kept at dissection table for reference.

IDENTIFY following landmarks on model of ear and dried skull: **external** and **internal acoustic meatus**, **mastoid** and **styloid processes**, **stylomastoid** and **jugular formina**, and **carotid canal**.

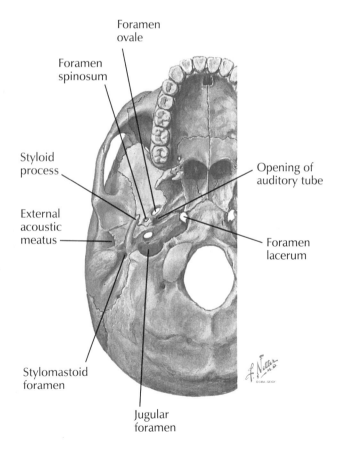

PLATE 5

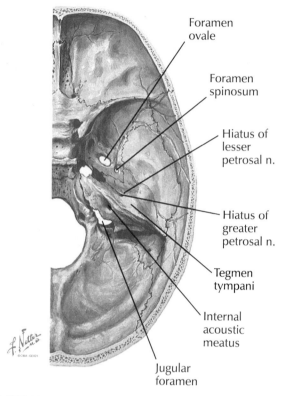

PLATE 7

IDENTIFY opening of **bony part** of **auditory tube**, **hiatuses** of **greater** and **lesser petrosal nerves**, **tegman tympani**, and **foramina lacerum**, **ovale** and **spinosum**.

IDENTIFY following parts of **auricle** on cadaver and fellow student: **lobule**, **helix** and **crus**, **antihelix** and **crura**, **scaphoid fossa**, **cymba** and **cavum** of **concha**, **tragus**, **antitragus**, and **intertragic notch**.

REMOVE (scrape) muscle fibers and fascia from external surface of squamous part of temporal bone.

INCISE anterior wall of external acoustic meatus to expose external surface of **tympanic membrane**.

POSITION cadaver so that bisected cranial cavity is upright in anatomical position.

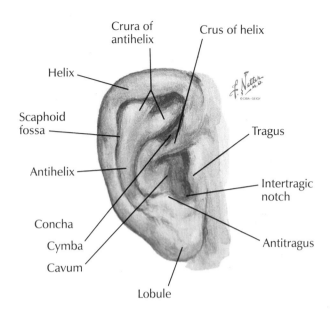

Crura of antihelix

Crus of helix

Helix

Scaphoid fossa

Tragus

Antihelix

Intertragic notch

Concha

Cymba

Antitragus

Cavum

Lobule

PLATE 88

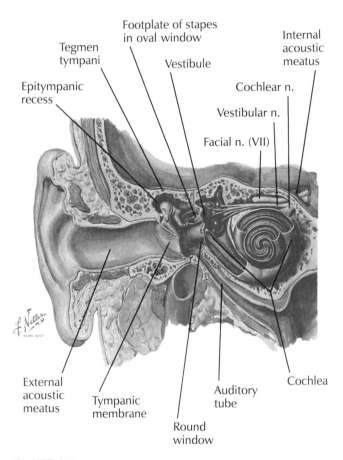

Footplate of stapes in oval window

Tegmen tympani

Internal acoustic meatus

Vestibule

Epitympanic recess

Cochlear n.

Vestibular n.

Facial n. (VII)

External acoustic meatus

Cochlea

Tympanic membrane

Auditory tube

Round window

PLATE 87

CAUTION During next step, protect greater petrosal nerve (*not shown*) as it exits its hiatus and traverses floor of middle cranial fossa and foramen lacerum.

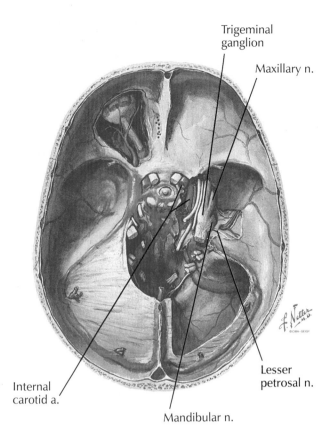

Trigeminal ganglion

Maxillary n.

Internal carotid a.

Lesser petrosal n.

Mandibular n.

PLATE 98

CAUTION Protect lesser petrosal nerve as it exits its hiatus crossing floor of middle cranial fossa to either foramen ovale or innominate foramen.

PEEL dura mater free from floor of middle and posterior cranial fossae.

LOCATE greater and **lesser petrosal nerves** exiting their namesake hiatuses.

REMOVE internal carotid and meningeal arteries, all venous dural sinuses, and trigeminal ganglion.

MARK incision line on floor of middle cranial fossa so that cut transects foramina ovale and lacerum through anterior edge of magnum.

SAW through floor of middle cranial fossa along marked line with Stryker saw (**Figure 42**).

SEPARATE wedge of temporal bone containing petrous part free from bisected head, cutting any attached tissue.

241

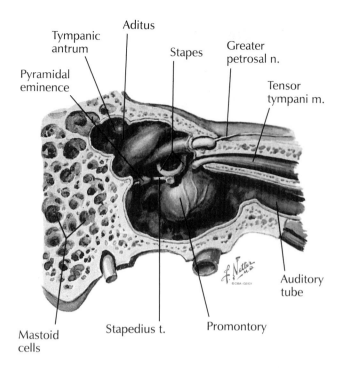

Aditus

Tympanic antrum

Stapes

Greater petrosal n.

Pyramidal eminence

Tensor tympani m.

Mastoid cells

Stapedius t.

Promontory

Auditory tube

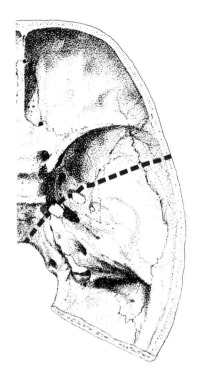

Figure 42

PLACE wedge of temporal bone containing petrous part into chelating fluid or 5% hydrochloric acid solution for 24 hours to decalcify bone.

NOTE that examination of facial nerve (VII) and middle ear should precede inspection of inner ear.

IDENTIFY **facial nerve (VII)** and **vestibulocochlear nerve (VIII)** as they enter internal acoustic meatus.

INSERT wire or thin probe into internal acoustic meatus to establish direction of horizontal component of facial canal.

INSERT wire into stylomastoid foramen to establish direction of vertical component of facial canal.

TRACE facial nerve (VII) within horizontal component of facial canal by shaving away roof of tegman tympani with a sharp scalpel. Begin by opening roof of internal acoustic meatus.

IDENTIFY **geniculate ganglion** and greater petrosal nerve extending anterior from it.

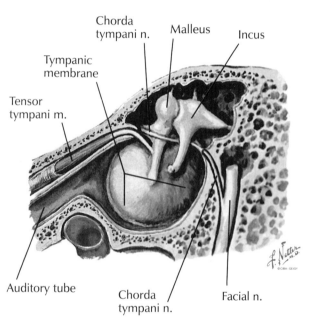

Chorda tympani n.

Malleus

Incus

Tympanic membrane

Tensor tympani m.

Auditory tube

Chorda tympani n.

Facial n.

PLATE 89

SHAVE away additional bone posterior to middle ear to expose **aditus** (*not labeled*) and **antrum of mastoid cells**.

SHAVE away additional bone lateral to geniculate ganglion to expose epitympanic recess of middle ear.

IDENTIFY head of **malleus** within epitympanic recess.

REMOVE entire roof of middle ear by careful shaving and flicking away of bone chips with scalpel.

REMOVE incus with forceps, but leave malleus and stapes *in situ*.

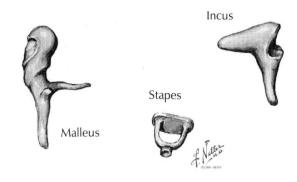

Incus

Stapes

Malleus

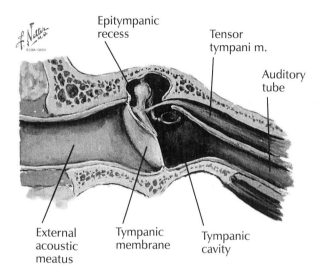

Epitympanic recess

Tensor tympani m.

Auditory tube

External acoustic meatus

Tympanic membrane

Tympanic cavity

PLATE 88

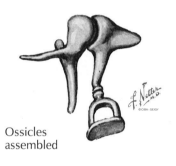

Ossicles assembled

PLATE 88

IDENTIFY chorda tympani nerve passing medial to handle of malleus internal to tympanic membrane.

IDENTIFY site of attachment of tendon of **tensor tympani** to malleus.

IDENTIFY stapes and tendon of **stapedius** extending from **pyramidal eminence** on posterior wall of middle ear.

REMOVE stapes with forceps.

LOCATE promontory formed by 1st turn of cochlea on medial wall of middle ear.

IDENTIFY oval (**vestibular**) and **round** (**cochlear**) **windows** on medial wall of middle ear.

INSERT wire, or thin probe, into opening of **auditory tube**, entering from nasopharynx.

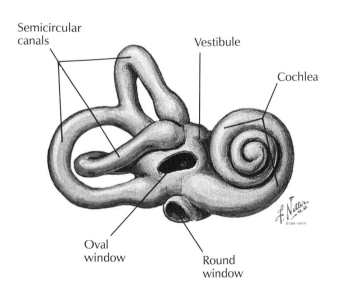

Semicircular canals

Vestibule

Cochlea

Oval window

Round window

PLATE 90

EXAMINE relationships of carotid canal and jugular foramen to middle ear.

DIRECT attention to entrance of vestibulocochlear nerve (VIII) into opened internal acoustic meatus.

TRACE cochlear nerve toward cochlea by shaving away roof of tegman tympani medial to geniculate ganglion with a sharp scalpel.

SHAVE away additional bone to expose cochlea.

TRACE vestibular nerve toward **vestibule** by shaving away more bone.

SHAVE away additional bone to expose parts of **semicircular canals**.

REINSPECT auditory ossicles and all above landmarks on model of ear to study position and relationships of structures within both middle and inner ears.